EMERGENCY NURSING
Examination
REVIEW

FOURTH EDITION

2015

SENIOR EDITORS

Laura Gasparis Vonfrolio RN, PhD
www.GREATNURSES.com

Lee Taylor-Vaughan JD(c), MSN, RN, ACNP, CCRN-CSC,
CEN, NREMT-P, LNC
www.CardiacEd.com

Lauren Bohacik-Castillo JD(c), BSN, RN, CEN, LNC
www.TaylorCastillo.com

EMERGENCY NURSING EXAMINATION REVIEW

Fourth Edition

Copyright 2015 Education Enterprises

ISBN: 1-888315-08-3

Cover Design:
Laura Gasparis Vonfrolio RN, PhD
Pamela LoCascio

Copy Editors:
Lee Taylor-Vaughan JD(c), MSN, RN, ACNP, CCRN-CSC, CEN, EMT-P, LNC
Kevin Kern, MICP, EMT-P

Published by:
EDUCATION ENTERPRISES
1-800-331-6534
www.GREATNURSES.com

Dear Emergency Department Colleagues:

Welcome to the 4ᵗʰ Edition of the **Emergency Nursing Examination Review Book!** You are going to love this book – it is easy to read, informative, and jam packed with lots of information written by nurses current in their field of expertise.

In order to provide you with more information, there are over 1,000 questions with answers and appropriate rationale.

This book is set up according to Emergency Nurses Association's Emergency Nursing Core Curriculum. The following areas are covered: Abdominal, Cardiovascular, Eye, Ear, Nose, Throat, Environmental, Facial, General Medical, Genitourinary, Gynecologic, Neurologic, Obstetric, Organ Donation, Orthopedic, Psychiatric, Psychological, Respiratory, Shock, Toxicology, Substance Abuse, Surface Trauma, Professional Issues, and more...

This book is an excellent review for those nurses preparing for the CEN® examination; as well as for nurses wanting to update, enhance, and validate their current knowledge of bedside emergency nursing.

I wish you lots of luck in your quest of emergency care knowledge and the pursuit of your Emergency Nursing certification!

Join me at one of my seminars, and if you need a vacation, look into our yearly vacation getaways!

Laura Gasparis Vonfrolio PhD, RN
www.GREATNURSES.com

CONTRIBUTORS

Alice Belcher, RN, BSN, CCRN
Mary Blum, RN, MSN
Lauren Bohacik-Castillo, JD(c), BSN, RN, CEN, LNC
Carol A. Botin, RN
Patrice Case, RN, MA
Elizabeth Connelly, RN, MS, CCRN
Kathy Daly, RN, MS, CCRN
Marcia Downs, RN, CEN
Vincent J. Ferragano, MD
Heather A. Foley, RN
Deborah S. Gough, RN, MSN, CCRN, CEN
Stephanie Higie, RN, BSN, CEN
Catherine T Kelly, RN, MSN, EMT-P, CCRN, CEN
Lori Kelty, MSN, RN, CCRN, CEN, NE
Kevin Kern, MICP, EMT-P
Linda Anne Laner, RN, MSN CS, CEN, CCRN
Joanne Lapidus-Graham, RN, MA
Lisa Mayercilc, RN, BSN
Marilyn McDonald, RN, MA
Kathleen McMahon, RN, MSN, CEN
Elizabeth Mizerek, MSN, RN, CEN, CPEN, FN-CSA
Patricia Murphy, MD
Theresa Nauta, RN, MSN
Janet A. Neff, RN, MN CCRN, CEN
Nell Nepola, MD
Joanne Noone, RN, MSN, CCRN, CEN **(Past Editor)**
June L. Olsen, RN, MS
Catherine Paradiso, RN, MSN, CCRN, CEN
Linda Reese, RN, MA
Deborah Reilly, RN, MSN, CEN
John P Reilly, MD
Nancy J. Reselman, BSN, RN, LNC
Patricia Robertazza, RN, MSN, CCRN
Susan Schulmerich, RN, MS, MA, CNA, CEN
Joanne Scotto, RN, BSN
Eva Scripps, RN, BSN, CCRN, CEN

Nancy C. Seddio, RN, CS, PhD
Maureen Sheehy, RN, CCRN, CEN
Lee Taylor-Vaughan, JD(c), MSN, RN, ACNP, CCRN-CSC, CEN, NREMT-P, LNC
Patricia Tooker, RN, MSN, CCRN
Debra Toth, RN, BSN,
David Tinkle, RN, CCRN, CEN
Charles T Vonfrolio, MD
Laura Gasparis Vonfrolio, RN, PhD, CCRN, CEN
David Weaver, Esq.

TABLE OF CONTENTS

ABDOMINAL EMERGENCIES

1. A patient arrives in the emergency department (ED) with an ice pick protruding from his left lower abdominal quadrant. An appropriate nursing action would be to:

A. Immediately remove the object and apply firm pressure to the wound
B. Leave the object in place until the patient is taken to the operating room
C. Establish two large-bore IV lines, then remove the object
D. Obtain an abdominal X-ray, then remove the object

2. Which type of penetrating injury would the nurse document in the assessment findings for a patient with a gunshot wound at the sixth intercostal space?

A. Chest
B. Abdominal
C. Thoracoabdominal
D. Pelvic

3. A patient with a gunshot wound to the left lower abdominal quadrant arrives at the ED with the following vital signs: blood pressure (BP) 110/70 mmHg, pulse rate 96 beats/minute, and respirations 24 breaths/minute. What would be the highest priority at this time?

A. Emergency exploratory laparotomy
B. Abdominal computed tomography (CT) scan
C. Diagnostic peritoneal lavage
D. Close observation in the ED over the next several hours

4. A patient arrives at the ED with a penetrating gunshot wound to the abdomen and hematuria. Which diagnostic test would the nurse expect the physician to order before surgery?

A. Diagnostic peritoneal lavage
B. Abdominal X-ray
C. Intravenous pyelography (IVP)
D. Abdominal CT scan

5. When assessing a patient for potential complications from a gunshot wound to the right upper abdominal quadrant, the nurse should observe the patient closely for injury to the:

A. Liver
B. Transverse colon
C. Stomach
D. All of the above

6. Which nursing action would the nurse expect to perform preoperatively for a patient with a penetrating abdominal wound?

A. Establishment of two large-bore IV lines
B. Serial abdominal examinations
C. Strict monitoring of patient's urinary output
D. All of the above

7. The nurse would expect to note early signs of shock in a young male patient who has sustained a penetrating abdominal wound after the patient has suffered a blood volume loss of:

A. 20%
B. 25%
C. 30%
D. 50%

8. All of the following injuries are considered penetrating except:

A. A stab wound to the right upper abdominal quadrant
B. A severe abdominal laceration caused by a fall
C. A gunshot wound to the left lower abdominal quadrant
D. A BB pellet to the lower abdomen

9. All of the following assessment findings would lead the nurse to suspect a perforated gastric ulcer except:

A. Absent bowel sounds
B. Hypotension and tachycardia
C. Anxiety and respiratory difficulty
D. Severe upper abdominal pain radiating to the jaw

10. Which of the following can cause chemical peritonitis in a patient with a perforated gastric ulcer:

A. Overuse of antacids
B. Salicylate ingestion
C. Gastric and intestinal content spillage
D. Sodium and calcium imbalance

11. Perforated ulcers occur most commonly in the:

A. Stomach
B. Jejunum
C. Duodenum
D. Ileum

12. The nurse knows that such abdominal emergencies as obstruction, perforation, and acute intractable hemorrhage are typically treated by:

A. Surgery
B. Fluid and blood replacement
C. Antacids, anticholinergics, and sedatives
D. Stress reduction and dietary changes

13. The most common causes of upper GI bleeding include:

A. Neoplasms, gastritis, and duodenal ulcers
B. Peptic ulcers, acute mucosal lesions, and esophageal varices
C. Esophagitis, gastric ulcers, and hematologic disorders
D. Mallory-Weiss tears, peptic ulcers, and vascular anomalies

14. The nurse recognizes which is a common cause of esophageal varices?

A. Abnormal circulation within the splenic artery
B. Portal hypertension
C. Excessive use of ibuprofen, alcohol, tobacco, or spicy foods
D. An existing esophageal carcinoma

15. Nursing care of the patient with a three-lumen, double-balloon esophageal tube includes all of the following except:

A. Maintaining constant observation during balloon inflation
B. Ensuring that the balloon pressures are kept at the levels required to control bleeding
C. Remaining alert for any complaints of chest pain
D. Placing the patient in a supine position to prevent shock

16. Of the following history findings, the most likely cause of pancreatitis is:

A. Excessive alcohol intake
B. Excessive fat intake
C. Heredity
D. Stress

17. The nurse knows that pancreatitis also may occur as a complication of a perforated duodenal ulcer when:

A. Serum amylase is elevated to dangerous levels
B. The perforation erodes into the pancreas
C. The patient's alcohol intake is high
D. The pancreatic duct is obstructed

18. Which nursing diagnosis is most appropriate for a patient at risk for complications from pancreatitis?

A. Potential for injury related to seizures
B. Risk for impaired perfusion due to cardiac related hyperkalemia and induced arrhythmia
C. Altered thought processes related to hypoglycemia
D. Impaired gas exchange related to pulmonary edema

19. The nurse normally assesses a patient with acute pancreatitis for elevated levels of serum:

A. Cholesterol
B. Amylase
C. Potassium
D. Calcium

20. The nurse should assess the patient for all of the following symptoms of hemorrhagic pancreatitis except:

A. Jaundice
B. Extreme epigastric or umbilical pain extending to the back or flank
C. Shock
D. Hypertension

21. Nursing interventions for a patient with acute hemorrhagic pancreatitis include all of the following except:

A. Administration of large volumes of colloid and electrolyte solutions
B. Administration of calcium gluconate
C. Monitoring of central venous pressure and urine output
D. Administering a clear liquid diet

22. Over the course of several months of caring for various patients with pancreatitis, the nurse would expect the physician to order broad-spectrum antibiotics:

A. Frequently
B. Only when surgery is required
C. Rarely
D. Never

23. The patient is being admitted to the medical-surgical unit for further treatment and observation. Which dietary regimen would the nurse expect for a patient with pancreatitis?

A. Low fat, no-alcohol, no-caffeine
B. Low fat, low-cholesterol
C. Low-salt, low-sugar, no-alcohol
D. No-alcohol, no-caffeine, no-sugar

24. Which assessment finding is characteristic of acute appendicitis?

A. Rovsing's sign
B. Leukopenia
C. Abdominal distention
D. Audible borborygmi

25. When compared with older children and adults, young children have a higher incidence of perforation of the appendix with ensuing peritonitis because they typically have:

A. Difficulty describing symptoms
B. A greater pain tolerance
C. A weaker appendiceal wall
D. Less resistance to infection

26. Which internal organ is typically injured in a patient with a blunt abdominal trauma?

A. Pancreas
B. Spleen
C. Small intestine
D. Gallbladder

27. Which type of solution would the nurse expect to infuse to restore circulatory dynamics in a patient with blunt abdominal injury?

A. Hypertonic
B. Hypotonic
C. Isotonic
D. Hypo-osmolar

28. Which statement regarding the spleen is false?

A. The normal spleen is palpable below the lower left costal margin
B. The spleen is injured more frequently than any other abdominal organ
C. The high incidence of splenic complications is directly related to the organ's high vascularity
D. Approximately 50% of patients with splenic bleeding exhibit a positive Kehr's sign

29. The nurse would suspect splenic injury in the patient with an injury to the:

A. Bladder
B. Sternum
C. 11th or 12th rib on the right side
D. 8th, 9th, or 10th rib on the left side

30. The nurse understands that bowel obstruction occurs most commonly in extremely young and old patients and that the hallmark signs and symptoms include:

A. Pain, distention, vomiting, and prolonged constipation
B. Absence of pain, nausea and vomiting, and prolonged constipation
C. Loss of bowel sounds, distention, constipation, and nausea
D. Hyperactive bowel sounds, diarrhea, vomiting, and cramping

31. A 74-year-old man is brought to the hospital by his nephew after complaining of severe abdominal cramping and swelling. He claims to have had a stomach virus for the past few days. His symptoms include nausea, anorexia, mild discomfort, and constipation. Within the last 12 hours, his pain has increased in intensity, and he has vomited small amounts of greenish liquid several times. The physician diagnoses his condition as a possible bowel obstruction. An appropriate nursing diagnosis for this patient would be:

A. Fluid volume deficit related to fluid shifting and vomiting
B. Decreased cardiac output related to impaired myocardial contractility
C. Fluid volume excess related to decreased renal perfusion
D. Fluid volume excess related to increased water absorption from stool

32. Which condition is the primary cause of large-bowel obstruction in an adult?

A. Adhesions
B. Volvulus
C. Carcinoma
D. Diverticulitis

33. While the nurse is completing the initial physical assessment and history of a patient with abdominal pain, the patient becomes increasingly restless and confused. The nurse obtains a second set of vital signs and notifies the physician. The vital signs: BP 90/58 mmHg, weak peripheral pulses at a rate of 134 beats/minute, temperature 96.6° F (35.9° C) with a cool skin surface, and respirations 16 breaths/minute and shallow. The nurse would know that this is likely development of:

A. Cerebrovascular accident
B. Congestive heart failure
C. Shock
D. Anxiety

34. Which is the correct sequence for assessing and evaluating a patient's abdomen:

A. Auscultation, percussion, inspection, and palpation
B. Auscultation, inspection, percussion, and palpation
C. Inspection, auscultation, percussion, and palpation
D. Inspection, auscultation, palpation, and percussion

35. A 38-year-old stockbroker is brought to the ED by a coworker after experiencing an episode of severe weakness after a business luncheon. Although the patient claims to have no medical or surgical history, he admits to taking large amounts of liquid antacids to calm his stomach. He has had several episodes of bloody vomitus within the past 3 to 4 days. The physician diagnoses the patient as having upper GI bleeding. Which nursing intervention would be most helpful in determining the cause of the patient's bleeding?

A. Inserting an NG tube to measure the pH of gastric fluids
B. Collecting blood specimens for a complete blood count, type and screen, and coagulation profiles
C. Prompt scheduling of an endoscopy
D. Obtain a thorough history and perform a physical exam

36. In assessing the patient's health status, the nurse should know that hematemesis is most commonly caused by:

A. Malignant tumors
B. Peptic ulcers
C. Blood dyscrasias
D. Esophageal varices

37. Anticholinergic drugs, commonly used to treat peptic ulcer disease, typically produce which pharmacologic action:

A. Decreased patient responsiveness
B. Increased gastric emptying
C. Inhibited histamine formation
D. Blockage of the effects of vagal nerve impulses on smooth muscles

38. Which diagnostic test would the nurse anticipate for a patient with lower gastrointestinal bleeding?

A. Angiography
B. Abdominal CT scan
C. Esophagogastroduodenoscopy
D. Colonoscopy

39. An elderly man is brought to the ED by his daughter after an episode of rectal bleeding. After initial treatment in the ED, the patient will probably be:

A. Prepared for emergency surgery
B. Admitted to the intensive care unit
C. Sent directly to the endoscopy unit
D. Sent home with referral to a specialist

40. In a patient with prolonged bleeding, anemia is a potential complication. The nurse assesses for anemia by noting signs of pallor in the patient's:

A. Lips
B. Gums
C. Sclera
D. Nail beds

41. Which condition is the most common cause of lower GI bleeding?

A. Diverticulitis
B. Hemorrhoids
C. Ischemic bowel disease
D. Neoplasm

42. When a patient is undergoing emergency endoscopy, the nurse should assess for all of the following potential complications except:

A. Cardiac arrhythmias
B. Perforation
C. Aspiration
D. Paralytic ileus

43. Lower GI bleeding is characterized by bleeding from:

A. The colon
B. Any source below the ligament of Treitz
C. Any source below the appendix
D. Diverticula

44. A patient is admitted to the ED after a high-speed, head-on automobile accident. He is conscious and alert; his skin is cool and dry. Vital signs are: BP 110/70 mmHg, pulse rate 100 beats/minute, and respirations 24 breaths/minute. The on-scene paramedic reports severe front-end damage to the car and a broken steering wheel. After assessing the patient's airway, breathing, and circulation, the nurse's primary concern would be to:

A. Ask the patient when he ate his last meal
B. Establish two large-bore IV lines
C. Insert an indwelling urinary catheter
D. Insert an NG tube

45. Which assessment finding is the earliest indication of impending shock?

A. Tachycardia
B. Hypotension
C. Narrowing pulse pressure
D. Cool and clammy skin

46. The patient's BP suddenly drops to 88/60 mmHg and his pulse increases to 130 beats/minute. After administration of 500 mL of Lactated Ringer's solution, the patient's BP increases to 100/70 mmHg and his pulse rate decreases to 100 beats/minute. The nurse's priority at this time would be to:

A. Prepare the patient for an IVP
B. Prepare the patient for an emergent CT scan
C. Prepare the patient for surgery
D. Immediately transfuse the patient with O-positive or O-negative blood, depending on availability

47. Results of a diagnostic peritoneal lavage may be falsely negative in a patient with a:

A. Splenic hemorrhage
B. Diaphragmatic rupture
C. Bladder tear
D. Retroperitoneal hematoma

48. Which sign is not an indication for IVP?

A. Blood at the urinary meatus
B. A high-riding prostate on rectal examination
C. Hematuria
D. Frequent urinary tract infections

49. During a patient assessment, the nurse notes a large mass in the left upper abdominal quadrant, displacement of the stomach, and associated rib fractures in the left lower thorax. These signs are consistent with injury to the:

A. Liver
B. Small intestine
C. Spleen
D. Colon

50. During the assessment, the nurse notes a large mass in the left upper abdominal quadrant, displacement of the stomach, and associated rib fractures in the left lower thorax. The nurse identifies the patient's primary nursing diagnosis as:

A. Potential for infection related to abdominal contamination
B. Impaired gas exchange related to respiratory trauma
C. Fluid volume deficit related to blood loss
D. Decreased cardiac output related to cardiac trauma

51. A 61-year-old man is transferred to the ED by ambulance from his physician's office with a diagnosis of a possible abdominal aortic aneurysm. When eliciting the patient's history, the nurse keeps in mind that one of the most common factors predisposing a patient to abdominal aortic aneurysm is:

A. Diabetes
B. Congestive heart failure
C. Renal disease
D. Abdominal carcinoma

52. Which assessment finding would be typical for a patient with an abdominal aortic aneurysm?

A. Hoarseness
B. Abdominal distention
C. Difficulty swallowing
D. Mid-scapular back pain

53. The patient's abdominal X-ray reveals a fusiform infrarenal non-dissecting aortic aneurysm. Which nursing diagnosis would be the highest priority for this patient?

A. Altered renal tissue perfusion related to decreased blood flow to the kidneys
B. Impaired gas exchange related to blood loss
C. Decreased cardiac output related to decreased preload
D. Altered peripheral tissue perfusion related to decreased arterial blood flow

54. While in the ED, which is the best parameter for evaluating expected patient outcomes for the above nursing diagnosis:

A. Urine output studies
B. Respiratory rate measurements
C. Arterial blood gas studies
D. Femoral pulse assessments

55. Which of the following signs is a symptom of peritonitis?

A. Psoas sign
B. Blumberg sign
C. Obturator sign
D. Currant jelly stool

ABDOMINAL EMERGENCIES: RATIONALE

1. **B** The appropriate nursing action in this situation would be to leave the object in place. The object should be removed in the operating room, where hemorrhage can be surgically controlled. Removing the object in the emergency department may cause further exsanguination and the development of shock.

2. **C** The diaphragm, which separates the chest (thoracic cavity) from the abdomen, rises to the level of the sixth intercostal space on respiratory exhalation. Therefore, a gunshot wound at the sixth intercostal space is considered a thoracoabdominal injury because a bullet may enter both the abdomen and the chest.

3. **A** Emergency exploratory laparotomy is the highest priority for a patient with a gunshot wound to the left lower abdominal quadrant. This procedure is necessary to determine which structures the bullet has penetrated so that hemorrhage can be controlled. Abdominal computed tomography (CT) scan and peritoneal lavage cannot help to identify the extent of injury to vessels. These procedures or observation in the ED could take considerable time, thereby predisposing the patient to hemorrhage.

4. **C** The nurse should expect the physician to order all the tests except for an intravenous pyelography (IVP). Although it would be useful to know if the patient has at least one kidney is functioning in case the patient must undergo nephrectomy, the patient would die from hemorrhage long before the test was completed. It is possible that and IVP could be done in the OR, however that is the decision of the surgeon. The existence of hematuria signifies that renal trauma may have resulted from the gunshot wound. Diagnostic peritoneal lavage, abdominal X-

ray, and abdominal CT scan will provide information on organ structure discovering the degree of injury.

5. **D** Once a bullet entered the abdomen, it is impossible to predict the organs affected. Therefore, the nurse must closely observe the liver, transverse colon, and stomach for signs of penetration.

6. **D** The nurse would expect to perform all of the nursing actions preoperatively. Establishing two large-bore IV lines provides access for administration of fluids and blood products. Performing serial abdominal exams would help to detect a change in the patient's physical assessment. Strict monitoring of a patients urinary output of less than 30 mL/hour indicates hypo-perfusion of the kidneys and likely shock.

7. **A** The nurse would expect to note the early signs of hypovolemic shock, especially tachycardia and orthostatic hypotension, after a patient sustains a blood loss of 15%. Significant hypotension (below 90/60 mmHg or a 30 mmHg drop from the patient's baseline) typically occurs after a blood loss of 25%. Irreversible shock, which does not respond to treatment and leads to cardiac arrest, is common after a blood loss of 40% to 50%.

8. **B** All injuries that penetrate the surface of the skin classified as penetrating, with the exception of abrasions or lacerations. Injuries that are caused by blunt trauma are not classified as penetrating.

9. **D** A patient with a perforated gastric ulcer does not typically complain of severe upper abdominal pain radiating to the jaw. Patients may complain of severe upper abdominal pain radiating to the neck, which is caused by irritation of the

diaphragm and phrenic nerves. Other signs of perforated gastric ulcer include absent bowel sounds, hypotension, tachycardia, anxiety, and respiratory difficulty.

10. **C** Chemical peritonitis, the inflammation of a portion or all of the parietal and visceral surfaces of the abdominal cavity, results from the rapid escape or spillage of gastric and intestinal contents after perforation. The peritoneum's primary response to injury includes edema in the subperitoneal tissues, bowel hypermotility, and an outpouring of plasma like fluid from the extracellular, vascular, and interstitial compartments into the peritoneal space. Overuse of antacids, sodium, and calcium imbalance are not associated with perforated ulcer. Salicylate ingestion may initiate ulcer formation but does not cause the resulting chemical peritonitis that occurs after perforation.

11. **C** The most common site of a perforated ulcer is the duodenum, constituting approximately 80% of all ulcers. The remaining 20% are considered gastric and occur in the stomach. Duodenal ulcers typically manifest in those between ages 30 and 50. Gastric ulcers are more common in those over age 50. The jejunum and the ileum are not sites of ulcer formation.

12. **A** Surgery usually is indicated in life-threatening and acute intractable hemorrhage. Other forms of treatment - including fluid and blood replacement, antacids, anticholinergics, sedatives, stress reduction and dietary changes - may be indicated for less serious abdominal illnesses.

13. **B** The most common causes of upper GI bleeding are peptic ulcers, acute mucosal lesions (resulting from gastritis, esophagitis, or Mallory-Weiss tears), and esophageal or gastric varices. Neoplasms, hematologic disorders, and vascular anomalies rarely cause upper GI bleeding.

14. **B** Esophageal varices are dilated-tortuous veins found in the submucosa of the lower esophagus. Varices may extend throughout the esophagus and into the stomach. Nearly always caused by portal hypertension, varices result from obstruction of the portal venous circulation or cirrhosis of the liver (from excessive alcohol intake). Abnormal circulation within the splenic artery or superior vena cava may also cause esophageal varices; however, such abnormalities are not the most common cause. Frequent intake of alcohol, tobacco, or spicy foods may lead to esophageal carcinoma; however, this is not directly related to the development of esophageal varices.

15. **D** Placing the patient in a supine position is not a part of the normal nursing care of a patient with a three lumen, double-balloon esophageal tube. The tube helps to control esophageal bleeding through the inflation of gastric and esophageal balloons. During inflation, the nurse must maintain the head of the bed in a slightly elevated position, unless the patient is in shock, in which case a supine position may be necessary. Such elevation helps prevent gastric regurgitation and diminishes nausea and gagging. The nurse must observe the patient closely for signs of airway obstruction from migration of the esophageal balloon into the trachea. The nurse should also ensure that balloon pressures are kept at levels required to control bleeding and should remain alert for any signs of chest pain, which may indicate that the balloon pressures are excessive and causing tissue ischemia.

16. **A** The most common cause of pancreatitis is excessive alcohol intake, which typically causes toxic effects on the pancreas or a backup of pancreatic juices into the pancreas. Biliary tract disease, another common cause of pancreatitis, typically causes pancreatic duct obstruction, a backup of pancreatic juices, and cholecystitis (which is caused by reflux

of bile components into the pancreatic duct). Although decreasing fat intake and reducing stress can help to reduce symptoms of pancreatitis, fat intake and stress are not necessarily precipitating causes. Heredity is also not a causal factor.

17. **B** Pancreatitis may result as a complication of a perforated duodenal ulcer when the perforation erodes through the pancreatic wall and into the pancreas. An elevated serum amylase level is a sign, not a cause, of pancreatitis. Alcohol levels and pancreatic duct obstruction are not associated with ulcer perforation.

18. **D** The most appropriate nursing diagnosis for a patient at risk for complications from pancreatitis is impaired gas exchange related to pulmonary edema. Adult Respiratory Distress Syndrome (ARDS) is an associated pulmonary complication of pancreatitis. ARDS may result from the pancreatitis itself, from ensuing sepsis or hypovolemia. Researchers theorize that pancreatic exudate destroys surfactant, which leads to the development of ARDS. The other diagnoses would be inappropriate because seizures are not associated with pancreatitis. Common complications of pancreatitis are hypokalemia and hyperglycemia, not hyperkalemia and hypoglycemia.

19. **B** Within a few hours after onset of acute pancreatitis, serum amylase levels rise and remain elevated for about 3 days. After 24 hours, serum lipase levels also rise and remain elevated for up to 10 days. Serum levels of cholesterol, potassium, and calcium reveal nothing about acute pancreatitis.

20. **D** Hypertension is not a symptom of hemorrhagic pancreatitis. Jaundice is caused by common bile duct

obstruction, which occurs as a result of pancreatic edema. Shock develops when trypsin, a chemical found in the inflammatory fluid that spills into the peritoneum and causes pancreatitis, activates kinin, a vasodilator. Hemorrhage occurs when activated elastase dissolves the fibers of surrounding blood vessels. The pooling of blood caused by vasodilation compounded by blood loss leads to the development of signs of shock, such as hypotension. Pain results from distention of the pancreatic capsule, ductal spasm, or increased secretion of enzymes after eating.

21. **D** Administering a clear liquid diet would be inappropriate in this situation. A patient with acute hemorrhagic pancreatitis should receive nothing by mouth (NPO) but should have a nasogastric tube inserted and attached to low suction, to drain gastric secretions and prevent further pancreatic stimulation. The nurse normally administers large quantities of volume expanders, such as colloid and electrolyte solutions, to combat shock and also administers calcium gluconate to correct the hypocalcemia that commonly occurs in acute pancreatitis. Central venous pressure and urine output should be monitored hourly to assess for impending shock and its treatment.

22. **C** Antibiotics are rarely used to treat pancreatitis, except when infection has been established. In cases of infection, broad-spectrum antibiotics, such as ampicillin and gentamicin sulfate, may be ordered to help combat the bacteria, which readily multiply in necrotic tissue.

23. **A** The nurse would expect the physician to order a low fat, no-alcohol, no-caffeine diet for a patient with acute pancreatitis. Limiting fat intake and avoiding alcohol helps prevent pancreatic stimulation. Avoiding caffeine prevents stimulation of gastric acid secretion, which activates pancreatic activity.

Although a low-cholesterol, low-sodium, and low-sugar diet is beneficial, it does not affect stimulation of the pancreas or gastric acid secretion.

24. **A** Rovsing's sign, which is pain in the right lower abdominal quadrant that intensifies when pressure is applied to the left lower abdominal quadrant, is characteristic of acute appendicitis. Other classic signs include a slightly elevated temperature (99°F to 101°F, or 37.2°C to 38.3°C) and moderate leukocytosis (an elevated white blood cell count). The patient may also have anorexia, nausea, and vomiting. Abdominal distention and audible borborygmi are commonly associated with bowel obstruction.

25. **A** Young children have a higher incidence of perforated appendixes with ensuing peritonitis because they typically have difficulty describing symptoms. Also, the abdominal omentum (the peritoneal fold extending from the stomach to adjacent organs) is not well developed in children, allowing for rapid development of peritonitis because infection cannot be easily contained. Such children invariably have pain, although they may be unable to articulate the location or degree of pain. Appendicitis should be suspected in any child over age 2 who demonstrates symptoms of persistent abdominal pain, as early recognition can prevent rupture and other serious complications. Also, young children do not have a weaker appendiceal wall.

26. **B** Some abdominal organs are more susceptible to injury than others. The spleen, liver, and kidneys are the three most commonly injured organs in blunt abdominal trauma.

27. **C** The nurse should expect to administer an infusion of an isotonic solution, such as Lactated Ringer's or normal saline

solution, to restore circulatory dynamics in a patient with a blunt abdominal injury and suspected injury to internal organs. This type of solution maintains the same osmotic pressure as blood serum and ensures that cellular constituents remain unchanged until surgery can be performed. Hypertonic solutions are better suited for treating electrolyte imbalances, such as dilutional hyponatremia in which the patient has an excess of free water. Hypotonic solutions, which are hypo-osmolar, are indicated in such electrolyte imbalances as hypernatremia to dilute the excess sodium load.

28. **A** The spleen, which is located in the left upper abdominal quadrant under the diaphragm and near the abdominal wall, is partially protected by the lower left ribs and cannot be palpated until triple its normal size. This organ is injured more frequently than any other abdominal organ. The high incidence of splenic complications is directly related to the fact that the spleen is the most vascular organ in the body. Splenic lacerations and ruptured hematomas are notorious sources of persistent bleeding into the peritoneal cavity. Kehr's sign, which is referred pain to the left shoulder from blood irritating the diaphragm, is evident in many patients with splenic bleeding.

29. **D** Because the spleen is located in the left upper abdominal quadrant, the nurse should suspect splenic injury in fractures involving the 8th, 9th, or 10th rib on the left side.

30. **A** The hallmark signs and symptoms of intestinal obstruction include abdominal pain, distention, vomiting, and prolonged constipation (obstipation). All four signs and symptoms are not necessarily present in every case, and the severity varies with the level and type of obstruction. When an obstruction is high in the small intestine, the patient may have copious vomiting early with minimal abdominal distention.

When obstruction is low in the colon, the patient may have marked distention with no vomiting. Constipation may be overlooked because the patient may have two or three bowel movements early in its initial stages, until the bowel, distal to the point of obstruction, is evacuated. On physical examination, bowel sounds typically are high-pitched and occur in rushes. Regardless of the degree of abdominal distention, the abdomen is not tender, unless the bowel is ischemic.

31. **A** An appropriate nursing diagnosis for a patient with bowel obstruction is fluid volume deficit related to fluid shifting and vomiting because of the loss of fluid through shifting in the intestinal lumen and vomiting. Myocardial contractility usually is not impaired in bowel obstruction. Although decreased renal perfusion may result from hypovolemia, acute renal failure is not a common complication. Although excess water is reabsorbed from impacted stool, it is not enough to cause fluid volume excess.

32. **C** The primary cause of large-bowel obstruction in an adult is carcinoma. Diverticulitis is the second leading cause, volvulus the third. Adhesions are a less common cause of bowel obstruction. Cancer of the colon and rectum accounts for more than 50,000 deaths annually, the second highest death rate in the United States for any type of cancer. Men are affected more commonly than women. The highest incidence occurs in people in the fifth decade of life. The 5-year survival rate is 40% to 50%, the best of the visceral cancers.

33. **C** Shock, a condition in which effective circulating blood volume decreases, causes inadequate organ and tissue perfusion and can lead to derangements of cellular function. Clinical manifestations include decreasing arterial pressure (systolic pressure falls more rapidly than diastolic), tachycardia, cold and

clammy skin, circumoral pallor, altered mental status, and suppressed kidney function.

34. **C** The correct sequence for assessing and evaluating a patient's abdomen is inspection, auscultation, percussion, and palpation. Auscultation precedes percussion and palpation to prevent distortion of auscultatory findings related to pressure on the abdominal wall. Percussion precedes palpation to screen for an enlarged spleen before deep palpation.

35. **D** Because acute upper GI bleeding is a potentially life-threatening condition, the patient requires immediate assessment to determine the extent and cause of bleeding. Therefore, the most helpful nursing action would be to determine the patient's shock status, then obtain a detailed health history and perform a thorough physical examination. The history and subsequent physical examination help to identify the sequence of events that prompted the patient to seek aid and reveals specific information about the nature of current or previous bleeding episodes, associated symptoms or diseases, and drug use. Inserting a nasogastric tube, collecting blood specimens to evaluate the patient's hematologic status, and scheduling an endoscopy as necessary are all-important subsequent interventions.

36. **B** In approximately 80% of all patients, hematemesis (the vomiting of blood) is caused by peptic ulcers. Other common causes, in decreasing order of frequency, include gastric and duodenal ulcers, bleeding esophageal varices, and gastric carcinoma.

37. **D** Anticholinergic drugs, such as atropine sulfate, methantheline bromide (Banthine), and propantheline bromide (Pro-Banthine), are administered to suppress gastric secretions

and to delay gastric emptying by blocking the effects of vagal nerve impulses on smooth muscle. Sedatives are usually administered with anticholinergics to decrease the patient's level of responsiveness. H_2-receptor antagonists, such as cimetidine (Tagamet) and ranitidine (Zantac), inhibit the action of histamine, which causes gastric acid secretion.

38. **D** If the clinical findings suggest the lower bowel is the source of bleeding, proctoscopy should be the first diagnostic procedure. Proctoscopy will determine if the bleeding is from the rectosigmoid colon, rectum, or anal canal. Bleeding lesions commonly identified by proctoscopy include diffuse mucosal lesions (such as, ulcerative and ischemic colitis) and local vascular lesions (such as, hemorrhoids and tumors: polyps or cancer). An abdominal CT scan may be necessary as a follow-up to proctoscopy. Angiography is not indicated to evaluate GI bleeding. Esophagogastroduodenoscopy is useful in pinpointing the source of upper GI bleeding.

39. **D** The treatment for patients in the ED with lower GI bleeding depends on the extent and type of bleeding. If hemorrhoids or fissures cause bleeding, emergency admission is rarely necessary, and the patient may be referred to an outpatient clinic. If the bleeding is overt and from polyps, carcinoma, or ulcerative colitis, blood replacement may be necessary. This may be performed in the ED or on a medical unit. A patient with lower GI bleeding would rarely need emergency surgery, emergency endoscopy or admittance to the intensive care unit.

40. **D** When the amount of hemoglobin has been significantly reduced, the nail beds or palms will reveal anemia, unless the hand has been held in an awkward position or has been exposed to extreme cold or heat. Skin color, as in lips and gums, is an

unreliable index of the degree of anemia because of wide individual variations in the amount of melanin in the skin. The conjunctiva is typically evaluated for pallor, not the sclera.

41. **B** Hemorrhoids, the most common cause of lower GI bleeding, typically produce intermittent, minute amounts of bright-red blood on the outside of formed stool or on toilet tissue. Massive bleeding rarely occurs. Bleeding from the colon is much less common than from the stomach or duodenum; however, the blood loss may be abrupt. Perirectal diseases, such as hemorrhoids, fissures, diverticulitis, ischemia, and tumors, usually result in lower GI bleeding.

42. **D** Paralytic ileus is not a complication of endoscopy. Emergency endoscopy can be a useful diagnostic tool; however, its use may result in serious complications in certain situations. A patient who is uncooperative, unresponsive or who has esophageal obstruction is at high risk for perforation or aspiration. In addition, the patient may be at risk for cardiac arrhythmias because the endoscope increases airway resistance.

43. **B** Lower GI bleeding is characterized by bleeding from any source below the ligament of Treitz. The ligament of Treitz at the duodenojejunal junction is the dividing point for upper and lower GI bleeding.

44. **B** The nurse's primary concern after assessing the patient's airway, breathing, and circulation would be to establish two large-bore IV lines in the event that the patient develops hypotension or tachycardia secondary to hemorrhage and requires rapid fluid and blood replacement.

45. **A** The earliest indications of shock is tachycardia, a compensatory mechanism initiated by the sympathetic nervous

system in an attempt to maintain cardiac output and organ perfusion. Later signs include a narrowing pulse pressure, which indicates a falling cardiac output, followed by hypotension and cool, clammy skin.

46. **B** The nurse's priority at this time would be to prepare the patient for transport to radiology for a CT scan to determine whether the patient has internal bleeding. IVP may be necessary later if renal trauma is suspected. Neither immediate surgery nor blood replacement is warranted at this time.

47. **D** Because hemorrhage from retroperitoneal structures does not cause bleeding into the abdominal compartment, the results of a peritoneal lavage in a patient with a retroperitoneal hematoma may be falsely negative. A negative lavage typically yields less than 100,000 red blood cells/mm^3 in the drainage. After injury to the spleen, diaphragm, or bladder, bloody drainage (a positive result) is typically obtained.

48. **D** Frequent urinary tract infections is not an indication for IVP. Blood at the urinary meatus, lower abdominal crepitus, a high-riding prostate on rectal examination, and hematuria all indicate trauma to the genitourinary system. An IVP or abdominal CT scan may be necessary to diagnose the specific site of damage.

49. **C** The spleen, located in the left upper abdominal quadrant, is a highly vascular organ that normally cannot be palpated. However, when traumatized, intrasplenic bleeding may occur, resulting in a large mass that may be palpated in the left upper abdominal quadrant and displacement of the stomach. Fractured ribs in the left lower thorax may also signal a possible spleen injury. The liver, located in the right upper abdominal quadrant, cannot be palpated on the left side. Damage to the small

intestine or colon usually is associated with lower quadrant injuries.

50. **C** Because the assessment findings indicate an injury to the spleen, a highly vascular organ, the patient is at risk for fluid volume deficit related to blood loss. Potential for infection related to abdominal contamination would be an appropriate diagnosis for bowel perforation. Impaired gas exchange related to inspiratory trauma would be applicable if respiratory trauma were suspected. Decreased cardiac output related to cardiac trauma would be appropriate if cardiac trauma were evident.

51. **A** One of the most common factors predisposing a patient to abdominal aortic aneurysm in an older adult is a history of diabetes. Other risk factors include hypertension, male sex, advanced age, and smoking. Congestive heart failure, renal disease, and abdominal carcinoma are not considered risk factors for this condition.

52. **B** Abdominal distention, a pulsatile abdominal mass, and lower back pain are signs of an abdominal aortic aneurysm. Hoarseness, dysphagia, and mid-scapular back pain are signs of a thoracic aortic aneurysm.

53. **D** The highest priority nursing diagnosis for a patient with a fusiform infrarenal non dissecting aortic aneurysm, the most common type of abdominal aortic aneurysm, would be altered peripheral tissue perfusion related to decreased arterial blood flow. The other diagnoses are inappropriate because blood flow to the kidneys should not be impaired, and the patient's breathing and cardiac output should remain unaffected unless the aneurysm dissects.

54. **D** Femoral pulse assessments are the best parameter for evaluating tissue perfusion to the lower extremities. The other parameters are indirect measurements of tissue perfusion.

55. **B** Blumberg sign is a symptom of peritonitis and is assessed upon rebound tenderness. The psoas and obturator signs indicate irritation of the appendix and are elicited when the hips are flexed and internally rotated (the obturator sign) or when the examiner passively extends the right hip with the patient is lying on her left side (the psoas sign). Currant jelly stool, or stool that is composed of blood and mucus, is seen in patients with intussusception of the intestines.

CARDIOVASCULAR EMERGENCIES

1. A 68-year-old man arrives at the emergency department (ED) complaining of frequent episodes of substernal chest pain that have grown increasingly severe throughout the morning. He is alert and denies experiencing nausea, vomiting, or any radiation of the pain. The episodes, which began during the past month, typically occur at rest and last 10 to 15 minutes; they subside when the patient takes nitroglycerin sublingually. After initiating cardiac monitoring, the nurse administers oxygen 24% by facemask. The patient's electrocardiogram (EKG) demonstrates ST-segment elevation. Vital signs are blood pressure 130/90 mmHg, pulse rate 110 beats/minute, and respirations 24 breaths/minute. After reviewing the patient's history and EKG, the nurse determines that the findings are consistent with those of:

A. Stable angina
B. Preinfarction angina
C. Prinzmetal's angina
D. Angina decubitus

2. Appropriate nursing diagnoses for a patient with angina include all of the following except:

A. Knowledge deficit related to anginal pain
B. Potential for activity intolerance related to pain
C. Noncompliance related to life-style changes
D. Altered cardiopulmonary tissue perfusion related to coronary spasms

3. The nurse understands which EKG finding to be indicative of myocardial ischemia?

A. ST-segment depression
B. ST-segment elevation
C. T-wave elevation
D. U-wave appearance

4. The nurse recognizes that all of the following precipitating factors can contribute to the development of angina pectoris except:

A. Stress
B. Ingestion of heavy meals
C. Bed rest
D. Smoking

5. Which abnormality would the nurse detect during an angina attack:

A. Transient diastolic murmur
B. Transient abnormal point of maximal impulse
C. Pulsus paradoxus
D. Pericardial friction rub

6. The nurse understands the administration of propranolol to a patient with angina is contraindicated in all of the following circumstances except:

A. Heart block
B. Uncompensated congestive heart failure (CHF)
C. Tachycardia
D. Acute asthma

7. The triage nurse assesses an anxious and diaphoretic 54-year-old man who arrives at the ED complaining of severe, left-sided pressure like chest pain, and left arm numbness. The pain began 2 hours ago and is unrelieved by rest. He has no significant medical history. After initiating cardiac monitoring, the nurse administers oxygen at 2 liters/minute and establishes an IV line of dextrose 5% in water (D_5W) at a KVO rate. The patient's vital signs are blood pressure 120/60 mmHg, pulse rate 88 beats/minute and irregular, and respirations 20 breaths/minute. The cardiac rhythm shows normal sinus rhythm with occasional unifocal premature ventricular contractions (PVCs). The triage nurse suspects that this patient is exhibiting signs of a myocardial infarction (MI) because the chest pain:

A. Had not occurred previously
B. Is severe and radiating
C. Has lasted for 2 hours
D. Is accompanied by PVCs

8. The 12-lead EKG demonstrates ST elevation in leads V_1 through V_3. The nurse interprets this as an acute MI involving the:

A. Inferior wall
B. Anteroseptal wall
C. Lateral wall
D. Posterior wall

9. A patient's chest pain is unrelieved after the oxygen and sublingual nitroglycerin (1/150 grain every 5 minutes for three doses). Morphine sulfate has been ordered, because:

A. It is a powerful analgesic and decreases myocardial workload
B. It dilates coronary arteries when used with nitroglycerin
C. It produces sedation
D. It is an effective sedative and non-addicting when given in small doses

10. The physician orders Amiodarone (Cordarone) at a loading dose of 150 mg IV bolus over 10 minutes at 15 mg/min. Then a maintenance infusion of 360 mg over 6 hours at 1mg/min. Amiodarone (Cordarone) is indicated because it:

A. Lowers the fibrillation threshold
B. Decreases the heart's need for oxygen
C. Eliminates irritability within necrotic areas of the myocardium
D. Eradicates potentially dangerous PVCs

11. While awaiting transfer to the coronary care unit, your patient becomes tachycardic but his blood pressure remains stable. Which nursing action is most appropriate at this point?

A. Giving additional morphine and reassuring the patient
B. Prepare to give a beta-blocker by mouth
C. Auscultating the patient's lungs
D. Placing the patient in a low-Fowler's position

12. Which should be the nurse's primary goal when planning the care of a patient with an acute MI:

A. Preventing arrhythmias
B. Minimizing further cardiac damage
C. Decreasing the patient's oxygen needs
D. Alleviating the patient's anxiety

13. When caring for a patient with an MI, the nurse understands all of the following statements to be true except:

A. Most patients with inferior wall MIs develop life-threatening conduction disturbances
B. Arrhythmias associated with atrioventricular (AV) block usually are transient and not dangerous when they occur with an inferior wall MI
C. Severe nausea and vomiting are common with an inferior wall MI
D. Ventricular irritability, demonstrated by PVCs, is dangerous regardless of the type of MI

14. Upon auscultation, the nurse detects a new crescendo-decrescendo systolic murmur, which produces a blowing noise. This may be indicative of:

A. Aortic insufficiency
B. Papillary muscle dysfunction
C. Ventricular aneurysm
D. Early pericarditis

15. The nurse would suspect the development of a lateral wall MI in a patient who demonstrates:

A. Q waves in leads II, III, and aVF
B. Q waves in leads I, aVL, V_5, and V_6
C. Q waves in leads V_1 through V_4,
D. Tall R waves in leads V_1, and V_2

16. Which health history finding would not predispose a patient to developing an MI?

A. Diabetes
B. Hypertension
C. Hyperlipidemia
D. High estrogen levels

17. You assess a patient's blood pressure to be 90/60 mmHg and pulse rate 116 beats/minute and irregular. Based on the above vital signs, the nurse determines the patient's pulse pressure to be:

A. 30 mmHg
B. 50 mmHg
C. 70 mmHg
D. 75 mmHg

18. A 56-year-old woman is brought to the ED by emergency medical service personnel for evaluation of increasing shortness of breath. Her shortness of breath began 2 days ago and has become increasingly severe. She is pale and diaphoretic, and her skin is warm. Her respirations are 36 breaths/minute, and she exhibits increasing use of supraclavicular and abdominal muscles. The nurse detects bilateral crackles on auscultation. The nurse notes that the patient has a history of coronary artery disease and that she had an MI 2 years ago. After assisting the patient into a high Fowler's position, the nurse records the following vital signs: blood pressure 90/60 mmHg and pulse rate 116 beats/minute and irregular. The nurse notes that the patient's presenting symptoms and vital signs are consistent with:

A. Right ventricular failure
B. Left ventricular failure
C. Biventricular failure
D. Backward failure

19. The nurse understands that the physical assessment findings of a patient with right ventricular failure would typically include:

A. Gallop rhythm and pulsus alternans
B. Elevated pulmonary artery diastolic pressure and pulmonary capillary wedge pressure
C. Hepatosplenomegaly with or without pain
D. Cough, dyspnea, and crackles

20. Which intervention would the nurse know to be inappropriate for a patient with left ventricular failure?

A. Assessing the patient's fluid intake and output and electrolyte balance
B. Restricting the patient's fluid intake
C. Maintaining an infusion of normal saline solution
D. Maintaining the patient's intake of dietary sodium at 2 g/day

21. The nurse understands that the most common cause of right ventricular failure is:

A. Left ventricular failure
B. MI
C. Pulmonary hypertension
D. Cor pulmonale

22. Which nursing diagnostic category would be appropriate for a patient with CHF?

A. Decreased cardiac output
B. Impaired gas exchange
C. Activity intolerance
D. All of the above

23. The nurse understands that the rationale for administering inotropic and vasodilative drugs to a patient with CHF is to:

A. Decrease preload, increase afterload, and decrease contractility
B. Decrease preload, decrease afterload, and increase contractility
C. Increase preload, decrease afterload, and increase contractility
D. Increase preload, increase afterload, and decrease contractility

24. The nurse anticipates which diagnostic results to be expected findings in a patient with congestive heart failure?

A. Hypernatremia
B. Hyperkalemia
C. Elevated BUN and creatinine
D. Decreased BNP levels

25. The physician orders an ACE inhibitor to be added to the patient's medication regimen for treatment of congestive heart failure. The nurse understands the pharmacologic effects of ACE inhibitors to include:

A. Blocks the formation of angiotensin II, a potent vasoconstrictor
B. Limits the production of aldosterone thus increasing sodium and water excretion
C. Lowers arteriolar resistance and increases cardiac output
D. All of the above are correct statements

26. A patient receiving ACE inhibitors are at risk for developing which of the following adverse effects:

A. Hypokalemia
B. Hypertension
C. Persistent dry cough
D. Increased ventricular irritability

27. The nurse understands that ACE inhibitors should be used with caution in patients with:

A. Impaired renal function
B. Dehydration
C. Hypovolemia
D. All of the above conditions

28. Which nursing diagnostic category is most appropriate for a patient on ACE inhibitors whose condition has been stabilized?

A. Self-care deficit
B. Activity intolerance
C. Knowledge deficit
D. Sensory-perceptual alteration

29. Which EKG finding would the nurse expect for a patient whose potassium level is 6.5 mEq/L?

A. ST-segment depression
B. PVCs
C. Peaked T waves
D. Prominent U waves

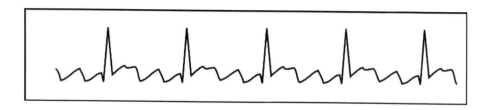

30. The nurse recognizes that the above EKG tracing is representative of:

A. Ventricular flutter
B. Atrial flutter
C. Atrial fibrillation
D. Paroxysmal atrial tachycardia with block

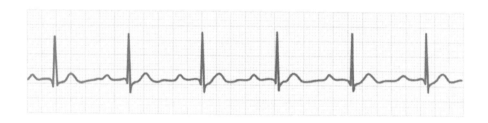

31. All of the following are consistent with the above EKG tracing except:

A. Inferior wall MI
B. Digoxin use
C. Hypokalemia
D. Organic heart disease

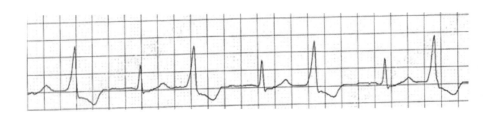

32. The above EKG tracing was taken from a patient who is asymptomatic. The pulse indicates perfusion of all beats. The nurse identifies this rhythm to be:

A. Pacemaker beats alternating with normal beats
B. Intermittent RBBB beats
C. Ventricular coupling
D. Ventricular bigeminy

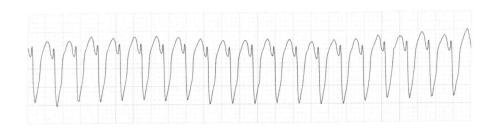

33. A patient who is experiencing an acute MI suddenly becomes unresponsive and pulseless while speaking with the nurse. The nurse notes the EKG rhythm above and responds by calling for help and:

A. Administering Amiodarone 300 mg IV
B. Defibrillating using 200 joules for biphasic and 360 joules for monophasic
C. Performing synchronized cardioversion using 100 joules
D. Administering repeated precordial thumps

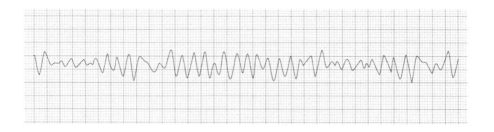

34. Which action should the nurse take first if she/he witnessed the patient's EKG rhythm shows the configuration above?

A. Administer 300 mg IV bolus of Amiodarone
B. Administer Vasopressin 40 units IV
C. Defibrillation
D. Perform synchronized cardioversion using 300 joules

35. The nurse observes a patient's cardiac rhythm converts to sinus bradycardia with a rate of 30 beats/minute and notes that he is exhibiting frequent PVCs. The patient complains of feeling lightheaded and nauseous. Which of the following is the treatment of choice in this situation?

A. Placement of a temporary pacemaker
B. Administration of a bolus of an appropriate antiarrhythmic agent
C. Administration of atropine sulfate IV
D. Infusion of isoproterenol (Isuprel)

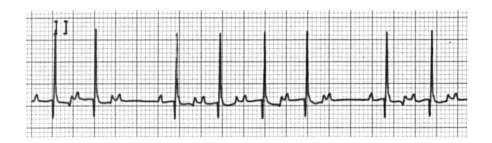

36. The nurse interprets the EKG tracing above as indicating:

A. Wandering atrial pacemaker
B. Second-degree AV block, Mobitz type I
C. Second-degree AV block, Mobitz type II
D. Third-degree heart block

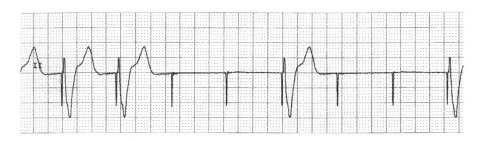

37. The nurse notes the rhythm above while monitoring a patient with a temporary pacemaker. Which nursing action would be unsafe in this situation?

A. Turn the patient on his side
B. Increase the pacemaker rate
C. Check the pacemaker connections
D. Turn up the output (mA) dial

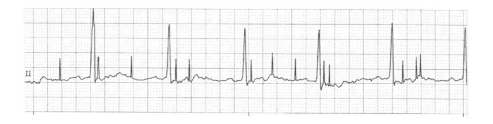

38. Which problem is represented by the EKG tracing above?

A. Runaway pacemaker
B. Loss of capture
C. Loss of sensing
D. Inadequate connection between the distal wire of the catheter and the negative terminal of the pulse generator

39. Aneurysms are classified according to all except:

A. Type
B. Shape
C. Consistency
D. Location

40. Which signs would the nurse typically note when assessing a patient with a proximal dissecting aortic aneurysm?

A. Hypotension, tachycardia, and radiating back pain
B. Hypotension, bradycardia, and EKG changes
C. Anterior chest pain, altered consciousness, and paraparesis
D. Hypertension, vomiting, and chest pain

41. The nurse understands that the most helpful studies in diagnosing aortic aneurysms include:

A. Complete blood count (CBC), electrolyte studies, and chest X-ray
B. CBC, lactic dehydrogenase (LDH) level, and chest X-ray
C. LDH level, aspartate aminotransferase (AST) level, and EKG
D. AST level, EKG, and echocardiography

42. A 63-year-old man arrives at the ED in an ambulance, complaining of a persistent, dull epigastric pain radiating to the interscapular region; the pain began 2 days ago. The nurse notes that he is alert and has good coloring and that his skin is warm and dry. Vital signs include right-arm blood pressure (BP) 120/60 mmHg, left-arm BP 220/100 mmHg, right radial pulse 2+, and left radial pulse 3+. The nurse notes bilateral basilar crackles and a systolic cardiac murmur at the second right intercostal space. The patient has a 33-year history of hypertension, for which he is taking medications. The physician prescribes an antihypertensive agent for the patient. The main objective of therapy is to maintain:

A. Systolic blood pressure at 100 to 120 mmHg
B. Systolic blood pressure at 140 to 160 mmHg
C. Diastolic blood pressure at 90 to 120 mmHg
D. Diastolic blood pressure at 130 to 150 mmHg

43. The nurse understands that most aneurysms usually occur in the:

A. Cerebral arteries
B. Aorta
C. Iliac artery
D. Popliteal artery

44. Which nursing diagnostic category is most appropriate for a patient with a dissecting aortic aneurysm and a blood pressure of 220/100 mmHg in the right arm and 140/100 mmHg in the left arm?

A. Altered tissue perfusion
B. Ineffective breathing pattern
C. Fluid volume deficit
D. Potential for infection

45. A 20-year-old man is admitted to the ED after being removed from a serious automobile accident. He sustained severe chest injuries as a result of not wearing his seat belt while driving. Chest x-rays reveal fractures to the second, third and fourth ribs on the left side. The physician diagnoses cardiac tamponade. The nurse should assess for which sign in a patient with suspected cardiac tamponade?

A. Pulsus alternans
B. Wide pulse pressure
C. Large R waves in V_1 to V_6
D. Restlessness

46. Initially, administering IV fluid to a patient with acute cardiac tamponade would:

A. Be very important to replace lost fluid volume
B. Increase preload, thereby temporarily increasing cardiac output
C. Increase afterload, thereby temporarily increasing blood pressure
D. Be contraindicated because of accompanying pulmonary edema

47. Which treatment would receive the highest priority in a patient with cardiac tamponade?

A. Thoracotomy
B. Administration of IV fluids
C. Pericardiocentesis
D. Administration of colloid fluids

48. The nurse understands that all of the following are common complications of pericardiocentesis except:

A. Ventricular perforation
B. Pneumothorax
C. Complete heart block
D. Ventricular fibrillation

49. Which is the most important nursing intervention during pericardiocentesis?

A. Preparing an infusion of isoproterenol (Isuprel)
B. Monitoring the patient's EKG tracings in the precordial leads V_1 through V_6
C. Positioning the patient flat, if possible
D. Encouraging the patient to perform Valsalva's maneuver, if possible

50. The nurse knows that the most common cause of acute cardiac tamponade is:

A. MI
B. Penetrating chest trauma
C. Blunt chest trauma
D. Cancer

51. A 50-year-old man arrives at the ED complaining of headache, nausea, vomiting, and blurred vision. His blood pressure is 210/144 mmHg. When asked about his medication history, the patient states that he usually takes clonidine hydrochloride (Catapres) but that he hasn't taken it for 2 days because he ran out of medication. Which assessment finding is least important in alerting the nurse to the patient's need for prompt medical attention?

A. Systolic blood pressure of 210 mmHg
B. Diastolic blood pressure of 144 mmHg
C. Headache and blurred vision
D. Nausea and vomiting

52. A 50-year-old man arrives at the ED complaining of headache, nausea, vomiting, and blurred vision. His blood pressure is 210/144 mmHg. When asked about his medication history, the patient states that he usually takes clonidine hydrochloride (Catapres) but that he hasn't taken it for 2 days because he ran out of medication. The nurse suspects this patient is in a hypertensive crisis, which is probably the result of:

A. Retention of sodium and water
B. Renal failure
C. Increased peripheral vascular resistance
D. Increased sympathetic stimulation from the brain

53. Nitroprusside sodium (Nipride) is commonly used in hypertensive emergencies. The nurse understands that this medication:

A. Must be administered slowly, through micro drip tubing
B. Has a direct vasodilating effect on the smooth muscles of arteries and veins
C. Has an onset of action of 2 to 3 minutes
D. Stimulates alpha-adrenergic receptors, producing sympathetic inhibition of blood pressure

54. The nurse understands that the most common cause of hypertension is:

A. Renal disease
B. Endocrine system dysfunction
C. Poor dietary habits
D. Idiopathic causes

55. A patient is brought into the ED by two EMTs, who are performing cardiopulmonary resuscitation (CPR). The patient is connected to a cardiac monitor and is receiving 100% oxygen by a hand-held resuscitation (Ambu bag). He has an endotracheal tube and a subclavian line in place. His EKG tracing shows that he is in ventricular fibrillation. He has been defibrillated two times by EMS, and one time by the ED, all attempts of defibrillation were unsuccessful. After the patient has been unsuccessfully defibrillated, the nurse should intervene by preparing an administration of:

A. Epinephrine hydrochloride (Adrenalin)
B. Calcium chloride
C. Amiodarone (Cordarone)
D. Sodium Bicarbonate

56. A patient's ventricular fibrillation continues. His arterial blood gas levels are pH 7.25, PCO_2 35 mmHg, PO_2 60 mmHg, and HCO_3^- 15 mEq/L. At this time, the nurse should expect to administer:

A. Sodium bicarbonate
B. Calcium chloride
C. Magnesium
D. All of the above

57. Which drug is usually infused after termination of ventricular fibrillation or ventricular tachycardia?

A. Vasopressin
B. Amiodarone
C. Verapamil hydrochloride (Isoptin)
D. Dopamine

58. The nurse understands that the treatable causes of persistent ventricular fibrillation may include:

A. Acute myocardial infarction
B. Hypoxemia and hypothermia
C. Hypovolemia
D. All of the above

59. Treatment of a patient with symptomatic complete heart block that is refractory to atropine typically includes:

A. Dopamine
B. Epinephrine
C. Isoproterenol
D. Transcutaneous pacing

60. The nurse understands that one of the therapeutic effects of propranolol is:

A. Increased myocardial contractility
B. Decreased cardiac output
C. Decreased myocardial oxygen supply
D. Prolonged AV conduction time

61. Which drug is commonly used to treat hypotensive shock in a cardiac patient?

A. Dopamine
B. Norepinephrine
C. Isoproterenol
D. Epinephrine

62. Which statement about dopamine is true?

A. It should be infused through a central line
B. The dose should be regulated through micro drip tubing
C. It is the drug of choice in treating uncontrolled arrhythmias
D. It may increase oxygen demand, when given in low doses

63. The nurse would expect to administer which of the following medications to a hypotensive patient in severe congestive heart failure?

A. Epinephrine
B. Dopamine
C. Dobutamine
D. Digoxin

64. The nurse understands that the most serious adverse effect of IV nitroglycerin therapy is:

A. Hypotension
B. Bradycardia
C. Congestive heart failure
D. Ventricular fibrillation

65. The nurse understands that a rapid IV infusion of nitroprusside may cause the patient to experience:

A. Hypertension and bradycardia
B. Chest pain and muscle twitching
C. Dyspnea and arrhythmias
D. Syncope and vomiting

66. The nurse understands that tPA (Activase) is used to:

A. Dissolve thrombi and reperfusion of blood flow to the heart muscle
B. Improve myocardial function
C. Limit the size of an infarction
D. All of the above

67. The nurse understands which statement about tPA to be false?

A. It is contraindicated for anyone with abnormal Q waves
B. Arrhythmias may occur during the infusion process
C. It should be administered within 6 hours of the onset of symptoms
D. It is contraindicated for anyone who has had recent major surgery

68. Which principle is most important to remember when administering tPA?

A. It should not be mixed in an IV line with any other medications
B. The patient should be monitored closely for changes in mental status
C. It should be infused along with a heparin drip to prevent re-thrombosis
D. All of the above

69. Which nursing action is least important during tPA administration?

A. Monitoring EKG tracings for reperfusion arrhythmias
B. Checking the patient's neurologic status frequently
C. Inspecting the skin for bruising and the urine for blood
D. Measuring QT intervals every 2 hours

70. The nurse understands which of the following routine medications will be given to patients receiving tPA therapy?

A. Antiplatelet treatment, antithrombotic therapy, adrenergic antagonists, and ACE inhibitors
B. Antithrombotic therapy, nitrates, calcium antagonists, and ACE inhibitors
C. Beta adrenergic antagonists, antiarrhythmic agents
D. IV nitrates, IV antiarrhythmia drugs, and magnesium

71. A patient has received successful tPA therapy, which EKG changes would the nurse expect to see?

A. Elevation of ST segments
B. Presence of Q waves
C. Increased T-wave inversion
D. Return of ST segments to the isoelectric line

72. A 32-year-old man, the driver of an automobile involved in an accident, is brought to the ED by ambulance. He is complaining of chest pain and shortness of breath. EKG tracings show sinus tachycardia with frequent PVCs. Based on the presenting signs and symptoms, the nurse suspects that the patient has:

A. An MI
B. Fractured ribs
C. Pericarditis
D. A cardiac contusion

73. The nurse understands that blunt chest trauma commonly results in damage to the:

A. Left ventricle
B. Right ventricle
C. Septum
D. Right atrium

74. Which therapy would be contraindicated for a patient with a myocardial contusion?

A. Nitroglycerin
B. Amiodarone
C. Morphine sulfate
D. Oxygen

75. A 32-year-old man, the driver of an automobile involved in an accident, is brought to the ED by ambulance. He is complaining of chest pain and shortness of breath. EKG tracings show sinus tachycardia with frequent PVCs. The nurse should monitor this patient for development of which complication?

A. Adult respiratory distress syndrome
B. Pulmonary embolism
C. CHF
D. Cardiomyopathy

76. Which drug would be contraindicated for a patient with complications from a myocardial contusion?

A. Heparin
B. Digoxin
C. Dopamine
D. Amiodarone

77. A 56-year-old man is being examined in the ED after complaining of chest pain and shortness of breath. His history reveals open-heart surgery, which occurred 1 month ago. He claims that, until today, he has been feeling fine. Pericarditis is diagnosed. During the initial assessment, the nurse would find first:

A. Cool to touch
B. Pericardial friction rub
C. Pulsus paradoxus
D. Kussmaul's sign

78. The nurse would expect a patient with pericarditis to exhibit which of the following signs and symptoms?

A. Further chest pain when leaning forward
B. Immediate relief of discomfort during deep inspiration
C. Bradycardia with ST-segment depression
D. Dyspnea and tachypnea

79. A 56-year-old man is being examined in the ED after complaining of chest pain and shortness of breath. His history reveals open-heart surgery, which occurred 1 month ago. He claims that, until today, he has been feeling fine. The nurse practitioner diagnoses pericarditis. The nurse understands that the administration of which drug classification may best relieve the patient's symptoms?

A. NSAIDs
B. Antibiotics
C. Nitrates
D. Inotropes

80. Which patient history finding would not predispose a patient to developing pericarditis?

A. Rheumatic fever
B. Post-myocardial infarction
C. Chronic obstructive pulmonary disease
D. Kidney disease

81. A 26-year-old man with a long history of IV drug abuse enters the ED complaining of fever, shaking, chills, and severe night sweats. The physician diagnoses his condition as endocarditis. Which procedure would be considered the nurse's lowest priority when assessing a patient with endocarditis?

A. Auscultating for S_3 heart sounds
B. Monitoring EKG tracings for PVCs
C. Monitoring the patient's temperature
D. Auscultating for crackles

82. The nurse would expect the laboratory studies of a patient with endocarditis to reveal:

A. Leukocytopenia
B. Elevated erythrocyte sedimentation rate
C. Polycythemia vera
D. Thrombocytosis

83. Which laboratory study is a definitive diagnostic tool and will guide patient treatment for a patient with diagnosed with endocarditis?

A. Blood culture
B. CBC with differential
C. Electrolyte studies
D. Clotting profile

84. A 32-year-old woman is admitted to the ED with complaints of sudden, severe pain in the right leg. After a thorough assessment, the physician diagnoses her condition as acute arterial occlusion of the right leg. Which history finding is atypical of a patient with acute arterial occlusion?

A. Atrial fibrillation
B. Postpartum status
C. Prosthetic valve replacement
D. MI

85. Which symptom would the nurse expect to assess in a patient with acute arterial occlusion?

A. A swollen affected extremity with trophic changes
B. Positive Homans' sign with nonpalpable pulses
C. A pale affected extremity that is tender to deep pressure
D. Paresthesias

86. An appropriate action for the ED nurse caring for a patient with an arterial occlusion is to:

A. Apply hot compresses to the extremity
B. Elevate the ischemic extremity
C. Infuse heparin, as ordered
D. Measure the patient's calf width

87. The nurse would anticipate preparing this patient for all of the following procedures except:

A. Arteriovenous shunt
B. Embolectomy
C. Thrombolytic infusion
D. Extraction of emboli with a balloon-tipped catheter

88. A patient is receiving intravenous nitroglycerin. The nurse understands that the mechanism of action of nitroglycerin is to:

A. Dilate arteries to increase systemic vascular resistance (SVR)
B. Dilate veins to increase blood return to the heart
C. Increase preload and afterload
D. Relax vascular smooth muscles

89. The nurse understands which of the following statements is false regarding unstable angina?

A. Episodes of chest pain occur at rest and low levels of exertion
B. The EKG shows persistent ST segment changes
C. 14% of patients with unstable angina will die within one year
D. Aspirin at a low dose will decrease the immediate risk of death in patients with unstable angina

90. The nurse understands which of the following 12 Lead EKG changes is strongly suggestive of high-risk unstable angina?

A. New left bundle branch block
B. Non-specific ST changes on EKG
C. Development of ST elevation in all the leads
D. ST segment depression

CARDIOVASCULAR EMERGENCIES: RATIONALE

1. **C** Based on the history and electrocardiogram (EKG), the nurse determines that the patient's findings are consistent with Prinzmetal's angina, a form of severe, non-effort-induced pain that occurs at rest. This type of pain occurs cyclically (commonly at the same time each day) and may be of a greater duration than the other types of anginal pain. Prinzmetal's angina, which is most common in women under age 50, is caused by spasms of a large coronary artery. Stable angina is characterized by chronic pain that shows no variance in duration, intensity, or frequency for at least 2 months; it may be debilitating or mild. Preinfarction angina, or unstable angina, is characterized by pain that increases in frequency, duration, and severity and usually develops into a myocardial infarction (MI). Angina decubitus is characterized by pain that occurs upon assuming a recumbent position.

2. **C** Noncompliance related to life-style changes would be an inappropriate nursing diagnosis because the ED nurse would not know whether the patient was compliant or not. All of the other diagnoses are appropriate because they identify specific treatable aspects of the patient's conditions.

3. **A** Transient myocardial ischemia, which produces the chest pain or discomfort characteristic of angina pectoris, may be identified by ST-segment depression or T-wave inversion on an EKG tracing. ST-segment elevation on an EKG tracing is typically associated with Prinzmetal's angina. T-wave elevation is common in patients with hyperkalemia. The appearance of U-waves on an EKG is associated with hypokalemia.

4. **C** The underlying cause of angina pectoris is disequilibrium between myocardial oxygen supply and demand, in which too little oxygen is available to meet the demands of the heart. Bed rest decreases myocardial oxygen demand and therefore poses no threat to equilibrium. Stress and ingestion of heavy meals increase oxygen demand; smoking decreases the blood and oxygen supply through vasoconstriction.

5. **B** During an angina attack, the nurse would be able to detect a transient abnormal point of maximal impulse. Other signs and symptoms of angina include anxiety, diaphoresis, pain or discomfort, cold and clammy skin, dyspnea, increased heart rate, pulsus alternans, atrial gallop (S_4), and a rare transient systolic murmur. Pulsus paradoxus may occur in a patient with cardiac tamponade or hypovolemic shock. Pericardial friction rub may be auscultated in a patient with pericarditis.

6. **C** Reflex tachycardia, which is induced by the use of nitrates, can be compensated by the bradycardic effects of beta blockade, resulting in a decrease in myocardial contractility, blood pressure, and heart rate. Beta-blockers, such as propranolol hydrochloride, usually are administered until the patient obtains relief or experiences adverse reactions. After abrupt cessation of propranolol, the patient may experience exacerbation of angina, which may induce an acute myocardial infarction (MI). Common relative contraindications to beta-blocker use include heart block, uncompensated congestive heart failure (CHF), and asthma.

7. **C** Any chest pain lasting longer than 45 minutes is probably caused by an MI. Chest pain associated with angina rarely lasts longer than 30 minutes and may also be severe and radiating, but it is usually relieved by rest. Premature ventricular

contractions (PVCs) may result from myocardial ischemia; they may occur during an angina episode.

8. **B** In this setting, ST-segment elevations are indicative of acute myocardial injury. Because leads V_1, V_2, and V_3 represent the anteroseptal wall of the left ventricle, the nurse would suspect that the patient is experiencing an MI involving the anteroseptal wall. Leads II, III, and aVF represent the inferior wall; leads I, aVL, V_5, and V_6 represent the lateral wall. ST-segment elevations are not characteristic of posterior wall MI; instead, mirror images (represented by ST-segment depression) would be present in leads V_1, V_2, and V_3, along with tall R waves.

9. **A** Morphine is a powerful analgesic. It reduces preload by causing peripheral vasodilation and reduces sympathetic activity, thereby decreasing myocardial workload. It has no direct effect on coronary arteries. Although morphine may produce sedation and is non addictive in small doses, it is not administered for these reasons.

10. **D** PVCs, which result from myocardial irritability, are dangerous in a patient with an acute MI because they are precursors to life-threatening ventricular arrhythmias. Amiodarone eradicates potentially dangerous PVCs. This medication has several actions which include: a delay in the rate at which the heart's electrical system recharges after the heart contracts; a prolongation in the electrical phase during which the heart's muscle cells are electrically stimulated; a slowing of the speed of electrical conduction through the heart; a reduction in the rapidity of firing of the electrical impulses in the heart; and a slowing of conduction through various specialized electrical pathways, called accessory pathways which can be responsible for arrhythmias. The ischemic area surrounding the

area of infarction, not the necrotic area, is the source of irritability, as necrotic tissue can neither generate nor transmit impulses.

11. **C** The most appropriate nursing action at this time would be to auscultate the patient's lungs to identify the cause of the tachycardia. Tachycardia is frequently the first sign of heart failure in the patient with an MI. It is a compensatory mechanism for low stroke volume or cardiac output. Tachycardia may also be caused by anxiety and chest pain. If heart failure were the cause of the tachycardia, a high Fowler's position would be the most comfortable for the patient. The nurse must assess the patient to determine the cause of tachycardia before administering morphine.

12. **C** The primary goal when planning the care of patient with an acute MI is to decrease the patient's oxygen needs. In an MI, the patient has an imbalance between myocardial oxygen supply and demand. Measures that reduce the body's need for oxygen, such as giving supplemental oxygen, promoting rest, and reducing the patient's anxiety, can decrease the occurrence of complications, such as arrhythmias, and prevent further myocardial damage.

13. **A** A patient with an anterior wall MI, not an inferior wall MI, is more likely to develop life-threatening conduction disturbances because the left anterior descending coronary artery supplies the His bundle and bundle branches as well as the anterior wall of the left ventricle. Such a patient should be closely monitored because second-degree heart blocks, especially Mobitz type II, are more likely to progress to complete heart block and cardiac arrest. First-degree atrioventricular (AV) blocks and second-degree AV (Mobitz type I, or Wenckebach) blocks are common in patients with an

inferior wall MI, and are caused by vagus nerve stimulation and AV node ischemia and edema, these blocks are transient and are not considered dangerous to the patient; progression to more dangerous blocks rarely occurs.

14. **B** This murmur is characteristic of a papillary muscle dysfunction, namely mitral valve insufficiency. When a papillary muscle becomes infarcted, improper valve closure results in regurgitation of blood from the left ventricle into the left atrium, producing a blowing sound. Aortic insufficiency produces a diastolic murmur, and pericarditis produces a friction rub. Various murmurs can accompany ventricular aneurysm, depending on the aneurysm's location. Alone, none of these is diagnostic.

15. **B** Q waves are indicative of myocardial necrosis. Therefore, Q waves in leads I, aVL, V_5, and V_6 which represent the lateral wall of the left ventricle, would lead the nurse to suspect that the patient is experiencing a lateral wall MI. Leads II, III, and aVF represent the inferior wall; leads V_1, V_2, the anterior wall. Tall R waves in leads V_1 and V_2 reflecting mirror images of Q waves are characteristic of a posterior wall infarction.

16. **D** Estrogen is thought to decrease lipoprotein levels and help coronary arteries resist atherosclerosis. For this reason, MI rarely occurs in women of childbearing age, as these women typically have high estrogen levels. However, when women reach menopause, estrogen levels decrease and their chance of developing coronary artery disease approaches that of men. Diabetes, hypertension, and hyperlipidemia are considered predisposing factors for the development of an MI.

17. **A** Pulse pressure is the difference between the systolic and diastolic blood pressures; therefore, a patient with a blood

pressure of 90/60 mmHg would have a pulse pressure of 30 mmHg. If arterial pressure falls and sympathetic compensatory vasoconstriction occurs, the pulse pressure is narrowed. Stroke volume and peripheral resistance influence the pulse pressure. A narrow pulse pressure indicates a low stroke volume (decreasing systolic pressure) or high peripheral resistance (increasing diastolic pressure).

18. **B** A falling blood pressure and narrowing pulse pressure are ominous signs of left ventricular failure, or forward failure. CHF can be described as right-sided or left-sided, although failure of both sides may occur simultaneously (biventricular failure) or one may progress to the other. In left-sided heart failure, fluid accumulates in the pulmonary bed, whereas in right-sided heart failure, fluid accumulates in the systemic circulation. CHF can also be described according to the direction of the main force of blood flow. Cardiac output is decreased in forward failure. Backward failure occurs when blood accumulates in one or both ventricles and the venous system, thus decreasing cardiac output,

19. **C** Hepatosplenomegaly, with or without pain, is characteristic of a patient who exhibits signs of right ventricular failure. The signs of right-sided heart failure are a result of venous congestion. With systemic vascular engorgement, the pressure in the capillaries of the abdominal organs will rise, resulting in edema. The edema produces a sense of fullness in the abdomen and may cause anorexia, nausea, and vomiting. Liver congestion causes tenderness over the hepatic area. The liver should be palpated for tenderness and engorgement. (Normally, the liver cannot be palpated.) Gallop rhythm, pulsus alternans, an elevated pulmonary artery diastolic pressure and pulmonary capillary wedge pressure, dyspnea, and crackles are

seen in left ventricular failure. Cough is not associated with right or left ventricular failure.

20. **C** In this situation, maintaining an infusion of normal saline solution is inappropriate because this would worsen the patient's CHF. Appropriate nursing interventions include monitoring the patient's blood pressure and closely monitoring the patient's fluid and sodium intake. Although the patient's serum sodium concentration level may be low, dilution from excessive fluid retention may be masking the underlying problem of sodium excess. Fluid restriction is necessary to allow the sodium concentration to reach a normal level. Maintaining the patient's intake of dietary sodium at 2 g/day is necessary to control thirst and water intake.

21. **A** The most common cause of right ventricular failure is left ventricular failure. This occurs as an increase in pulmonary venous and arterial pressures that is seen in left ventricular failure strains and increases the preload on right ventricular tissue. Other causes of right ventricular failure include intrinsic lung disease, valvular disease, right ventricular infarction, and pulmonary hypertension. Cor pulmonale is right ventricular failure that occurs from prolonged pulmonary hypertension.

22. **D** All of the diagnostic categories are appropriate because a patient with CHF has decreased cardiac output, impaired gas exchange, and activity intolerance—all problems the nurse can identify and treat.

23. **B** The aim of inotropic and vasodilative drug therapy in a patient with CHF is to decrease left ventricular demand and increase myocardial oxygen supply. This is accomplished by decreasing preload, decreasing afterload, and increasing contractility.

24. **C** Hyponatremia is seen in severe congestive heart failure and is due to a dilutional hyponatremia from fluid retention. Hypokalemia is present if the patient is taking diuretics. An elevated BUN and creatinine is present from decreased renal perfusion. The BNP is elevated, as BNP is an endogenously generated peptide activated in response to ventricular volume expansion.

25. **D** An ACE inhibitor is a pharmaceutical drug uses primarily for the treatment of hypertension and congestive heart failure. Frequently prescribed ACE inhibitors include captopril, enalapril, lisinopril and ramipril. ACE inhibitors reduce the activity of the renin-angiotensin-aldosterone system. The result of blocking the conversion of angiotensin I to angiotensin II, lowers the arteriolar resistance and increase venous capacity; increase cardiac output, lowers renovascular resistance. Aldosterone will decrease, thus there is a decreased absorption of sodium and excretion of potassium.

26. **C** ACE inhibitors may cause hyperkalemia. Suppression of angiotensin II leads to a decrease in aldosterone levels, which is responsible for the excretion of potassium. Hypotension is another adverse effect as ACE inhibitors block the conversion of angiotensin I to angiotensin II, a powerful vasoconstrictor. ACE inhibitors also reduce the plasma norepinephrine levels, which may reduce the prevalence of malignant cardiac arrhythmias. A persistent dry cough is a common adverse effect believed to be associated with the increased bradykinin levels produced by ACE inhibitors.

27. **D** Since renal impairment is a significant adverse effect of all ACE inhibitors caution must be used especially in those patients with impaired renal function. ACE inhibitors may reduce the glomerular filtration rate, a marker of renal function.

Please note that there is great concern if a patient is concomitantly taking an NSAID and a diuretic, as these three drugs taken together, predisposes the patient to a very high risk of renal failure. With ACE inhibitor use, the production of angiotensin II is decreased, thus leading to a decreased blood pressure.

28. **C** The most appropriate nursing diagnostic category for a patient on ACE inhibitors, whose condition has been stabilized, would be knowledge deficit. Using the category allows the nurse to formulate an appropriate diagnosis that enables him/her to determine the patient's current knowledge level regarding his health status, assess the patient's cognitive and emotional readiness to learn, recognize barriers to learning, assess the patient's learning needs, establish short and long-term goals, and encourage the patient's significant others to reinforce correct information regarding the diagnosis and therapies to the patient. The desired outcome of this diagnosis is that the patient participates in the learning process and communicates an understanding of his current health status and therapies.

29. **C** A potassium level greater than 5 mEq/L results in hyperkalemia, a condition represented by peaked T waves, prolonged PR intervals, and widened QRS complexes on EKG. A potassium level less than 3 mEq/L results in hypokalemia, a condition represented by ST-segment depression, PVCs, prominent U waves, and flattened T waves.

30. **B** This EKG tracing represents atrial flutter, which is characterized by an atrial rate of up to 300 beats/minute, a sawtooth pattern of flutter waves, and normal QRS complexes. In the given strip, a 2:1 ratio is represented. Atrial fibrillation is characterized by an atrial rate of 350 to 600 beats/minute and indistinguishable P waves. QRS complexes are normal in

configuration but occur in an irregular rhythm. Paroxysmal atrial tachycardia with block is characterized by an atrial rate of 150 to 250 beats/minute. Although P waves precede each QRS complex, they are not conducted when a block occurs. The P waves, which may be buried in preceding T waves, are often different in configuration because they arise from an ectopic focus.

31. **C** This EKG tracing represents first-degree AV block, in which the PR interval is greater than 0.20 seconds. Prolongation of the PR interval is associated with hyperkalemia, not hypokalemia. First-degree AV block is a common finding in inferior wall MI because of AV-node ischemia. The effects of digoxin and organic heart disease can cause delayed conduction through the AV node, thus prolonging the PR interval.

32. **D** Beware of PVCs in slow rhythms as they may be an escape focus. If they perfuse, do not give anti-arrhythmic agents. The nurse should check oxygen saturation, electrolytes such as potassium and magnesium, and blood pressure. In a patient with low-grade ectopy, including bigeminy, with no underlying cardiac, drug or metabolic cause, can usually be managed with reassurance.

33. **B** This EKG tracing represents ventricular tachycardia. The nurse would respond appropriately by calling for help and defibrillating the patient, followed by administration of Amiodarone 300 mg IV. However, if the nurse had been able to detect a pulse, synchronized cardioversion would be indicated. In this case, the defibrillator would be synchronized with the cardiac monitor so that the electrical impulse is discharged on the QRS complex (depolarization) and not on the T wave, which can cause the rhythm to deteriorate.

34. **C** If the patient goes into ventricular fibrillation, as represented in this EKG tracing, the nurse would respond correctly by immediately defibrillating the patient. Resume BLS immediately after each shock attempt. Administer epinephrine 1 mg IV bolus (repeat every 3 - 5 minutes while patient is in ventricular fibrillation). Vasopressin 40 units IV is an acceptable alternative to the 1st or 2nd dose of Epinephrine, but only as a one-time dose. Because the rhythm is chaotic, without evidence of P waves or QRS complexes, synchronized cardioversion cannot be used.

35. **C** The patient's PVCs may be a symptom of hypoxia caused by the bradycardia. If this is the case, increasing the oxygen could eliminate the PVCs; hence, they should not be treated with an antiarrhythmic. The initial treatment of choice for symptomatic bradycardia and bradycardia associated with PVCs (after oxygen) is administration of a 0.5 mg - 1 mg bolus of atropine sulfate IV, which may be repeated every 3- 5 minutes, as necessary, to a maximum dose of 3 mg. Should atropine be ineffective then a transcutaneous pacing should be applied. Other options are an infusion of either epinephrine or dopamine. Afterward, treatment may include the placement of a temporary or permanent pacemaker.

36. **B** This EKG tracing represents second-degree AV block, Mobitz type I (Wenckebach), which is characterized by a recurring sequence in which each PR interval becomes progressively wider until a QRS complex is finally dropped. Wandering atrial pacemaker is characterized by P waves that vary in size and configuration, as well as by PR intervals that vary, depending on the distance of the pacemaker to the AV node. Second-degree AV block, Mobitz type II, is characterized by constant PR intervals and unpredictable dropping of QRS complexes. In third-degree heart block, no relationship exists

between the P waves and QRS complexes. The atria and ventricles beat independently; the atrial rate may be 60 to 100 beats/minute, with regularly occurring P waves. The ventricular rate may be 20 to 60 beats/minute, depending on whether the impulse originates in the AV node or the ventricles (the rate is slowest when the impulse arises from the ventricle).

37. **B** Increasing the pacemaker rate would be unsafe for a patient whose temporary pacemaker is signaling loss of capture (no ventricular complex following a pacemaker spike), as depicted in this EKG tracing. Although the pacemaker is sensing the patient's slow rate and firing appropriately, the pacing spikes are not followed by QRS complexes. Increasing the pacemaker rate will not solve the problem; it will only produce more spikes. Possible causes of capture loss include an inadequate amount of energy (measured in milliampere [mA]) and displacement of the catheter tip. Turning up the output (mA) dial will increase the amount of electrical energy delivered by the pacemaker to the myocardium. Turning the patient on either side may cause the catheter to move back toward the endocardium. Another possible cause is disconnection of the negative terminal of the pulse generator from the distal wire of the pacing catheter. Since the distal electrode delivers the energy that paces the heart, checking the pacemaker connections would be in order.

38. **C** This EKG tracing depicts loss of sensing, in which the pacemaker fails to sense the cardiac rhythm and continues to fire at a preset rate even though the patient's heart rate is higher. Pacemaker spikes normally do not appear when the patient's own rate is consistently higher than that set for the demand pacemaker. Their appearance signals that the patient's own pacemaker and the temporary pacemaker are competing for control of the heart. Pacemaker spikes that occur on T waves,

which represent the repolarization (vulnerable) phase of the cardiac cycle, are dangerous because they may result in ventricular fibrillation. Runaway pacemaker, the firing of the pacemaker at a rate faster than that of the pacemaker setting, commonly results from battery depletion. The absence of pacemaker spikes will occur if an inadequate connection between the pacemaker wire and generator exists.

39. **C** Aneurysms usually are described according to shape and identified according to type and location. Their shape may be fusiform (in which the aneurysm appears as a uniform, round arterial dilatation) or saccular (in which the aneurysm appears as a vascular outpouching with a small neck attached to the arterial wall). A true aneurysm refers to a dilatation enclosed by at least one intact arterial wall. A false aneurysm (or pseudoaneurysm) refers to an extravascular accumulation of blood from a disruption of all three layers of the arterial wall. A dissecting aneurysm is one that results from a separation of arterial layers, in which blood accumulates in the middle layer secondary to a tear in the inner lining.

40. **C** A patient with a proximal dissecting aortic aneurysm typically experiences anterior central chest pain that rarely radiates to the back. The patient may also have signs of a neurologic deficit (such as cerebral apoplexy, paraparesis, or peripheral neuropathy) and altered mental status. Another common finding is blood pressure variations between the arms and pulse deficits. Hypertension typically occurs in a patient with a distal dissecting aortic aneurysm.

41. **B** The most common signs of a dissecting aortic aneurysm are an elevated lactic dehydrogenase (LDH) level, leukocytosis, and a widened aorta; therefore, the most helpful diagnostic studies include a complete blood count (CBC), an LDH level,

and a chest X-ray. Other helpful diagnostic tools include: EKG monitoring—to detect left ventricular hypertrophy, angiography—the most definitive diagnostic procedure to determine the location and extent of dissection and to evaluate the status of the renal, mesenteric, and iliac circulations. Emergency anteroposterior and lateral lumbosacral spinal X-ray studies or ultrasonography—to determine the exact size and location of the aneurysm (if the aneurysm is small and the patient is symptomatic, ultrasound studies should be performed approximately every 6 months to monitor size and determine need for surgery).

42. **A** The initial therapy and treatment of choice for all types of dissecting aneurysms is drug therapy, the primary objective of which is to decrease the systolic pressure to 100 to 120 mmHg for 24 to 48 hours, thereby controlling blood pressure. Another important objective of drug therapy is to decrease cardiac contractility; therefore, diuretics may be given concurrently. Drug therapy hastens the fibrotic phase of the healing process, reduces edema, and reduces bleeding in subsequent surgery. Once pain is relieved and blood pressure controlled, aortography is performed to enable the physician to select the appropriate, definitive therapy.

43. **B** Most aneurysms develop in the aorta, although they also may occur in the left ventricle after an acute MI, in the cerebral arteries, and in other central and peripheral arteries. Aortic aneurysms are categorized according to location, such as thoracic-ascending, transverse, descending, thoracoabdominal, and abdominal. Ascending thoracic aneurysms are located in the area of the aorta that is closest to the heart. Aneurysms of the transverse arch include the carotid, subclavian, and upper vertebral arteries. Aneurysms of the descending thoracic aorta are found in the proximal part of the descending aorta.

Abdominal aneurysms are found below the arteries of the kidney and above the bifurcation of the iliac arteries. Thoracoabdominal aneurysms extend from immediately above the diaphragm to the area immediately below it and are typically associated with decreased blood supply to the celiac, superior mesenteric, and renal arteries.

44. **A** An appropriate nursing diagnostic category for a patient with a dissecting aortic aneurysm would be altered tissue perfusion, as this occurs as a result of impaired blood flow secondary to a narrowed aortic lumen.

45. **D** Restlessness is a common sign of cardiac tamponade and results from hypoxia caused by a decreased cardiac output. Other common signs include a narrowing pulse pressure, pulsus paradoxus, and decreased amplitude of QRS complexes. Pulse pressure narrows because of a decrease in systolic pressure caused by the drop in cardiac output; diastolic pressure rises because of peripheral vasoconstriction. Pulsus paradoxus, the exaggerated decrease in systolic pressure during inspiration, is noted by the absence of heart sounds for a period greater than 10 mmHg while the blood pressure cuff is being slowly deflated. The amplitude of the QRS complexes typically decreases as a result of fluid accumulation, which increases the distance of the heart from the chest wall, thereby interfering with EKG recording.

46. **B** Preload refers to the stretching force of the ventricle immediately before contraction. According to Starling's law, an increase in the left ventricular volume will increase the volume pumped out during systole. Beyond a certain point, however, this mechanism no longer works. Therefore, increasing the circulating volume can temporarily support the patient's cardiac output until measures can be instituted to relieve the pressure of

the tamponade. Large amounts of blood are seldom lost when tamponade occurs quickly. As little as 100 mL of blood in the pericardial space is enough to cause a severe decrease in cardiac output. Patients with cardiac tamponade usually do not have pulmonary edema. They typically have normal chest X-rays, although a widened cardiac silhouette may be apparent. Afterload refers to the force against which the left ventricle must pump (peripheral vascular resistance).

47. **C** Pericardiocentesis, the aspiration of blood or fluid through an intracardiac needle inserted into the pericardial sac, is the priority treatment for cardiac tamponade. This procedure allows the physician to withdraw a minute amount of blood to reduce myocardial compression and increase cardiac output; removing as little as 20 mL of blood may save the patient's life. After hemodynamic stability is restored, the patient may be taken for a thoracotomy, if indicated. Administration of IV fluids may temporarily increase cardiac output.

48. **C** Heart block is not a complication of pericardiocentesis. Ventricular perforation can occur if the needle is advanced too far. Pneumothorax can occur if the needle is accidentally introduced into the pleural space. Ventricular fibrillation can result from the needle making contact with the myocardium. Although not a common complication, heart block could occur if damage to the heart's conduction system occurred due to injury from the needle being advanced into the wrong area of the myocardium.

49. **B** The most important nursing intervention during pericardiocentesis is to monitor the patient's EKG tracings in leads V_1 through V_6 because a precordial (V lead) lead is normally attached to the hub of the intracardiac needle. Any contact between the needle and the myocardium results in a

current of injury pattern, which is represented by an ST-segment elevation on the EKG. During the procedure, an awake patient may be placed in a high Fowler's position for maximum comfort. Isoproterenol (Isuprel) and Valsalva's maneuver are not indicated in the treatment of pericardial tamponade.

50. **B** Penetrating chest trauma is the most common cause of acute cardiac tamponade; blunt trauma is the second most common cause. Tamponade is also a rare but serious complication that can result from a transmural MI. Chronic fluid accumulation in the pericardial sac can result from various disorders, such as cancer, autoimmune disease, and uremia. Because these effusions occur chronically, the pericardium has a chance to stretch to accommodate as much as 1,500 mL of fluid. In this situation, the onset of symptoms is much more gradual and less immediately life-threatening.

51. **A** A systolic blood pressure of 210 mmHg would be the least important assessment finding in this situation. Hypertensive crisis is characterized by a diastolic pressure greater than 130 mmHg. When symptoms such as headache, visual disturbances, nausea, and vomiting accompany a critically elevated diastolic pressure, hypertensive encephalopathy should be suspected. Hypertensive encephalopathy is a medical emergency and occurs when arterial spasm and cerebral edema produce neurologic symptoms. Other symptoms of this syndrome include papilledema, transient hemiparesis, disorientation, and convulsions. If untreated, hypertensive encephalopathy can lead to death.

52. **D** In this situation, the nurse would suspect that the patient's hypertensive crisis is probably the result of increased sympathetic stimulation from the brain, resulting from the

discontinuation of clonidine hydrochloride (Catapres). Clonidine lowers blood pressure by acting directly on alpha-adrenergic receptors in the central nervous system, thereby causing a decrease in sympathetic outflow from the brain. Abrupt discontinuation of this drug can cause a withdrawal reaction leading to severe rebound hypertension. This may occur within 12 to 48 hours. Clonidine does not have any effect on sodium and water balance and is not known to have any direct effect on the peripheral vasculature. Nothing in the patient's history warrants suspicion of renal failure.

53. **B** Nitroprusside has a powerful, direct vasodilating effect on the smooth muscle of arteries and veins. This medication should always be administered through an infusion pump. Onset of action is 30 to 60 seconds. Profound hypotension can occur quickly in response to this medication; therefore, the patient's blood pressure must be closely monitored, preferably with the use of an arterial line.

54. **D** Although various factors predispose an individual to hypertension, most patients have no known medical problems directly causing hypertension and their condition is attributed to idiopathic causes. Predisposing factors include old age, elevated cholesterol levels, heredity, obesity, and sedentary life-style. Minorities of patients have secondary hypertension in which there is an identifiable cause. These include the use of tobacco, alcohol, caffeine, and certain drugs; cardiovascular disorders, such as coarctation of the aorta; endocrine disorders, such as pheochromocytoma and disorders of the adrenal cortex; neurologic disorders, such as increased intracranial pressure; kidney disorders, such as renal artery stenosis, acute or chronic renal failure, and renin-secreting tumors; and pregnancy.

55. **A** Epinephrine hydrochloride (Adrenalin), an endogenous catecholamine with both alpha- and beta-adrenergic actions, is the drug of choice in this situation. During resuscitation, epinephrine elevates perfusion pressure generated during chest compression, improves myocardial contractility, and increases the vigor of ventricular fibrillation. Recommended dose of epinephrine is 1 mg of a 1:10,000 solution. Because of its short duration of action, it may be necessary to repeat the dose at 3-5 minute intervals. Epinephrine should not be added to an alkaline solution because that may result in inactivation. Amiodarone (Cordarone) is the antiarrhythmic agent of first choice for VT/VF and given after epinephrine administration. Calcium chloride is no longer recommended as an advanced life-support medication because research studies have shown no therapeutic effects from its use. Sodium Bicarbonate is generally not indicated for the first 5 - 10 minutes of an arrest, unless the patient had a severe preexisting metabolic acidosis.

56. **A** In this situation, the nurse should expect to administer sodium bicarbonate, an extracellular buffer responsible for controlling acid-base balance. During cardiac resuscitation, the body is in a state of ventilatory failure, which leads to respiratory acidosis and circulatory failure. Metabolic acidosis is the result of these events. Efficient lung ventilation is essential to eliminate carbon dioxide and provide adequate oxygenation. The need for therapy must be guided by evaluation of arterial blood gas studies and is appropriate only if metabolic acidosis exists. Sodium bicarbonate is administered at a dose of 1 mEq/kg.

57. **B** If converted out of ventricular fibrillation or ventricular tachycardia, Amiodarone is the first choice. Give a 300 mg IV bolus for cardiac arrest. May give repeat boluses of 150 mg IV as needed for persistent ventricular fibrillation 10 minutes after

the initial 300 mg bolus. The maximum cumulative dose is 2,200 mg over 24 hours. Follow the Amiodarone bolus by maintenance IV infusion at a rate of 1 mg per minute for 6 hours and then at a rate of 0.5 mg per minute for the next 18 hours.

58. **D** The treatable causes of persistent ventricular fibrillation center around finding a cause that can be reversed in approximately a 10 minute period, and include the Hs and Ts: Hypovolemia, Hypoxis, Hydrogen Ion Acidosis (pH), Hyper/Hypo-kalemia, Hypoglycemia, Hypothermia, Tension Pneumothorax, Cardiac Tamponade, Toxins (overdose), Trauma, Thrombosis Pulmonary, and Thrombosis Acute Coronary Syndromes.

59. **D** Atropine 0.5 mg IV is given every 3 - 5 minutes up to 3 doses while the pacing is being setup. The treatment for unstable third degree AV block is transcutaneous pacing. If pacing is ineffective then Epinephrine 2 - 10 mcg per minute or Dopamine 2 - 10 mcg/kg per minute may be given. Isoproterenol is a pure beta-adrenergic agent possessing positive inotropic and chronotropic properties that increases cardiac output and heart rate. The recommended infusion rate is 2 to 10 mcg per minute titrated to maintain a heart rate of 60 beats/minute. Extreme caution must be exercised when the drug is used to treat MI because isoproterenol may enlarge ischemic and infarcted areas. Additionally, Isuprel is rarely used and can be helpful in those patients that have undergone a heart transplant. Heart transplant patients no longer have their vagus nerve connected to their heart and therefore require some form of sympathetic stimulation to the SA and AV node in the heart.

60. **D** One of the therapeutic effects of propranolol administration is prolonged AV conduction time. A beta-

blocker is used for beta-adrenergic blockade in the treatment of angina pectoris, cardiac arrhythmias, and hypertension. Beta-blockade action is useful in controlling the ventricular response to atrial flutter or fibrillation and in preventing recurrences of paroxysmal supraventricular tachycardia, as it decreases AV conduction. Propranolol also decreases myocardial contractility, which results in decreased myocardial oxygen demand. A decrease in cardiac output would not be a therapeutic effect.

61. **A** Dopamine, an endogenous catecholamine, is an important agent to treat various types of shock, such as hypotensive shock, because it directly increases cardiac output and renal blood flow. The hemodynamic effects depend on the dosage. At dosages less than 10 mcg/kg/minute, increases in cardiac output, myocardial contractility, and renal blood flow predominate; little or no vasoconstriction occurs. At dosages higher than 10 mcg/kg/minute, alpha-adrenergic effects predominate, leading to peripheral vasoconstriction and an increase in mean arterial pressure. Dobutamine hydrochloride (Dobutrex), norepinephrine, and epinephrine are inappropriate in this situation.

62. **A** Dopamine should be infused through a central line by an infusion pump. This drug is contraindicated in patients with uncontrolled arrhythmias or pheochromocytoma and in those receiving monoamine oxidase inhibitors; it may cause or exacerbate cardiac arrhythmias. At high doses, dopamine increases myocardial oxygen demand and may result in the extension of ischemic areas in those with coronary artery disease.

63. **C** Dobutamine is the preferred drug to treat severe heart failure. It produces a greater increase in cardiac output, a lessened increase in heart rate and peripheral vascular

resistance, and fewer cardiac arrhythmias than equivalent doses of dopamine. Adverse effects of dobutamine include nausea, headache, dyspnea, and angina. Epinephrine and digoxin increase myocardial oxygen consumption and are therefore inappropriate in treating severe heart failure.

64. **A** Adverse effects from the use of IV nitroglycerin include headache, methemoglobinemia, bradycardia, and hypotension. Hypotension is the most serious effect and can result in ischemia to organs that are dependent on perfusion pressure, such as the heart, kidneys, and brain. Hypotension can be treated with fluid administration. Bradycardia can be corrected with the use of atropine. Continuous nitroglycerin infusion is initiated at 10 to 20 mcg/minute and increased by 5 to 10 mcg/minute until desired hemodynamic or clinical results are achieved. Congestive heart failure and ventricular fibrillation are not adverse effects of IV nitroglycerin therapy.

65. **B** Nitroprusside is a potent vasodilator, decreasing preload and afterload. Rapid infusion of IV nitroprusside results in profound hypotension, apprehension, restlessness, muscle twitching, palpitations, and chest and abdominal pain. Treatment consists of titrating the infusion rate. The dose of nitroprusside should be regulated by an infusion pump, because of its potency and rapid onset of action. Thiocyanate levels should be monitored if high doses of nitroprusside are infused for longer than 48 hours. Rapid infusion of this drug does not cause hypertension, bradycardia, dyspnea, arrhythmias, syncope, or vomiting.

66. **D** Tissue plasminogen activator (tPA) (Activase) is indicated in the management of acute MI to dissolve thrombi obstructing coronary arteries; thereby improving blood flow,

improve myocardial ventricular function, reduce the incidence of CHF; and limit the size of the infarction.

67. **A** tPA is not contraindicated in patients with abnormal Q waves because the appearance of Q waves does not necessarily indicate completed infarction. Reperfusion arrhythmias, a complication resulting from coronary thrombolysis, may occur within 1 hour after administration of tPA therapy. These arrhythmias, such as sinus bradycardia, accelerated idioventricular rhythm, PVCs, and ventricular tachycardia, are not different from those often seen in the ordinary course of an acute MI and may be managed with standard antiarrhythmic measures. Lysis of coronary artery thrombi has been documented in 71% of patients treated with tPA within 6 hours of the onset of symptoms. Because bleeding is the most common complication encountered during tPA therapy, tPA is contraindicated for anyone who has had recent (within 10 days) major surgery or who has any condition in which bleeding constitutes a significant hazard.

68. **D** tPA is intended for administration by intravenous infusion only, via a volumetric infusion pump to ensure a precise flow rate. It should be administered in a separate IV line with no other medications. Heparin may be administered concomitantly with tPA to reduce the risk of re-thrombosis. Because the patient is at risk for bleeding, the mental status of the patient should also be carefully monitored.

69. **D** Measuring the QT interval is unnecessary because tPA does not affect this EKG parameter. During tPA administration, the nurse should closely monitor the patient's EKG tracings for the appearance of reperfusion arrhythmias. The nurse should remain with this patient at all time throughout the procedure to check the patient's neurologic status frequently for signs of

hypotension and to inspect his skin for bruising and his urine for blood because of the increased risk of abnormal bleeding.

70. **A** Administration of tPA therapy would also include: antiplatelet treatment such as Aspirin and clopidogrel; antithrombotic therapy such as low molecular weight heparins; and beta-adrenergic antagonists. ACE inhibitors improve survival rate in patients who have reduced left ventricular ejection fraction. Routine use of intravenous or oral nitrates does not improve outcomes in patients with STEMI. Nitrates may be used for pain relief. There is no role for the routine use of calcium antagonists, intravenous magnesium, or antiarrhythmic agents.

71. **D** Serial EKG tracings should be monitored throughout the course of tPA therapy. The nurse would expect to note several EKG changes if the drug has been successful, one of which is the return of ST segments to the isoelectric baseline. If the ischemia is abolished, T waves should return to their normal position. Deep Q waves are evidence of myocardial necrosis. If tPA has been effective, the extent of myocardial necrosis may be limited; therefore, Q waves should be absent or decreased in size.

72. **D** In this situation, the nurse would suspect that the patient has suffered a cardiac contusion, which commonly occurs after blunt chest trauma, such as steering wheel injuries. Myocardial edema and hemorrhage result in myocardial ischemia and necrosis. The signs and symptoms of cardiac contusion are similar to those of an MI: chest pain, shortness of breath, EKG changes (ST-segment elevation, T-wave inversion, and Q-wave formation), and cardiac enzyme elevation. However, because the precipitating event is have traumatic, rather than coronary artery, origin, the nurse would not suspect an MI.

73. **B** The right ventricle is the most common area of damage after a cardiac contusion because it is situated directly behind the sternum.

74. **A** nitroglycerin is not indicated in the treatment of cardiac contusion because the pain is not of coronary artery origin and dilation of the coronary arteries would not relieve it. Morphine sulfate is the analgesic of choice for the pain associated with cardiac contusion. Oxygen should be given to improve the oxygen supply to the damaged myocardium. Amiodarone is indicated in the treatment of ventricular dysrhythmias associated with cardiac contusion.

75. **C** The nurse should monitor the patient for development of CHF, one of several complications of cardiac contusion that results from damage to the myocardium from edema and microscopic hemorrhage. Other complications include ventricular arrhythmias, pericarditis, cardiac tamponade, and cardiogenic shock.

76. **A** Anticoagulants, such as heparin, are contraindicated in cardiac contusion because of the microscopic hemorrhage that occurs after the trauma. Hemopericardium, or bleeding into the pericardium, may result if heparin is administered. Digoxin and dopamine may be indicated if CHF develops. Amiodarone may be indicated if the ventricular arrhythmias are present.

77. **B** During the initial assessment of a patient with pericarditis, the nurse would likely find a pericardial friction rub before other findings. Further assessment typically would reveal pulsus paradoxus rub; however, this finding would likely not be appreciated before listening to the heart and lungs. Moreover, unless a manual blood pressure cuff was used, pulses paradoxus would likely not be detected. Additionally, these

findings do not help in evaluating the severity of the condition. An elevated temperature is not a constant finding. Kussmaul's sign, which is paradoxic inspiratory neck vein filling, is rarely seen in an acute setting. Pericarditis, or inflammation of the pericardial sac, may occur alone or with myocardial inflammation.

78. **D** A patient with pericarditis typically exhibits dyspnea and tachypnea. The pain associated with this condition is typically augmented with deep inspiration, trunk rotation, or lying flat. Palliative measures include sitting upright or leaning forward. A severe pleuritic substernal chest pain usually evidences pericarditis with widespread ST-segment elevation on EKG.

79. **A** Treatment for pericarditis involves the use of drug therapy to relieve pain and resolve acute inflammation. Anti-inflammatory drugs, such as aspirin, indomethacin (Indocin), or steroids, are commonly used. If pericarditis results from an infection, antibiotics, such as penicillin, would also be used; here, there are no facts to support an infection. In this situation, the patient has a recent history of open-heart surgery; therefore, the pericarditis probably is an autoimmune reaction to pericardial injury, and indomethacin would be prescribed. Nitrates or inotropes have no anti-inflammatory properties.

80. **C** Chronic obstructive pulmonary disease is not associated with pericarditis. The causes of pericarditis are multiple. Medical histories include viral infections; inflammatory processes, such as systemic lupus erythematosus, rheumatic fever, and scleroderma; and hypersensitivity or autoimmune responses, such as post-myocardial infarction (Dressler's syndrome). Other causes of pericarditis include certain metabolic disturbances (such as uremia or myxedema), kidney disease, and blunt or penetrating trauma.

81. **B** Monitoring EKG tracings for PVCs would be the nurse's lowest priority when assessing a patient with endocarditis because PVCs are rarely associated with infective endocarditis. Most patients with endocarditis present with sudden fever, the most essential feature of this disease, along with septicemia, and CHF. Therefore, priority-nursing procedures include monitoring the patient's temperature and assessing for symptoms of CHF, which includes auscultating for S_3 heart sounds and crackles. The patient should be placed on a cardiac monitor for assessment of heart rate because the tachycardia is frequently out of proportion to the patient's temperature.

82. **B** The nurse would expect the patient's laboratory studies to show an elevated erythrocyte sedimentation rate, the most common finding in endocarditis. Other common findings include leukocytosis (an increased white blood cell count) and anemia.

83. **A** Blood cultures are of prime diagnostic importance for a patient with endocarditis. Culture specimens from several sites should be obtained as the fever is climbing. Culture media and techniques for identifying fungi and anaerobic bacteria should be used, as should the standard techniques for aerobic strains. Once cultures define the type of bacteria, then appropriate antibiotic therapy can be narrowed. Although a nonspecific test, measurement of the erythrocyte sedimentation rate is useful in a negative sense; that is, if the rate is not elevated, a diagnosis of bacterial endocarditis becomes most unlikely. It is highly unlikely that the results of a cultures will be resulted in the ED (typically 24-72 hours), however, the care in the ED will continue through the patients stay in the hospital; hence being of prime importance. Although an elevated WBC with presence of neutrophils on the differential will indicate an acute

infection, it will not, however, reveal the species of bacteria and antibiotic susceptibility.

84. **B** A postpartum patient may be predisposed to a venous occlusion, not an acute arterial occlusion. Patients who develop acute arterial occlusion commonly have a medical history that predisposes them to mural thrombi formation. This may occur in rheumatic valvular disease, atrial fibrillation, MI, and previous cardiac surgery, such as prosthetic valve replacement.

85. **D** Physical examination of a patient with acute arterial occlusion typically reveals a pale or cyanotic affected extremity that is cold to the touch, nonpalpable pulses distal to the occlusion, paresthesias, and trophic changes, such as thin, shiny, and hairless skin. Swelling and tenderness in the affected extremity and a positive Homans' sign are symptoms of a venous occlusion.

86. **C** In this situation, administering an infusion of heparin, as ordered, would be an appropriate action. Other appropriate nursing interventions for a patient with acute arterial occlusion include providing warm environmental temperature to relieve arterial spasms (heat is never applied to the extremity) and elevating of the head of the bed or stretcher on 8 to 10 inch (20 to 25 cm) blocks so that gravity will augment flow of blood to the ischemic extremity (the affected extremity should never be elevated).

87. **A** The nurse would not anticipate preparing the patient for an arteriovenous shunt. Such a shunt may be surgically placed in a patient requiring hemodialysis. The nurse would anticipate preparing the patient for possible embolectomy, thrombolytic infusion, or extraction of emboli with a balloon-tipped catheter.

88. **D** The mechanism of action of nitroglycerin is to relax vascular smooth muscle causing vasodilation. Vasodilation of arteries results in a decrease in SVR and afterload. Vasodilation of veins results in a decrease in blood return to the heart and preload. The combined effects of venous and arterial dilation produced by nitroglycerin decrease the workload of the heart reducing its oxygen demand.

89. **B** Unstable angina is characterized by episodes of chest pain at rest or at low levels of exertion that are increasing in frequency, intensity or duration and by the absence of persistent segment elevation on EKG. Up to 7% of patients will die or have a myocardial infarction within seven days and up to 14% will die within one year. Aspirin at low doses has been shown to reduce death, MI, and stroke in hospitalized patients.

90. **D** ST segment depressions and T wave inversions are strongly suspicious for myocardial ischemia and high-risk unstable angina. The development of a new left bundle branch block and ST elevation are often seen with myocardial injury.

EYE, EAR, NOSE, AND THROAT EMERGENCIES

1. A 5-year-old child who recently underwent adenotonsillectomy is brought to the ED because of profuse bleeding from the nose and mouth. The child is weak, pale, tachycardic, and hypotensive. Which nursing action holds the highest priority?

A. Clearing any blood clots from the nose and mouth
B. Placing a postnasal packing
C. Drawing a blood sample for hemoglobin and hematocrit testing and a type and cross-match
D. Administering IV Lactated Ringer's solution

2. A 22-year-old woman with a recent history of an upper respiratory tract infection is being examined in the emergency department (ED). She complains of hoarseness that has lasted 3 days, along with pain on speaking, nasal congestion, and dysphagia. Assessment findings reveal a purulent nasal discharge, erythematous posterior oropharynx, and a temperature of 101° F (38.3° C). Which condition is indicative of this patient's assessment findings?

A. Acute laryngitis
B. Chronic laryngitis
C. Laryngeal carcinoma
D. Vocal cord polyps

3. A 22-year-old woman with a recent history of an upper respiratory tract infection is being examined in the emergency department (ED). She complains of hoarseness that has lasted 3 days, along with pain on speaking, nasal congestion, and dysphagia. Assessment findings reveal a purulent nasal discharge, erythematous posterior oropharynx, and a temperature of 101° F (38.3° C). Which instructions would the nurse include in the discharge plan for this patient:

A. Voice rest, with whispering permitted
B. Complete voice rest
C. Swishing and gargling with an alcohol-based astringent
D. Gargling with aspirin and salt water

4. Which nursing action would be most effective in providing comfort for a patient with laryngitis?

A. Administering metaproterenol (Alupent)
B. Applying an ice bag to the patient's throat
C. Instructing the patient to gargle with an antiseptic solution
D. Instructing the patient to swish and swallow a topical anesthetic solution of lidocaine (Xylocaine) before eating

5. An 18-year-old man arrives at the ED complaining of being suddenly awakened by a feeling of something moving in his ear. On physical examination, the nurse notes a large, live cockroach in his external auditory canal. The nurse would anticipate the initial treatment for this patient to include:

A. Removing the insect with forceps
B. Spraying lidocaine 10% in the auditory canal
C. Irrigating the ear with warm water
D. Instilling warm mineral oil into the ear

6. After an insect is successfully removed from a patient's ear, subsequent management would include:

A. Administering 500 mg of ampicillin (Amcill) orally to prevent infection
B. Irrigating the ear canal with peroxide and applying a dry, sterile dressing
C. Packing the ear canal with iodoform gauze
D. Instilling antibacterial drops into the ear and packing the ear canal with 1/4" gauze strips

7. A 65-year-old man with a history of chronic obstructive pulmonary disease and laryngeal carcinoma is being examined in the ED. He is currently undergoing radiation therapy and has symptoms of acute respiratory distress. Assessment reveals inspiratory stridor, dyspnea, increasing apprehension, and facial flushing. The most appropriate nursing action would be to:

A. Obtain samples for arterial blood gas evaluation and administer 100% oxygen via facemask
B. Prepare for a tracheotomy
C. Prepare for intubation
D. Call for a chest X-ray

8. A patient is not intubated successfully, the nurse would expect to:

A. Obtain a smaller endotracheal tube
B. Assemble necessary equipment for a tracheotomy
C. Obtain a cricothyroidotomy tray
D. Order an X-ray of the patient's lateral neck

9. A 40-year-old man is brought to the ED after a mugging incident with blood oozing from his left ear. The nurse practitioner diagnoses a ruptured tympanic membrane. The nurse anticipates the initial treatment for this patient to include:

A. Removing blood clots and packing the ear canal
B. Administering antibacterial otic drops
C. Administering 50 mg of ampicillin orally
D. Administering tetanus toxoid

10. During discharge teaching for a patient with a ruptured tympanic membrane, the nurse would stress the importance of:

A. Gentle nose blowing
B. Avoiding heavy lifting
C. Rinsing the ear canal with warm water daily
D. Retaining packing in the ear canal for 1 week

11. A 26-year-old male is examined in the ED for complaints of ear pain. He has a 2-day history of itchiness in his ear, diminished hearing, and fever. He informs the physician that he has been swimming in a public pool during the previous week. Based on the above findings, which condition would the nurse suspect the child to have?

A. Acute otitis externa
B. Acute otitis media
C. Ruptured tympanic membrane
D. Ear canal cellulitis

12. The treatment plan for a patient with an ear infection and fever includes all of the following except:

A. Administration of acetaminophen (Tylenol)
B. Administration of an oral antibiotic
C. Administration of an otic antibiotic
D. Application of ice packs to the ear

13. The nurse is aware that a patient with acute otitis externa commonly demonstrates:

A. Upper respiratory tract infection
B. An elevated temperature above 102° F (38.9° C)
C. Otalgia
D. Periauricular lymphadenopathy

14. Which otic emergency is more common in children than adults?

A. Acute otitis externa
B. Acute otitis media
C. Meniere's disease
D. Bullous myringitis

15. If otitis media is not treated aggressively, all of the following serious complications may result except:

A. Meningitis
B. Ototoxicity
C. Mastoiditis
D. Permanent hearing loss

16. Aftercare instructions for a patient with a ruptured tympanic membrane have been effective if patient states:

A. "I should instill the antibiotic drops into the ear canal as prescribed."
B. "I should use a Q-tip to gently apply antibiotics to the affected ear."
C. "I should place a cotton ball coated in petroleum into the ear to protect/repel fluids from entering the ear."
D. " I may lose all hearing in the ear temporarily until it is healed."

17. The triage nurse examines a 54-year-old man with a history of alcohol abuse. He complains of having difficulty breathing through his nose after having fallen the previous night. His symptoms include a lacerated bridge of the nose, periorbital edema, and dried blood in his nares. The most serious cause of this patient's breathing difficulty can be attributed to:

A. Blood clots in the nares
B. Edema of the nose
C. Deviated septum
D. Septal hematoma

18. The triage nurse examines a 54-year-old man with a history of alcohol abuse. He complains of having difficulty breathing through his nose after having fallen the previous night. His symptoms include a lacerated bridge of the nose, periorbital edema, and dried blood in his nares. Which nursing intervention is appropriate in caring for this patient?

A. Asking the patient to blow his nose to help loosen and remove the clot
B. Inserting an intranasal packing
C. Examining the nasal bone for mobility
D. Administering tetanus toxoid, as ordered

19. Treatment for a linear facial fracture with nasal bleeding may include:

A. Nasal packing and establishment of an IV line
B. Administration of a decongestant and a vasoconstrictor
C. Application of a cold pack to the bridge of the nose
D. All of the above

20. Which nursing action is inappropriate for a patient with an anterior epistaxis?

A. Pinching the patient's nose for 4 to 5 minutes
B. Alleviating patient apprehension
C. Placing the patient in a semirecumbent position with his head tilted forward
D. Administering IV fluids

21. A 19-year-old man is brought to the hospital by emergency medical service after an automobile accident. He has multiple facial lacerations, nasal deformity, and cheek flattening, as well as diplopia and difficulty opening his mouth. The nurse suspects that, based on the assessment findings, the patient has a:

A. Mandibular fracture
B. Maxillary fracture
C. Zygomatic fracture
D. Temporomandibular joint dislocation

22. A 19-year-old man is brought to the hospital by emergency medical service after an automobile accident. He has multiple facial lacerations, nasal deformity, and cheek flattening, as well as diplopia and difficulty opening his mouth. An inappropriate nursing action during the immediate care of this patient would be to:

A. Prepare the patient for definitive treatment of fracture by the physician
B. Observe for potential airway obstruction
C. Assess the patient's level of consciousness
D. Evaluate the patient for cervical or spinal trauma

23. Which nursing action is considered unsafe when assisting the patient with suspected facial fractures to maintain optimal airway clearance?

A. Positioning the patient on his side
B. Inserting a nasopharyngeal airway
C. Placing the patient in semi-Fowler's position
D. Having tracheotomy equipment available

24. After assessment of this patient, which diagnostic procedure would the nurse expect the physician to order?

A. Water's view X-rays
B. Submental-vertex X-rays
C. Cervical spine X-rays
D. All of the above

25. After the patient's condition stabilizes and the physician rules out spinal injury and neurologic deficits, the nurse would expect to ensure the patient's comfort by performing all of the following except:

A. Administering narcotics or analgesics, as ordered
B. Positioning the patient with the head of the bed elevated
C. Applying cold compresses to the fracture site
D. Taping the bridge of the patient's nose to stabilize the bones

26. The triage nurse assesses a 25-year-old male carpenter. He complains of severe right eye pain, a gritty sensation in the eye, and sensitivity to light. He angrily claims that his symptoms began suddenly while he was hammering a nail and states that he is going to sue his boss. Which question is of least priority when obtaining a history from this patient?

A. "Describe your visual acuity before this incident; did you have any previous eye disease?"
B. "Were you wearing goggles or glasses and did any damage occur to them?"
C. "What caused the injury, and what was its trajectory and distance to your head?"
D. "Are you currently seeing halos around lights?"

27. The triage nurse assesses a 25-year-old male carpenter. He complains of severe right eye pain, a gritty sensation in the eye, and sensitivity to light. He angrily claims that his symptoms began suddenly while he was hammering a nail and states that he is going to sue his boss. Which nursing action would least effectively relieve the patient's pain?

A. Instilling a fluorescein stain
B. Applying topical analgesics
C. Covering the eye with an occlusive patch
D. Irrigating the eye with normal saline solution

28. The triage nurse examines a 60-year-old woman after having sustained blunt trauma to her right eye during a fall. Her only complaint is blurred vision in the right eye. The physician diagnoses hyphema. Which is the most important information to collect from this patient during the initial assessment:

A. The mechanism of injury
B. The patient's history of ocular disorders
C. The patient's symptoms before her arrival at the ED
D. The patient's use of medications, especially aspirin

29. Which nursing action should be included in the plan of care for a patient with hyphema?

A. Maintaining the patient in a supine position
B. Patching the patient's eyes during the acute phase
C. Irrigating the eye frequently with normal saline solution during the acute phase
D. Applying gentle finger massage to the eye

30. Which instruction should not be included in patient teaching, with hyphema, before discharge?

A. Avoid coughing and performing Valsalva's maneuver
B. Remain on strict bed rest for 2 weeks
C. Elevate the head of the bed to a 30-degree angle
D. Reduce stress and physical strain

31. A 29-year-old man is brought to the hospital via ambulance after sustaining a chemical burn to his eyes. He had been involved in a fight during which lye was thrown in his face. Which nursing action has the highest priority for this patient?

A. Checking the pH of the patient's eyes with litmus paper
B. Instilling antibiotic eye drops
C. Flushing the eyes with a sodium bicarbonate solution
D. Continuously irrigating the eyes with copious amounts of normal saline solution

32. All of the following statements regarding chemical burns of the eye are true except:

A. Alkaline burns are the most destructive
B. Acid burns are extremely irritating
C. An acid substance continues to dissolve soft tissue in the eye until it is removed
D. The principles of management for alkaline and acid burns are similar

33. What is the best indication that treatment has been effective for a patient with a chemical burn to the eyes?

A. Slight evidence of corneal whitening
B. A pH value of 7.0 on a litmus paper reading
C. Extraocular movements
D. Visual acuity limited to light perception

34. Which of the following is not a symptom of retinal detachment?

A. Eye pain
B. Loss of central vision
C. Seeing floaters
D. Photopsia

35. A healthy appearing three-year-old child arrives in the ED with a six-day history of a purulent, blood-tinged, foul-smelling discharge from the right nostril. The left nostril is clear. Mother notes frequent sneezing but the child is not coughing or febrile. He seems mildly agitated because he can only breathe through one nostril. The most likely reason for these findings is

A. Sinus infection
B. Uncontrolled allergic rhinitis
C. Foreign body in the right nostril
D. Viral upper respiratory tract infection (URTI)

EYE, EAR, NOSE, AND THROAT: RATIONALE

1. **A** Bleeding after adenotonsillectomy must be treated with utmost urgency. The priority action always includes clearing any blood clots from the nose and mouth to ensure a patent airway. IV fluids, such as Lactated Ringer's or normal saline solution, should be started promptly because children become hypovolemic much faster than adults, and the patient must be ready to go to the operating room immediately. Tonsillar sponges may be used to apply pressure to the tonsils, but a physician must place postnasal packing to control adenoidal bleeding.

2. **A** A recent history of an upper respiratory tract infection, hoarseness, fever, and erythematous oropharynx are indicative of acute laryngitis. Patients with vocal cord polyps have hoarseness but no upper respiratory tract infection, whereas those with laryngeal cancer may have hoarseness and difficulty breathing only if the lesion is large. Laryngeal cancer usually occurs in older men with a long history of smoking and alcohol abuse.

3. **B** Treatment for acute laryngitis involves complete voice rest, with no whispering permitted. Smoking, alcohol, and aspirin may cause further irritation, inflammation, edema, and pain; therefore, gargling with an alcohol-based astringent or a mixture of aspirin and salt water is never recommended. Saline solution gargles and topical anesthetics, however, may be helpful.

4. **B** The most effective comfort measure for the patient with acute laryngitis is the application of an ice bag to the throat. Metaproterenol (Alupent) treatments and antiseptic gargles are

inappropriate. Swishing and swallowing an anesthetic solution before eating is unsafe because aspiration may occur.

5. **B** Recent studies indicate that insects may be removed from the ear by spraying a topical neuro stimulant, such as lidocaine, into the external auditory canal. If this is unavailable, the insect should be immobilized and drowned in mineral oil, then removed with minute forceps. Irrigation with water may cause the insect's body to swell or may push the insect closer to the tympanic membrane.

6. **D** Subsequent management would include instilling antibacterial drops into the ear and packing the ear canal with gauze strips. Because insects are potential disease carriers, a topical otic antibiotic may be used prophylactically to prevent infection caused by bites or scratches. Attempts to remove foreign objects from the ear produce trauma, which may result in further swelling and even bleeding of the ear canal walls. A light packing of gauze strips may control bleeding. Oral antibiotics and iodoform gauze are unnecessary.

7. **C** The most appropriate nursing action would be to prepare the patient for immediate intubation to establish an airway. Patients undergoing radiation therapy to the head and neck are subject to complications, including edema of the upper airway, severe dryness of the oral cavity, and skin burns. Arterial blood gas studies are not an immediate priority in this situation. Administration of oxygen higher than 30% should be used with caution in a patient with COPD, as the patient breathes on an oxygen drive and higher levels would decrease the respiratory rate. However, one should never withhold oxygen to a patient in acute respiratory distress. Tracheotomy should not be performed in a patient with laryngeal cancer because this may lead to stomal carcinoma via direct extension of the tumor.

8. **C** If the immediate action, intubation, is unsuccessful, the next step would be to obtain a cricothyroidotomy tray for an emergency cricothyroidotomy. This procedure is indicated when the patient's edema or tumor is so great that an endotracheal tube cannot be passed initially and subsequent attempts would cause further swelling.

9. **A** When a patient has a ruptured tympanic membrane and basal skull fracture has been ruled out, bleeding from the ear may be controlled by removing blood clots and packing the ear canal. The packing may be removed when bleeding has stopped. Tympanic membrane rupture does not require antibiotics; a healthy exposed middle ear mucosa is especially vulnerable to ototoxicity from eardrops. The tympanic membrane should heal in 1 to 2 weeks.

10. **B** During discharge teaching, the patient must be encouraged to avoid heavy lifting and straining from Valsalva's maneuver for 1 to 2 weeks. Other activities to avoid include nose blowing, swimming, and any activity that might involve exposing the ear canal to water. Packing should be retained in the ear canal until the bleeding has stopped.

11. **A** Swimming in a public pool is a common source of contamination, especially for the ears, producing an inflammatory disorder of the auricle and external auditory canal known as acute otitis externa. It is most commonly caused by bacterial or fungal infections, particularly Pseudomonas. Predisposing factors include moisture in the ear canal, which may occur in a warm, moist climate or as a result of swimming, and trauma resulting from attempts to clean or scratch an itchy ear.

12. **D** Applying ice packs to the ear is inappropriate in this situation. Appropriate treatment includes administering analgesics, antibiotics (oral, otic, or topical), and antipyretics and applying hot, moist compresses to the affected ear.

13. **D** Periauricular lymphadenopathy is a common manifestation in patients with acute otitis externa. A history of an upper respiratory tract infection, a temperature of 102 F (38.8 C) or higher, and otalgia that increases with prone position are manifestations of acute otitis media.

14. **B** Acute otitis media is more common in children than adults because of children's narrower eustachian tubes, which are prone to occlusion. The condition is commonly preceded by an upper respiratory tract infection or childhood disease, such as measles or scarlet fever. This is because of the proximity and connection of the eustachian tube to the upper respiratory tract.

15. **B** Ototoxicity is an adverse reaction to salicylates or antibiotics, such as kanamycin (Kantrex) and streptomycin; it is not a complication of otitis media. Common complications that result when otitis media is not treated aggressively include meningitis, mastoiditis, intracranial abscess, and permanent hearing loss.

16. **A** Antibiotic therapy via drops is the preferred treatment for a ruptured tympanic membrane. Never instruct patients to put objects such as cotton swabs in the ear. The ear should be protected from getting wet, but petroleum should not be used as it could cause a blockage and impair antibiotic drop effectiveness. Any worsening or loss of hearing should be reported to the physician.

17. **D** In nasal trauma, a collection of blood develops under the septal mucosa, forming a septal hematoma, a bulging mass that causes serious breathing difficulty in both nares. Blood clots in the nares, edema of the nose, and a deviated septum also may cause breathing difficulty, but these are less serious conditions.

18. **D** Because the patient sustained a nasal laceration, the appropriate nursing action would be to administer a tetanus toxoid, a routine precaution for any open wound. Further treatment involves cleaning the nose with such agents as povidone-iodine solution and peroxide, followed by irrigation with normal saline solution. Before applying intranasal packing or blowing the nose, cerebrospinal fluid (CSF) rhinorrhea must be ruled out. This is accomplished by observing for drainage from the nose and testing any drainage for glucose (60% of CSF is serum glucose).

19. **D** Treatment for a linear nasal facture with nasal bleeding includes packing the nasal cavity, establishing an IV line, administering decongestants and vasoconstrictors, and applying cold packs to the bridge of the nose to decrease bleeding. Establishing an IV line is necessary to infuse fluids because of lost blood volume.

20. **D** Administering IV fluids to a patient with an anterior epistaxis would be inappropriate. Active bleeding from an anterior epistaxis can be controlled temporarily by pinching the nose for 4 to 5 minutes. If bleeding persists, cauterization with silver nitrate sticks or electrocautery should be attempted. If bleeding still is not controlled, the physician will anesthetize the nasal chamber and insert nasal packing. Whenever nasal packing of any sort is used, the patient should be placed on broad-spectrum antibiotics until packs are removed. Alleviating the patient's apprehension and placing the patient in a

semirecumbent position with his head tilted forward are appropriate measures.

21. **C** Nasal deformity, cheek flattening, difficulty in opening the mouth, and diplopia most likely indicate a zygomatic fracture. This type of facial fracture is associated with asymmetry of the face, painful jaw movement, limited movement of lower jaw, and visual disturbances. Zygomatic fractures are most commonly caused by automobile accidents and fights and are frequently associated with orbital floor fractures, also referred to as "blow-out fractures."

22. **A** The immediate management of a patient who sustained a zygomatic fracture would not include preparation for definitive treatment of the fracture by a physician. Definitive treatment may require semi-open reduction, open reduction, or internal wire fixation, which may be performed later. Appropriate immediate nursing actions aim to maintain a patent airway by examining for potential obstruction from blood clots, saliva, and loose teeth. The nurse should also assess the patient's level of consciousness to establish a baseline by which deterioration in neurologic status from associated head trauma can be recognized. The patient also should be evaluated for possible cervical or spinal trauma. Subsequent actions include controlling bleeding from facial lacerations and applying cold compresses to prevent facial edema. Prompt application of compresses will permit fractures to be tended sooner.

23. **B** Nursing interventions to ensure airway patency are of the utmost importance in a patient with a zygomatic fracture. However, the insertion of a nasopharyngeal airway is inappropriate and unsafe in such a patient because of the risk of further trauma and bleeding. Appropriate interventions include placing the patient in a side-lying or semi-Fowler's position for

optimal airway clearance and having emergency suction equipment on hand. Aspiration of teeth, bony fragments, blood clots, and vomitus must be prevented. Emergency intubation or tracheotomy equipment should also be accessible to ensure the immediate establishment of an airway, if necessary.

24. **D** Diagnostic procedures are essential for determining the extent of injuries and formulating a plan of care based on the patient's needs. Water's view X-rays permit evaluation of malar or zygoma eminence, and submental-vertex view permits evaluation of the zygomatic arch. Cervical spine X-rays, which are in many cases neglected because the facial deformities are not striking, must be obtained to evaluate fractures or dislocations that may result from the trauma.

25. **D** Taping the bridge of the patient's nose is not indicated. Appropriate interventions to ensure patient comfort include administering narcotics or analgesics as ordered, elevating the head of the bed, and applying cold compresses to the fracture site to decrease edema.

26. **D** Asking the patient whether he sees halos around lights is the least important information to elicit at this time. This symptom usually is associated with glaucoma, not extraocular foreign body emergencies. Because this type of trauma may be associated with future compensation, the nurse must conduct a comprehensive interview. Information obtained must include the time elapsed since the occurrence, the circumstances of the injury, the type and condition of safety apparatus worn at the time of injury, treatment before arrival, the patient's medical history, including his current medications, the date of his last tetanus immunization, any known allergies, and his visual status before the accident, and the time the patient last took any food or fluid by mouth.

27. **A** Instilling a fluorescein stain into the eye is a diagnostic procedure; it would be the least effective measure to relieve the patient's pain. Effective pain-relief interventions include irrigating the eye gently with a normal saline solution and applying topical analgesics. Photosensitivity is common in ocular injuries; therefore, the eye should be covered with an occlusive patch.

28. **D** The most important information to collect from the patient during the initial interview is the patient's use of medications, especially aspirin. Hyphema is a condition in which the blood vessels in the iris bleed into the anterior chamber of the eye. Prior use of any medications that may increase bleeding and decrease clotting time must be known. If bleeding is not minimized, severe ocular problems and loss of vision may ensue. Other important information to gather during the interview includes the nature of the specific injury, the mechanism by which the injury occurred, the time elapsed since the occurrence, the patient's symptoms and treatment before arrival in the ED, any changes in the patient's clinical status (such as visual changes; the patient's description of the pain), and the patient's history of ocular disorders.

29. **B** Patching the patient's eyes during the acute phase is part of the initial treatment for a patient with hyphema. To minimize recurrent bleeding, the patient's activities are restricted. Typically, the patient is put on bed rest in a semi-Fowler's position, with bathroom privileges only. Sedation may be given judiciously. Hyphema usually clears in 5 to 6 days.

30. **B** Discharge teaching for the patient with hyphema would not include remaining on strict bed rest for 2 weeks, as this has no therapeutic importance. A patient should be on limited activity during recovery (i.e. on bed rest with bathroom

privileges, but not strict bed rest). Appropriate discharge instructions would include telling the patient to avoid coughing and performing the Valsalva maneuver because these activities increase intraocular pressure, to maintain the head of the bed at a 30-degree angle to decrease intraocular pressure, and to try to reduce stress and physical strain during the recovery period.

31. **D** The highest priority in this situation would be to continuously irrigate the eyes with copious amounts of normal saline solution, preferably with a continuous irrigation setup. Checking the pH of the eye with litmus paper and instilling antibiotic drops are appropriate after complete irrigation. Steroids are also applied after irrigation, to reduce local inflammation. Flushing the eyes with sodium bicarbonate would be inappropriate because of the bicarbonate's alkalinity.

32. **C** An acid substance does not continue to dissolve soft tissue in the eye until it is removed. Acid chemicals cause a coagulation necrosis of the cornea; the extent of damage to the eye is limited by the coagulation formed in the process. Alkaline burns are the most destructive and are therefore considered an ocular emergency. The most destructive chemicals to enter the eye are alkaline substances, which include lye, ammonia, and plaster. Alkaline chemicals cause necrosis of the conjunctiva and cornea, which will continue to react with ocular tissues, producing severe damage All traces of the chemical must be removed to halt its corrosive action. Acid burns are usually not as devastating to the eye as are alkaline burns. Similar principles of management apply to alkaline and acid burns of the eye.

33. **B** A pH value of 7.0 on a litmus paper reading is the best indication that treatment has been effective. This finding verifies adequate irrigation and absence of chemical in the eye.

Whitening of the cornea and visual acuity limited to light perception result from ocular tissue damage, which produces varied degrees of vision loss.

34. **A** Eye pain is not a symptom of retinal detachment. Patients experience painless changes in vision, such as the loss of central vision, seeing floaters or cobwebs in the field of vision, and appearances of flashes of light (photopsia). If retinal detachment is confirmed during a fundal exam, the patient should be referred to a retinal surgeon for the repair.

35. **C** A thick, foul-smelling nasal discharge from only one nostril is highly suggestive of a foreign body. Young children often place small objects inside their nose or ears. When unnoticed, the body produces a discharge around the foreign body, which becomes foul smelling after a prolonged period of time. Although purulent drainage and nasal obstruction can be seen with a sinus infection, it is bilateral and associated with antecedent cold symptoms. In addition, sinusitis is not common at this age. An URTI is usually associated with other symptoms such as malaise, cough, sneezing, headache, scratchy throat, and watery eyes. Allergies are associated with bilateral nasal symptoms, itchy/reddish eyes, and a previous history of similar symptoms that usually flares up seasonally.

ENVIRONMENTAL EMERGENCIES

1. A patient is brought to the emergency department (ED) complaining of burning, tingling, and numbness of the fingers of both hands after an afternoon of shoveling snow. On examination, the nurse notes that the tissue is soft and the fingers fail to "pink up" after blanching. These assessment findings are characteristic of which condition:

A. Raynaud's phenomenon
B. Superficial frostbite
C. Deep frostbite
D. Chilblains

2. When planning the care of a hypothermic patient, the nurse should keep in mind that the major areas of heat loss from the body are the:

A. Hands and feet
B. Head and back of the neck
C. Head and chest
D. Exposed chest and abdomen

3. The nurse knows that frostbite is a traumatic condition caused by ice crystals forming and expanding in the:

A. Extracellular space
B. Intracellular space
C. Intravascular space
D. Subcutaneous tissues

4. The burned appearance of frostbitten tissue is a sign of:

A. Shrinkage of the cells due to vasoconstriction
B. Histamine release with decreased capillary permeability
C. Red blood cell (RBC) aggregation and microvascular occlusion
D. Rewarming

5. Which nursing intervention would be most appropriate to rewarm frostbitten digits?

A. Giving the patient alcohol to promote vasodilation
B. Rubbing the affected areas with crushed ice to promote circulation
C. Allowing the digits to thaw indoors, spontaneously and gradually
D. Rewarming the digits rapidly in a water bath at 100° to 105° F (38° to 40.5° C)

6. Which information should be included in the discharge teaching for a patient with frostbite?

A. Smoking is permissible
B. Children and elderly people are at a lower risk for frostbite
C. Any insulating effect is diminished when clothing becomes wet
D. The new insulating fabrics, such as those in a down jacket, are better than multiple clothing layers

7. A woman is brought to the ED by her husband. She had been burned when a pot of boiling water spilled down the front of her body. Which nursing action would be inappropriate for this patient?

A. Removing all of the patient's jewelry
B. Removing the patient's wet clothing and covering her with sterile towels
C. Flushing the burned areas with tepid water
D. Applying ice to the burned areas

8. After ensuring airway patency, obtaining baseline vital signs, and establishing an IV of Lactated Ringer's solution, the patient's condition stabilizes. Because airway obstruction may still occur, the nurse must assess frequently for airway patency. How long after injury should frequent airway assessments be made?

A. 12 hours
B. 24 hours
C. 36 hours
D. 48 hours

9. An adult patient has partial-thickness and full-thickness burns over one half the anterior chest and abdomen, the perineal area, and the anterior aspect of both legs and feet. Based on the Rule of Nines, the closest estimate of total body-surface area (BSA) involved would be:

A. 18%
B. 28%
C. 40%
D. 50%

10. The nurse recognizes which IV fluid will best treat the acidosis associated with a burn injury?

A. Dextrose 5% in water
B. Colloid
C. Lactated Ringer's
D. Normal saline

11. Admission assessment of a 54.4 kg patient shows partial-thickness and full-thickness burns over one half the back, the perineal area, and the posterior aspect of both legs and feet. Based on the standard fluid replacement formula, what is the maximum fluid the patient will receive over the first 24 hours based on this presentation?

A. 2,460 mL
B. 6,100 mL
C. 13,400 mL
D. 61,100 mL

12. Which parameter is commonly used as a guideline for adequate fluid replacement?

A. Half the fluid should be given in the first 8 hours
B. Mean Arterial Pressure (MAP) equal to 50 mmHg or less
C. Urine output should be between 30 and 50 mL/hour
D. Pulse rate should be less than 100 beats/minute

13. The phases of burn injury are emergent/resuscitation/burn shock, acute, and rehabilitative. During the acute phase of a burn injury, the capillaries seal and electrolytes remobilize with the fluid. At this time, the nurse should assess the laboratory results for:

A. Elevated hematocrit (hemoconcentration)
B. Elevated red blood cell count and hypokalemia
C. Hypernatremia and hypokalemia
D. Hyponatremia and hyperkalemia

14. Which statement best describes the rationale for keeping a patient from ingesting food or liquids (NPO status) while in the ED after a burn?

A. A danger of esophageal edema exists because of the burn injury
B. Keeping the patient NPO will prevent aspiration from nausea and vomiting
C. Burn patients are prone to developing paralytic ileus
D. Keeping the patient NPO will prevent bowel infarction

15. Cold, pain, apprehension, and episodes of infection potentiate a catabolic state in the burn patient. The nursing care plan should address appropriate nutritional support, which requires large amounts of:

A. Sodium
B. Lipids
C. Protein
D. Glucose

16. Elderly people are at risk for hypothermia because of:

A. Impaired hypothalamic function
B. Impaired thyroid function
C. Impaired circulation
D. Higher use of vasoactive medications

17. A 72-year-old man is admitted to the ED after an automobile accident. He had been trapped in the wreckage for 3 hours; the air temperature was 30° F (1° C). Although his fingers and toes were not frostbitten, he is stuporous. His pulse rate is 52 beats/minute and his respiratory rate is 8 breaths/minute. His core temperature is 81°F (27.2°C). An appropriate nursing diagnosis for this patient would be:

A. Fluid volume excess related to increased antidiuretic hormone secretion
B. Decreased cardiac output related to decreased chronotropic effect.
C. Decreased cardiac output related to hypermetabolic state
D. Potential fluid volume deficit related to hemorrhage

18. Which statement regarding hypothermia is false?

A. The myocardium is depressed and irritable, which may cause arrhythmias
B. Decreased retention of water and sodium causes generalized dehydration (cold diuresis)
C. Insulin release is increased, lowering the serum glucose levels
D. Hepatic function is altered, increasing metabolism of substrates or drugs

19. Which of the following would not be indicated for a patient with a core body temperature of 81°F (27.2°C):

A. Electrocardiographic monitoring, taking core temperature and urine output measurements, and performing a neurologic check
B. Warming IV fluids, checking the blood pressure frequently, and monitoring arterial blood gas measurements
C. Monitoring serum electrolyte and glucose measurements
D. Repositioning the patient frequently to enhance rewarming

20. After re-warming treatment is initiated, the nurse evaluates the hypothermic patient for after drop (or after fall), which refers to:

A. Drooping of the fingers or toes after rewarming
B. Temporary gait impairment after rewarming of the lower extremities
C. Continued drop of core temperature after the cause of hypothermia has been removed
D. Microcirculatory sludging, which may result in renal or hepatic failure

21. Which rewarming method is least effective for a hypothermic patient?

A. Applying hypothermia blankets to the entire body
B. Administering warm peritoneal dialysis
C. Administering warm enemas and IV infusions
D. Administering warm humidified oxygen

22. Which patient is least likely to have been exposed to radiation?

A. A cancer patient complaining of fatigue, vomiting, and diarrhea
B. A firefighter who suffered smoke inhalation 2 days ago during a warehouse fire and now complains of vomiting
C. A nuclear power plant worker who complains of weakness and epistaxis but who was not involved in a plant accident
D. A 55-year-old female bank employee with fever, chills, and malaise

23. Which finding would the nurse expect to occur in a patient exposed to 100 to 2,000 rad?

A. Tremors
B. Alterations in bone marrow function
C. Convulsions
D. Death

24. After the decontamination process, the Geiger counter readings show no reduction in the amount of external radiation. The nurse would interpret these findings to mean that:

A. The patient may have internal contamination
B. Convulsions and death will soon follow
C. This is a common and normal reaction
D. The patient should receive additional body scrubs

25. After radiation exposure, leukopenia and thrombocytopenia may be detected:

A. Immediately
B. Anywhere from 1 to 5 weeks after exposure, depending on the amount of exposure
C. 2 months after exposure
D. None of the above

26. Which two nursing diagnoses would be appropriate for a patient with leukopenia and thrombocytopenia secondary to a radiation exposure:

A. Potential for infection related to diminished immunity and potential for fluid volume deficit related to bleeding
B. Impaired gas exchange related to decreased oxygen-carrying capacity of the blood and altered microcirculatory tissue perfusion related to enhanced coagulation
C. Decreased cardiac output related to impaired myocardial contractility and potential for injury related to seizures
D. Altered cerebral tissue perfusion related to thrombotic event and potential for injury related to seizures

27. Which finding would the nurse expect when assessing a patient with heatstroke:

A. Anxiety
B. Elevated temperature above 106° F (41.1° C)
C. Blood pressure of 160/110 mmHg
D. Respiratory rate of 8 breaths/minute

28. The nurse assesses two runners and an 83-year-old man who had been observing the running race; all of them have signs and symptoms of heatstroke. Which differences would the nurse expect to note between the runners and the elderly man:

A. The runners' will continue to sweat
B. The runners' skin will be hot and flushed
C. The runners' will have bradycardia
D. The runners' will have lower temperatures than the elderly man

29. Which laboratory finding would the nurse expect for a patient with heatstroke:

A. Elevated serum glucose
B. Low serum blood urea nitrogen
C. Respiratory acidosis
D. Elevated hematocrit

30. All of the following nursing interventions are appropriate in caring for a patient with heatstroke except:

A. Applying ice packs to the axillae and groin
B. Instituting measures to prevent shivering
C. Stopping all cooling measures when the patient's body temperature reaches 100° F (37.8° C)
D. Instituting ice baths

31. The nurse is assessing several patients in the ED who had attended or participated in an annual Fourth of July marathon. The physician diagnoses heatstroke. The nurse explains to one runner how to prevent heatstroke when participating in future marathons. Which response indicates that the patient understands the information given?

A. "Running in the rain is good because it will keep me cool"
B. "I should keep hydrated by drinking beer before the race"
C. "I should run shorter distances in the same weather for several days before the race so that my body is prepared"
D. "I should try to run sprints during the race so that I don't have to run so long"

32. During treatment of a patient suffering from heat stroke, which laboratory test would be of least importance during the early stages?

A. CK
B. CBC
C. Clotting studies
D. BNP

33. The American Burn Association (ABA) recommends that all of the following burn injuries be referred to a burn center except:

A. Partial-thickness burns covering more than 2% of total body surface area (TBSA)
B. Burns involving face, hands, feet, genitalia, perineum, or any major joints (elbow, knee, hip, shoulder, etc.)
C. Lightening injuries
D. Inhalation burns

34. A patient has been burned with hydrochloric acid. Which of the following would be indicated as the treatment for this chemical burn?

A. Silvadene
B. Irrigation
C. Calcium gluconate
D. Antibiotic ointment, such as neomycin or bacitracin

35. A patient has been burned to the following areas: Anterior right leg-superficial partial thickness, entire left leg-superficial and partial thickness, and anterior chest-partial thickness. Using the rule of 9s, which of the follow is the total surface area burned?

A. 98%
B. 27%
C. 18%
D. 26%

36. A 29-year-old patient presents to the ED with signs and symptoms of anaphylaxis, after walking through a fire ant hill. Which of the following is the recommended treatment after receiving 1 dose of epinephrine 0.3mg, with minimal relief. ?

A. Antibiotics
B. Steroids
C. Anti-histamine
D. Additional dose of epinephrine

37. Friends bring a 22-year-old male to your ED. The friends leave immediately, however, the patient is confused, has generalized muscle weakness, and blue spray paint around the lips. The ED technician has applied a non-rebreather. The nurse must now:

A. Obtain an ABG
B. Administer calcium gluconate
C. Establish an IV
D. Draw blood specimens

38. A 50-year-old arrives at your ED complaining of nausea, vomiting, diarrhea, and weakness that began about 90 minutes ago. The patient reports that he was eating at a seafood restaurant and the symptoms began shortly after eating there. Which of the following is the likely cause of this patient symptoms?

A. Bacterial food poisoning
B. Dehydration
C. Mercury poisoning
D. Botulism

39. A 45-year-old male arrives at the ED after a night out with his friends. The patient is shivering. His body temperature is 95°F (35.3°C). Which of the following is an appropriate intervention?

A. Place the patient on Cardio Pulmonary Bypass (CPB) with a rewarming circuit
B. Place a force warm air blanket on the patient
C. Perform Peritoneal lavage with warm fluid
D. Use a form of passive rewarming

40. A drug of choice for a suspected organophosphate poisoning would be:

A. Amiodarone
B. Naloxone
C. Flumazenil
D. Pralidoxime

1. **B** Burning, tingling, and numbness of digits that are soft and fail to "pink up" after blanching are signs and symptoms of superficial frostbite. Deep frostbite is characterized by whitish tissue that is cold and solid to the touch and that turns pink or purplish blue and causes pain. Blisters typically form after thawing. Raynaud's phenomenon is characterized by intermittent attacks of pallor and cyanosis after exposure to cold or emotional stimuli. Chilblains, which results from intermittent exposure to temperatures ranging from 33° to 60° F (1° to 15° C), is characterized by edematous tissue with reddish-blue patches that itch and burn.

2. **B** The major areas of heat loss from the body are the head and the back of the neck because of the large amount of blood flowing near the surface of these areas. The other areas mentioned are considered minor areas of heat loss.

3. **A** Frostbite occurs when ice crystals enlarge in the extracellular space, compressing the cells and resulting in cell membrane rupture.

4. **C** As ice crystals enlarge and cells rupture, enzymatic and metabolic activity becomes interrupted. Such interruption results in histamine release and increased capillary permeability with resultant red blood cell aggregation and micro vascular occlusion, which causes the burned appearance of frostbitten tissue. Rewarming frostbitten tissue has nothing to do with its burned appearance.

5. **D** The treatment of choice for rewarming frostbitten digits is rapid rewarming in a water bath, no warmer than 106° F (41°

C). No mechanical friction, such as rubbing, should be used, nor should the affected part touch the bottom of the basin. Analgesics may be used to control pain. Nurses should use sterile technique, administer tetanus prophylaxis, and provide a bed cradle to prevent pressure and friction, as thawed tissue is extremely sensitive to trauma and infection. Giving the patient alcohol, rubbing the affected areas with crushed ice, and allowing the digits to thaw spontaneously and gradually are inappropriate measures that were formerly used but found to be ineffective in preserving tissue.

6. **C** When preparing discharge teaching for a patient with frostbite, the nurse should mention that cold conduction is enhanced by wet clothing and that any insulating effect is diminished when clothing becomes wet. The patient should be warned to take extra garments whenever he expects to be in the cold for an extended period. Multiple layers of clothing offer more effective insulation than a single garment, even a down jacket. Smoking causes peripheral vasoconstriction, resulting in decreased blood flow. Vasoconstriction promotes the development of frostbite because blood is less available to keep the extremities warm. Children, with a smaller body mass, and elderly persons with peripheral vascular disease are at increased risk for frostbite.

7. **D** Applying ice to already compromised tissue would be inappropriate because this could cause frostbite. Appropriate nursing actions in a burn situation would be to remove all of the patient's jewelry as soon as possible and to cover the patient with sterile towels or sheets to conserve heat that is paradoxically lost from damaged microcirculation. Covering burned areas also protects exposed nerves and minimizes the risk of wound infection. Flushing the burned areas with cool

water may be necessary if the skin is still hot from the burn or from hot jewelry.

8. **D** Frequent airway assessments are necessary during the first 48 hours after injury. Although a burn victim may not suffer mechanical airway obstruction as a result of the burn, the patient will have edema as fluid shifts from plasma to the interstitial spaces. This shifting occurs because of endothelial cellular swelling and disruption of the capillaries, which allows escape of colloidal and isotonic fluid. Fluids must be replaced during the first 24 to 48 hours to prevent hypovolemic shock. Such fluid replacement can add to the edema, thereby decreasing lung compliance. After about 48 hours, a burn patient enters the diuretic phase, characterized by increased urine output and decreased edema, and the danger of airway obstruction decreases. If burn injuries occur in an enclosed environment, the toxic products of combustion can cause deterioration of pulmonary function.

9. **B** Using the Rule of Nines, a method of estimating the body-surface area (BSA) of a burn patient in which the total BSA equals 100%, the estimated area of involvement would be 28%: the anterior chest and abdominal area is 18%, so one half equals 9%; the perineal area equals 1%; the anterior aspect of one full leg is 9%, so two legs equal 18%.

10. **C** Lactated Ringer's solution, which contains no dextrose and closely approximates the composition of extracellular fluid, should be infused during the first 24 hours after a severe burn injury. In the severely burned patient, dextrose significantly increases the blood glucose level and produces osmotic diuresis. Normal saline solution may be used selectively in patients with electrolyte imbalances. Colloids are not used at this stage except in small children or in patients with burns

covering 50% of BSA, because the albumin will leak into the tissue.

11. **B** Using the standard fluid replacement formula, the approximate amount of fluid that a 120 lb (54.4 kg) patient should receive is 6,100 mL. The standard fluid replacement formula is: 4 mL Lactated Ringer's x body weight (kg) x % BSA burned = the amount of fluid given in 24 hours. Therefore: 4 mL x 54.4 kg x 28 = 6,093 or 6,100 mL.

12. **C** A urine output of 30 to 50 mL/hour is the parameter commonly used as a guideline for adequate fluid replacement. Because evaporative losses from wounds are difficult to estimate, fluid replacement is titrated so that the patient achieves a serum sodium level of 135 to 145 mEq/L, a urine output of 30 to 50 mL/hour, a pulse rate between 60 and 140 beats/minute, a systolic blood pressure between 100 and 140 mmHg, and a clear sensorium. The goal is to perfuse vital organs as fully as possible without overloading the circulatory system and causing cardiac and respiratory complications. Half the fluid is usually given over the first 8 hours; however, this does not always indicate adequate fluid placement. A MAP equal or less then 50 mmHg and a pulse rate under 100 beats/minute do not reflect adequate fluid status.

13. **C** After the initial shock phase of a burn injury, the nurse should assess for hypernatremia and hypokalemia. Hypernatremia can result because interstitial fluid, with its high sodium content, now shifts intravascularly, resulting in evaporative losses at the wound site. Hypokalemia occurs because of potassium losses incurred from damaged tissue and destroyed RBCs along with the selective renal excretion of potassium that occurs with high aldosterone levels. Hemoconcentration and sludging of RBCs occur with the early

fluid shift to interstitial tissues, resulting in decreased intravascular volume and slowed blood flow. Hemodilution occurs with a drop in hematocrit and RBC count.

14. **C** Patients with massive burns frequently develop gastric distention and paralytic ileus from the stress of the injury; therefore, the patient should be prevented from ingesting food or liquids (NPO status) while in the ED. A nasogastric tube should be inserted, and gastric output should be measured and recorded. The aspirate should be checked for occult blood, and pH should be measured every 2 hours. Cimetidine (Tagamet) or ranitidine (Zantac) may be ordered. A sliding-scale antacid coverage may be ordered for a gastric pH less than 5.0. If the pH is 3.0, then 60 mL of an antacid is given; if pH is 4.0, then 30 mL of an antacid is given.

15. **C** Nutritional support for a burn patient requires large amounts of protein. Extensive burns produce a hypermetabolic response, which increases caloric and protein requirements to two and one-half times the patient's pre-burn state. A positive nitrogen balance is maintained by an intake of 6,000 to 10,000 calories per day, depending on the burn size and the presence of any associated trauma. Sodium may need to be replaced as needed. Lipids usually are administered once daily to maintain adequate fat intake. Glucose is necessary for caloric intake to prevent further protein breakdown.

16. **A** Elderly people have impaired hypothalamic function, presumably because of atherosclerotic changes. They are at risk for hypothermia even without any predisposing causes, such as impaired thyroid function or circulation, or the use of vasoactive medications.

17. **B** An appropriate nursing diagnosis for this patient would be decreased cardiac output related to decreased chronotropic effect. The other nursing diagnoses would be inappropriate because the patient is more at risk for fluid volume deficit than overload because of sodium and water loss; however, he has no evidence of trauma and is not at risk for hemorrhage. Also, the patient is in a hypometabolic state, not a hypermetabolic one. The profound effects of hypothermia place the heart in a bradycardiac state; because the patient will be bradycardic their hemodynamics will be impacted, and will be at risk for ventricular arrhythmias, such as, ventricular fibrillation, ventricular tachycardia and asystole.

18. **C** Insulin release is suppressed in hypothermia; as a result, the serum glucose level may be elevated to 500 to 600 mg/dL. However, glucose uptake and insulin secretion return to normal during rewarming.

19. **D** To prevent ventricular fibrillation, extreme caution must be used when moving, transporting, manipulating, and intubating a hypothermic patient because defibrillation is ineffective below 86° F (30° C), and, at 85° F (29.4°) the heart will not respond to drug therapy. Therefore, repositioning the patient frequently to enhance rewarming would be contraindicated. Appropriate nursing interventions would include electrocardiographic monitoring, recording of core temperature, taking blood pressure readings, performing neurologic checks, and monitoring urine output, serum electrolyte and glucose levels, vital signs, and arterial blood gas measurements. Warming IV fluids before administering them is also therapeutic.

20. **C** After drop is a common phenomenon in patients in whom the core temperature continues to drop about 2°F degrees (1.1°C

degrees) after the cause of hypothermia is removed. Vasodilation and increased muscular activity return peripherally sequestered cold blood to the central circulation. Microcirculatory sludging does occur, but this is not referred to as after drop. Drooping of the fingers and toes and temporary gait impairment do not occur after rewarming.

21. **A** Applying hypothermia blankets to the entire body is the least effective method of rewarming a hypothermic patient. Unlike administering warm IV fluids, enemas, peritoneal dialysis, and humidified oxygen, this external method does not result in core rewarming and an even return to a normothermic state.

22. **D** The bank employee with fever, chills, and malaise is least likely to have been exposed to radiation. All of the other patients should be ruled out carefully, since they show signs of radiation exposure (vomiting, diarrhea, bleeding from mucous membranes, and weakness) and have a likely source of contamination. For example, the firefighter may have been exposed to radiation during a fire, the nuclear power plant worker may have become contaminated at work, and the cancer patient may have received radiation as a form of therapy.

23. **B** Alterations in bone marrow function is associated with most cases of radiation exposure, regardless of the amount of exposure. Tremors, convulsions, and death are associated with severe contamination (exposure to more than 2,000 rad).

24. **A** If the Geiger counter readings do not show a reduction in the amount of external radiation after the decontamination process, the patient probably has internal contamination. Additional body scrubs will not help. Body fluids (saliva, blood, and waste) must be tested. Gastric lavage, cathartics, or

emetics may be administered, as well as chelating or blocking agents, which prevent uptake of radioactive iodine by the thyroid gland. Convulsions and death can still be avoided if appropriate treatment is instituted promptly.

25. **B** Leukopenia (a decreased white blood cell count) and thrombocytopenia (a decreased platelet count) always occur in patients exposed to radiation and manifest anywhere from 1 to 5 weeks after the incident, depending on the amount of exposure. In cases of mild exposure (100 rad), these symptoms typically manifest 4 to 5 weeks later; moderate exposure (300 to 600 rad), 3 weeks later; and high exposure (more than 600 rad), 1 to 3 weeks later.

26. **A** The two most appropriate nursing diagnoses for a patient with leukopenia and thrombocytopenia would be potential for infection related to diminished immunity and potential for fluid volume deficit related to bleeding. Such a patient would have decreased protection against infection because of fewer white blood cells and would be at increased risk for bleeding because of fewer platelets. Anemia would be associated with impaired gas exchange related to decreased oxygen-carrying capacity of the blood. A low platelet count would not enhance coagulation or increase the risk of thrombosis. Seizures and impaired myocardial contractility are not associated with leukopenia or thrombocytopenia.

27. **B** When assessing a patient with heatstroke, the nurse would expect him to have a temperature above 106° F (41.1° C). Other common signs include tachypnea, hypotension, and lethargy or coma.

28. **A** Exertional heatstroke, which is common in athletes, occurs with exercise during periods of high heat or humidity.

Non-exertional heatstroke, which is not associated with activity, may also occur during periods of high heat and humidity or with overuse of a hot tub or sauna. Since exertional heatstroke, manifests differently than non exertional heatstroke, the nurse would expect the runners with exertional heatstroke to continue to sweat and their skin to appear moist and clammy. A patient with non-exertional heatstroke will have hot, flushed skin, but will not sweat. Both forms of heatstroke cause variations in pulse rate and either elevated or severely elevated temperatures.

29. **D** The nurse would expect a patient with heatstroke to have an elevated hematocrit and blood urea nitrogen (BUN) level from hemoconcentration. Other laboratory findings typically include a decreased serum glucose level, from depletion of glucose stores, and respiratory alkalosis, from hyperventilation a compensatory method of increasing heat elimination from the body.

30. **C** Stopping all cooling measures, such as the application of ice packs to the axillae and groin and the institution of ice baths, when the patient's body temperature reaches 100° F (37.8° C) is inappropriate because the body temperature will continue to drop even after the measures have been removed. Such measures should be stopped after the body temperature reaches 102° F (38.9° C). The patient should be prevented from shivering because this mechanism increases heat production, which increases the body temperature.

31. **C** "I should run shorter distances in the same weather for several days before the race so that my body is prepared" indicates that the runner understands the nurse's instructions on ways to prevent heatstroke. Running shorter distances in the same type of weather for several days before a race acclimatizes the body to the need for increased sweat production. Running in

the rain or in high humidity would be inappropriate because this decreases heat elimination from the body. Drinking alcohol before a race is also inappropriate because this promotes vasodilation, thereby decreasing heat elimination. Sprinting should also be avoided because this increases heat production, thereby raising the body temperature.

32. **D** BNP (B-type natriuretic peptide) is a test associated with the development of heart failure. A CK would be of importance in heat stroke due to the potential for the development of rhabdomyolysis from muscle breakdown. CBC with differential should be monitored to observe for WBC elevation. Clotting studies should be monitored for the development of DIC (disseminated intravascular coagulation), a potential complication of the development of heat stroke.

33. **A** A patient with 10% or greater TBSA burned should be evaluated at a burn center. B, C, and D are recommended for transfer to a burn center.

34. **C** Hydrochloric acid requires special treatment. The hydrochloric acid penetrates the skin and damages tissue and bone. Therefore, the treatment is calcium gluconate. Although Silvadene is used in many types of burns, it is not indicated in hydrochloric acid burns. The other options may be treatment later on, but the specific antidote is calcium chloride.

35. **B** Entire leg 18% + Anterior leg 9% = 27% superficial burns do not form part of this calculation.

36. **D** The patient is experiencing an anaphylactic reaction to fire ants venom (albeit, anaphylaxis is rare). Fire ants are known to attack, sting, and bite in unison.

37. **D** Inhaling can be common as provides a means for a quick and cheap high. After the ABCs have been secured the patient must have IV access to facilities drawing of any lab specimens, administration of medications, or administration of IV fluid.

38. **A** The rapid onset of this patient's symptoms rules out botulism and mercury poisoning. Mercury poisoning would typically have some neurological symptoms. There are no facts to support dehydration in this scenario; additionally, the signs and symptoms do not typically relate to dehydration. Bacterial food poisoning is the mostly likely cause.

39. **D** This patient is mildly hypothermic and he requires passive rewarming while preventing further heat loss. The patient should be placed in a warm room, any cold/wet clothing removed, and application of warm blankets. Other methods of rewarming would involve warmed oxygen (which can rewarm the patient by 1 degree Fahrenheit every hour. If the patient is warmed too quickly they will have aftershock. The other options are not valid for this setting or mild hypothermia.

40. **D** Pralidoxime is the drug of choice as it releases the insecticide poisoning from the cell. Atropine (not listed here) would ease the symptoms. Naloxone, Flumazenil, and Amiodarone are not indicated here.

FACIAL EMERGENCIES

1. A 22-year-old man is bleeding profusely from a facial laceration when brought to the emergency department (ED). A part of his nose is missing. As the patient screams for help, he shows the nurse the missing nose part in his hand. The priority nursing intervention at this time would be to:

A. Apply direct digital pressure to the bleeding vessels
B. Obtain arterial blood gas measurements to assess airway patency
C. Question the patient about cause of the trauma
D. Evaluate the amputated nose part for possible reimplantation

2. Which is the nurse's next appropriate step to handle an amputated nose:

A. Place it in a jar of sterile normal saline solution
B. Wrap it in a saline-dampened cloth and place it in a plastic bag
C. Place it on dry ice
D. Discard it because nose are always contaminated

3. Before a patient's facial lacerations are treated, the nurse should:

A. Irrigate the wounds
B. Scrub the wounds vigorously
C. Apply an aerosol anesthetic
D. Provide a mirror for the patient to assess the injury

4. One of a patient's lacerations extends through his left eyebrow. The nurse responds appropriately by:

A. Shaving the eyebrow
B. Applying adhesive skin closures
C. Leaving the eyebrow intact
D. Assessing for injury to the first cranial nerve

5. When suturing the patient's lacerations, the nurse practitioner orders lidocaine with epinephrine. However, when anesthetizing the nose wound, the NP requests lidocaine without epinephrine because:

A. Epinephrine is a vasodilator and will cause further bleeding
B. Epinephrine will cause further nasal discharge and contaminate the wound
C. Epinephrine is a vasoconstrictor and may cause tissue ischemia
D. Administering epinephrine so close to the respiratory tract may cause bronchospasms

6. After a patient's lacerations are sutured, the nurse questions the patient and learns he received a tetanus booster 8 months ago. Based on this information, the nurse would:

A. Not administer a tetanus prophylaxis because it is unnecessary
B. Administer half the usual dose of tetanus toxoid
C. Administer 0.5 mL of absorbed tetanus toxoid
D. Suggest that the patient have two tetanus booster shots 3 months apart

7. A 22-year-old man is bleeding profusely from a facial laceration when brought to the emergency department (ED). A part of his nose is missing. As the patient screams for help, he shows the nurse the missing nose part in his hand. During the discharge instructions, the nurse should tell the patient to:

A. Keep the incision moist with a wet dressing
B. Ignore any redness or swelling because this is normal
C. Return to the hospital in 4 to 5 days for suture removal
D. Avoid touching the incision because scarring will occur

8. A 35-year-old woman is admitted to the ED with ecchymotic areas over her face, malocclusion, and complaints of pain. She withdraws when the nurse attempts to palpate the mandible. Based on the patient's reaction, the nurse suspects a mandibular fracture. Which assessment finding is consistent with a mandibular fracture?

A. Subscleral hematoma
B. Numbness of the lower lips
C. Diplopia
D. Epistaxis

9. A patient states that her injury to her mandible resulted from falling in the bathtub. However, the nurse suspects that the patient's history is inaccurate because mandibular fractures most commonly result from:

A. Heavy weights or objects falling on the chin
B. Contact sports and diving accidents
C. Penetrating wounds from sharp instruments
D. Interpersonal altercations and vehicle accidents

10. The priority nursing diagnosis for a patient with a mandibular fracture would be:

A. Pain related to broken bones and altered tissue integrity
B. Body image disturbance related to facial trauma
C. Knowledge deficit related to wound care
D. Ineffective airway clearance related to aspiration

11. A patient with a mandibular fracture is being prepared for emergency surgery. The nurse attempts to control any preoperative pain by:

A. Performing range-of-motion exercises and providing a quiet environment
B. Providing multiple distractions, including music
C. Administering narcotics, as ordered, and encouraging verbalization
D. Applying ice packs and administering analgesics, as ordered

12. After the patient is sent to the operating room for a reduction and fixation of a mandibular fracture, the nurse calls the medical-surgical unit to prepare for the patient's arrival. Which item should the ED nurse suggest that the unit have on hand?

A. A blender
B. Mouthwash
C. Wire cutters
D. A tilt bed

13. A 40-year-old man arrives at the ED with severe mid-facial trauma. He had been sitting in the front passenger seat of an automobile that crashed into a tree at 60 miles/hour. Because of the severe facial trauma and the report of the vehicular accident, the nurse's first priority would be to:

A. Call the patient's family to come to the hospital
B. Notify the police about the accident
C. Perform a drug screening on the patient
D. Maintain alignment of the spine

14. A 40-year-old man arrives at the ED with severe mid-facial trauma. He had been sitting in the front passenger seat of an automobile that crashed into a tree at 60 miles/hour. During the physical assessment, the nurse notes clear drainage from the patient's nose. The nurse should:

A. Report the finding on the assessment form
B. Test the nasal drainage for cerebrospinal fluid (CSF)
C. Assume that the patient has a respiratory infection
D. Suction the nose gently using a circular motion

15. The physician orders a Water's view X-rays to determine:

A. The presence of orbital floor fractures
B. The extension of fracture to the mastoid process
C. Whether external manipulation will fixate the fracture
D. The extension of the fracture to the mental protuberance

16. The radiologist reports that a patient's X-rays reveal a Le Fort II fracture, which involves:

A. The nasomaxillary segments of the zygomatic and orbital portions of the face
B. Displacement of facial bones from the cranium
C. A horizontal fracture line that separates the maxillary alveolus from the upper face
D. Compression of temporal bone fragments and lacrimal tears

17. The nurse assesses for function of the first cranial nerve by:

A. Observing the patient's facial expression
B. Asking the patient whether he recognizes a familiar odor
C. Asking the patient to follow finger movements
D. Checking for bilateral corneal reflexes

18. A 40-year-old man arrives at the ED with severe mid-facial trauma. He had been sitting in the front passenger seat of an automobile that crashed into a tree at 60 miles/hour. The orthopedic surgeon examines the patient and determines that an open reduction and internal fixation is required. When communicating the news to the patient's family, the nurse should:

A. Emphasize that the procedure will take several hours
B. Warn them that the surgical incision will be disfiguring
C. Reassure them that the patient will be able to talk soon
D. Discourage them from asking questions because the outcome cannot be predicted

19. A 16-year-old boy is admitted to the ED after being hit across the face with a baseball bat. He is complaining of pain, and bright red blood is draining from his nose. The physician determines that the patient has a zygomatic fracture. Which assessment findings are consistent with this type of fracture?

A. Restricted eye movement and a retinal tear
B. Periorbital ecchymosis and inferior orbit rim tenderness
C. Malocclusion and inability to close the mouth
D. Craniofacial detachment

20. A 40-year-old man arrives at the ED with severe mid-facial trauma. He had been sitting in the front passenger seat of an automobile that crashed into a tree at 60 miles/hour. The nurse documents that the patient also has trismus, which is characterized by:

A. Swelling over the fracture site
B. Purging in the ear when changing position
C. Contractions of the mastication muscles
D. Infraorbital hypoesthesia with loss of sensation

21. A patient with a nosebleed requires nasal packing. The nurse prepares a nasal packing tray by assembling all of the following except:

A. A catheter with a 30 mL balloon
B. Oxytetracycline-coated gauze
C. Gauze packing
D. Sterile gloves

22. The nurse informs the patient that nasal packing will be removed after 24 to 48 hours. The purpose of removing the packing at that time would be to:

A. Assess the degree of edema
B. Prevent scab formation
C. Obtain clear nasal X-rays
D. Prevent infection

23. A 40-year-old man arrives at the ED with severe mid-facial trauma. He had been sitting in the front passenger seat of an automobile that crashed into a tree at 60 miles/hour. After the surgeon informs the patient that an open reduction is necessary, the patient becomes agitated. The nurse responds appropriately by:

A. Obtaining an order for a minor tranquilizer
B. Listening to the patient's concerns to determine the source of anxiety
C. Restraining the patient to prevent removal of the nasal packing
D. Requesting that the surgery be postponed until a later time

24. When caring for a patient with a zygomatic fracture, the nurse should assess for a possible orbital floor fracture, which is indicated by:

A. Subcutaneous emphysema
B. Trismus
C. Vertical diplopia
D. Malocclusion

25. To evaluate the effectiveness of nursing care for a patient with a zygomatic fracture, the nurse would:

A. Check the X-ray report to determine bone alignment
B. Ask the patient to repeat the treatment plan
C. Observe patient to determine independent functioning
D. Compare the patient's length of stay in the ED with that of other patients treated for zygomatic fractures

26. The nurse is examining a 35-year-old man who is complaining of ear pain and pain on attempting to clench his teeth. The nurse notes that the patient cannot close his mouth completely and hears a click when he opens his mouth fully. The patient states that he recently stopped smoking and admits to frequent gum chewing as a substitute. Based on the assessment findings, the nurse suspects that the patient has:

A. Acute odontalgia
B. Temporomandibular joint (TMJ) dislocation
C. Bilateral malocclusion
D. Dental abscess of a wisdom tooth

27. A manual reduction of a patient's jaw is indicated. Which nursing intervention would best facilitate this procedure?

A. Administering diazepam (Valium) IV
B. Spraying a topical anesthetic on the mucous membranes of the mouth
C. Giving atropine sulfate IM to reduce oral secretions
D. Holding hot compresses to each side of the patient's face

28. Discharge instructions for a patient who has undergone a manual temporomandibular joint (TMJ) dislocation reduction should stress the importance of:

A. Frequent mouth exercises to strengthen muscles
B. Wearing a jaw brace while sleeping
C. Eating a soft diet for 3 to 4 days
D. Daily compliance with muscle relaxant therapy

29. A 40-year-old woman arrives at the ED with unilateral flaccid facial paralysis of acute onset. Physical examination reveals a lag on the affected side when closing the eyes, decreased lacrimation, and drooping of the mouth. The physician diagnoses Bell's palsy. To prevent development of corneal abrasions, the nurse should:

A. Administer 1% methylcellulose to the affected eye
B. Place an adhesive skin closure to maintain closure of the affected eye
C. Rinse the eyes with an antibiotic irrigating solution
D. Apply eye patches bilaterally until treatment is instituted

30. The nurse is examining a 35-year-old man who is complaining of ear pain and pain on attempting to clench his teeth. The nurse notes that the patient cannot close his mouth completely and hears a click when he opens his mouth fully. The patient states that he recently stopped smoking and admits to frequent gum chewing as a substitute. Discharge teaching for this patient should include instructions regarding:

A. Facial massage, exercises, and application of moist heat to the face
B. Techniques for corneal protection
C. Therapy with analgesics and steroids
D. All of the above

FACIAL EMERGENCIES: RATIONALE

1. **A** Because exsanguination is possible with facial artery lacerations, the priority nursing intervention in this situation would be to apply direct digital pressure to the bleeding vessels. Obtaining arterial blood gas measurements is unnecessary because the patient has a patent airway, as evidenced by his screaming. Questioning the patient about the cause of trauma and evaluating the amputated part for possible reimplantation are not priority interventions at this time; they should be included in the nurse's assessment once the bleeding is controlled.

2. **B** The next appropriate step would be to rinse the amputated part with normal saline solution, wrap it in a saline-dampened cloth, place the wrapped part in a plastic bag, and then place the bag on ice. Placing an amputated part directly in saline solution or on ice will macerate the tissue. Amputated parts should never be discarded until the surgeon has had time to evaluate any injury to the part and the amputated site.

3. **A** Before treating a facial laceration, the nurse should irrigate the wound until clean. If the area is large or extremely dirty, the lacerations may be irrigated with direct, hydraulic force, using a 30 mL syringe and a 22G needle. Scrubbing should be avoided if at all possible because mechanical force can further traumatize the tissue. Because repair of facial lacerations is painful, local anesthetics are injected into the involved area. Patients are typically distressed at the possibility of disfigurement after facial injuries. The visualization of the trauma site before suturing would not provide an accurate assessment of potential scarring and may further distress the patient.

4. **C** A lacerated eyebrow should be left intact. It should never be shaved, as it may not grow back properly. Also, the eyebrows serve as important landmarks for proper alignment when suturing. Bleeding will likely require suturing; therefore, adhesive skin closures would probably be inadequate. Assessment of the first cranial nerve is not specific to this injury, as injuries to this nerve typically occur with midface trauma.

5. **C** Epinephrine is a vasoconstrictor used on facial lacerations for hemostatic purposes; however, it would not be used in the nose because it may cause tissue ischemia. When administered with lidocaine, epinephrine produces localized effects, not the systemic effects needed to achieve the degree of anesthesia required for suturing a severe nose injury.

6. **A** According to guidelines established by the American College of Surgeons, tetanus prophylaxis is unnecessary in an immunized person who has received a booster within the previous 5 years. The usual dose for a patient who has never been immunized is 0.5 mL of tetanus toxoid.

7. **C** During discharge instructions, the nurse should tell the patient to return to the hospital in 4 to 5 days, as facial sutures usually can be removed at that time. Until then, the patient should try to keep the wound clean and dry. Any sign of infection, such as heat, redness, and swelling, should be reported. Infection may increase the possibility of scarring; however, advising the patient to avoid touching the incision is no guarantee that scarring will not occur.

8. **B** Assessment findings consistent with a mandibular fracture include paresthesia and numbness of the lower lip, swelling, sublingual edema, and tearing of gingival tissue with bleeding

around the teeth. Subscleral hematoma, diplopia, and epistaxis are signs of a zygomatic fracture. Although the patient may experience epistaxis with a mandibular fracture, it typically results from other facial trauma and not the fracture itself.

9. **D** Mandibular fractures most commonly result from interpersonal altercations involving direct blows to the mandible with a blunt object or fist and from vehicular accidents. Although falling in a bathtub could result in a mandibular fracture, the person would have to fall directly forward onto the chin to incur such an injury. Also, such a fall would probably result in bruises to the body; such bruises were not evident in this situation.

10. **D** A patient with a mandibular fracture is at risk for aspirating teeth, bone fragments, blood, and vomitus; maintaining a patent airway takes priority over every other problem. Therefore, the priority nursing diagnosis would be ineffective airway clearance related to aspiration. Appropriate interventions would include maintaining the patient in a side-lying position, having suction equipment ready, and being prepared to intubate if necessary.

11. **D** Mandibular fractures are painful injuries. Preoperative pain-control measures typically include the application of ice packs to control swelling and reduce discomfort and the administration of analgesics (particularly narcotics), as ordered, to decrease pain sensation. Because any movement of the fracture part will increase the pain, exercise and verbalization should not be encouraged. Although music may be an appropriate distraction, the nurse should keep in mind that a patient in pain typically cannot tolerate multiple stimuli or distractions; the environment should be quiet and restful.

12. **C** The ED nurse should suggest that the medical-surgical unit have wire cutters on hand. These should be kept at the patient's bed side at all times and carried by the patient as long as the jaw is wired shut. Keeping wire cutters on hand is a necessary precaution in the event that suctioning does not remove airway secretions and the patient goes into respiratory distress; the nurse would have to cut the wires and institute emergency intubation. A blender is unnecessary in this situation because, initially, the patient will be on a clear liquid diet; liquified foods are not indicated until after discharge. Most mouthwashes are contraindicated in patients with wiring of fractures. To prevent infection, patients are instructed to rinse with half-strength peroxide and water while wires are in place. After discharge, the patient may use mouthwash, water, or salt water to rinse the mouth. A tilt bed is unnecessary; a side-lying position is adequate to prevent aspiration.

13. **D** The nurse's first priority in this situation would be to maintain alignment of the patient's spine. A patient with a severe mid-facial injury probably has suffered a maxillary fracture. Such a fracture, when combined with a high-speed vehicular deceleration accident, may be accompanied by cervical spine injury. Alignment of the spine is necessary to prevent possible cord damage until cervical fractures are ruled out.

14. **B** Any rhinorrhea noted during assessment of a patient with mid-facial trauma should be checked for cerebrospinal fluid (CSF) because the patient may have a fracture of the cribriform plate, resulting in CSF leakage. The nurse can check for CSF as it contains glucose and respiratory secretions do not. After assessing for CSF, the nurse should report the finding on the assessment form. Nasal suctioning should be avoided; the nose may no longer be attached to other bones and suctioning may

produce further trauma to the area. If the patient has bloody drainage from the nose, the nurse should check for a clot with a yellow or clear ring (halo sign), indicating CSF.

15. **A** Water's view X-rays enable the visualization of the frontal, supraorbital, orbital floor, zygomatic, maxillary, and nasal areas. Although views determine the extension of a maxillary fracture, injuries to the mastoid and mandible (common in mid-facial trauma) are not extensions of a maxillary fracture and cannot be seen with these views.

16. **A** All mid-facial fractures are classified according to the Le Fort classification system. A Le Fort II fracture is one involving the nasomaxillary segments of the zygomatic and orbital portions of the face, which cause the nose to move with the dental arch. A Le Fort I fracture involves a horizontal fracture line that separates the maxillary alveolar process from the upper face. A Le Fort III fracture involves total displacement of the facial bones from the cranium. Temporal fractures do not involve the midface and are not classified as Le Fort fractures.

17. **B** Trauma to the midface sometimes results in damage to the first cranial nerve, known as the olfactory nerve. The nurse would assess for function of this nerve by asking the patient to identify a pungent odor. Assessment of the seventh cranial nerve, the facial nerve, involves observing the patient's facial expression and checking his sense of taste. Ocular movement is controlled by three cranial nerves—the third (oculomotor), fourth (trochlear), and sixth (abducens)—which may be assessed by asking the patient to follow finger movements. Damage to the fifth cranial (trigeminal) nerve, which controls corneal function, may be assessed by checking for bilateral corneal reflexes.

18. **A** Facial reconstruction procedures for Le Fort II fractures are complex, requiring internal wiring and bone grafting. When communicating news of the surgery to the patient's family, the nurse should emphasize that the procedure will take several hours. Aesthetic effects of the surgical incision are usually good, as the incisions are made along the skin folds of the lower eyelids. The patient's jaw will be wired during the procedure, making talking and eating difficult; therefore, reassuring the family that, the patient will be able to talk soon would be inappropriate. Families should never be discouraged from asking questions or expressing their concerns. Although no absolute predictions can be made, the patient's expected outcome can be discussed.

19. **B** Periorbital ecchymosis and tenderness over the inferior orbital rim are two of the most common clinical findings in a zygomatic fracture. Restricted eye movement does not result from a zygomatic fracture itself, but rather from other coexisting problems. Retinal tears do not occur with this type of fracture. Malocclusion and inability to close the mouth are indications of temporomandibular joint dislocation, not a zygomatic fracture. Craniofacial detachment is consistent with a midface fracture, not a zygomatic fracture.

20. **C** Trismus, which is characterized by tonic contractions of the mastication muscles, is a common assessment finding in patients with a zygomatic fracture as well as other types of trauma.

21. **D** Wearing gloves is a necessary precaution whenever body fluids are handled. However, because nasal packing is considered a medically aseptic and not a surgically aseptic procedure, sterile gloves are unnecessary. When preparing a nasal packing tray, the nurse should include gauze packing with

string, a catheter with a 30 mL balloon, oxytetracycline-coated gauze, forceps, and silk sutures. At the time of the packing, the provider decides whether to pack the nares with the oxytetracycline-coated gauze or the catheter.

22. **D** Nasal packing should never be left in place for over 48 hours because of the risk for infection and the possibility of compression necrosis. Edema can be assessed and X-rays taken with the packing in place.

23. **B** The idea of surgery, especially one that is unplanned, may be particularly distressing. Because the cause of distress will vary from patient to patient, the nurse must listen to the patient's concerns to determine the source of anxiety and intervene appropriately. The patient's anxiety may stem from fear of additional pain; fear of anesthesia, fear of separation from loved ones, or fear of the unknown. Before obtaining an order for a mild tranquilizer, the nurse should reassure the patient, provide honest and accurate explanations about the procedure, and attempt to strengthen the patient's coping skills. If the anxiety becomes severe, a mild tranquilizer may be used as an adjunctive therapy. Restraining the patient to protect himself from injury should always be a last resort. Postponing the surgery may be impractical or impossible; however, during the preoperative period, the nurse should attempt to prepare the patient physically and psychologically for the surgery.

24. **C** Vertical diplopia, the imposition of one image above another, occurs when a patient suffers a blowout fracture of the orbital floor. It is most apparent when the patient looks upward. Other common signs of orbital floor fracture include exophthalmos (bulging of the eye) or depression of the eye globe. Local swelling, not subcutaneous emphysema, may occur from a traumatic injury that results in a fracture.

Malocclusion does not occur with orbital floor fractures. Trismus, which occurs when a bone fragment from the zygomatic arch impinges on the temporalis muscle and the coronoid process of the jaw, is a common finding with zygomatic fractures and does not occur with orbital floor fractures.

25. **B** To evaluate the effectiveness of nursing care in this situation, the nurse should ask the patient to repeat the treatment plan. The nurse should never assume that the patient has understood explanations or instructions; traumatic stress and anxiety over the immediate future may interfere with the patient's ability to learn. Having the patient repeat the treatment plan allows the nurse to evaluate the patient's comprehension and identify knowledge deficits. Checking the X-ray report to determine bone alignment would be an appropriate measure to evaluate orthopedic surgical care, not nursing care. Independent functioning is a long-term patient goal, not an immediate, realistic goal applicable to ED nursing. A patient's length of stay in the ED is affected by multiple factors and is an inappropriate evaluation criterion of nursing care.

26. **B** Based on the assessment findings, this patient probably has temporomandibular joint (TMJ) dislocation, a condition characterized by jaw displacement in which spasms of jaw muscles prevent the condyles from returning to their normal position. TMJ dislocation, which may be unilateral or bilateral, usually is caused by trauma or opening the mouth too widely. It also may occur in individuals in high-stress occupations or constant chewers. On assessment, the patient typically cannot close his mouth completely and has referred pain to his teeth, temples, or ears.

27. **A** The administration of diazepam (Valium) IV facilitates manual reduction of the jaw by alleviating tension and anxiety, relaxing facial muscles, and increasing patient cooperation during the procedure. After the procedure, postreduction X-rays are necessary.

28. **C** Discharge instructions for a patient with TMJ dislocation should stress the importance of adhering to a soft diet for 3 to 4 days. A soft diet enables the patient to avoid excessive chewing or opening the mouth widely, which could place additional stress on the joint. Other important discharge information should include specific instructions on adhering to the medication regimen, if analgesics are prescribed. Frequent mouth exercises could precipitate a TMJ dislocation and therefore would not be included in the discharge plan.

29. **A** Appropriate nursing interventions to help prevent the development of corneal abrasions include administering a 1% methylcellulose (artificial tears) solution to the affected eye; performing gentle, manual closure of the eyelid periodically; instructing the patient to wear sunglasses; and applying an eye patch to the affected eye.

30. **D** Appropriate discharge teaching for a patient with Bell's palsy should include specific instructions on therapeutic aids, such as facial massage, facial muscle exercises, and the application of moist heat to the face, to speed recovery. Because Bell's palsy is thought to result from polyneuritis, steroids are beneficial; they decrease edema and inflammation. Analgesics may be given to decrease pain. Specific instructions on medication, such as analgesics and steroids, are essential to foster patient compliance. Techniques that promote corneal protection, such as wearing eye patches or sunglasses, should also be stressed.

GENERAL MEDICAL EMERGENCIES

1. A 70-year-old man was admitted to the hospital 2 months ago with a diagnosis of pulmonary embolism. He had been treated with heparin and discharged on warfarin sodium (Coumadin) therapy after the embolism resolved. Earlier today, he became confused and ingested 100 mg of warfarin. He is now being readmitted with hematemesis and bright-red rectal bleeding. During the initial assessment of this patient, the emergency department (ED) nurse should be particularly alert for:

A. Facial flushing
B. Petechiae
C. Pruritus
D. Hypertension

2. The nurse knows that a patient on long-term anticoagulant therapy must be carefully monitored for potential hemorrhagic complications that most commonly affect the:

A. GI tract
B. Genitourinary tract
C. Respiratory tract
D. Capillary vasculature

3. Which therapy would the nurse expect the physician to order for a patient who has overdosed on warfarin sodium (Coumadin)?

A. Peritoneal dialysis
B. Administration of vitamin K
C. Ethylenediaminetetraacetic acid (EDTA) chelation
D. Plasmapheresis

4. Which therapy would be inappropriate for a patient with hemorrhagic complications from oral anticoagulants?

A. Volume replacement
B. Administration of whole blood
C. Administration of fresh frozen plasma
D. Administration of protamine sulfate

5. The nurse would normally instruct a patient receiving anticoagulant therapy to:

A. Avoid excessive alcohol intake
B. Avoid using an electric shaver
C. Avoid using soft-bristled toothbrushes
D. Trim corns and calluses weekly

6. An appropriate nursing intervention for a patient receiving heparin therapy for deep vein thrombosis of the left calf would include:

A. Observing for hypertensive crisis and hematemesis
B. Monitoring the patient's prothrombin time (PT) to maintain therapeutic anticoagulant blood levels
C. Testing the patient's urine and stool for blood
D. Administering aspirin for leg pain, as needed

7. Which nursing action is inappropriate when administering heparin subcutaneously?

A. Changing the injection site with each dose
B. Using the iliac crest or abdominal fat layer as an injection site
C. Massaging the area after injection to facilitate absorption
D. Observing for bleeding at the injection site

8. Which statement regarding heparin administration is true?

A. Partial thromboplastin time (PTT) must be checked after each dose
B. Larger heparin doses are required during continuous infusion
C. Major bleeding episodes are more common with continuous IV infusions than with intermittent IV infusions
D. During continuous infusion, the drip rate must be accurately calculated and controlled

9. A 4-year-old boy is admitted to the ED with a sudden high fever. His mother notes that he has been weak and dyspneic and has had generalized pain and recurrent infections. He is found to have an elevated white blood cell count, anemia, thrombocytopenia, and tachycardia. The physician diagnoses acute lymphocytic leukemia. After which age is acute lymphocytic leukemia considered uncommon?

A. 20
B. 10
C. 5
D. ALL can occur at any age

10. A 4-year-old boy is admitted to the ED with a sudden high fever. His mother notes that he has been weak and dyspneic and has had generalized pain and recurrent infections. He is found to have an elevated white blood cell count, anemia, thrombocytopenia, and tachycardia. The physician diagnoses acute lymphocytic leukemia. Which nursing diagnosis would be appropriate for this patient?

A. Altered tissue perfusion related to enhanced coagulation from thrombocytosis
B. Altered tissue perfusion related to increased blood viscosity from polycythemia vera
C. Potential for infection related to immunosuppression
D. Potential for injury related to seizures

11. The nurse would expect to treat a leukemic patient with an elevated temperature with:

A. Aspirin
B. Acetaminophen (Tylenol)
C. Azathioprine (Imuran)
D. Antibiotics

12. The nurse explains to the patient, in age-appropriate terms, that chemotherapy is used to treat leukemia because it:

A. Destroys abnormal leukemic cells
B. Causes bone marrow recovery
C. Increases the patient's immunologic defense mechanisms
D. Produces granulocytosis

13. Which assessment finding is most significant in a patient with DIC?

A. Leukopenia
B. Maculopapular rash
C. Abnormal bleeding
D. Severe hypertension

14. The nurse would expect to observe bleeding from which site in a patient with DIC?

A. Mucous membranes
B. Venipuncture sites
C. GI tract
D. All of the above

15. The nurse understands which obstetric incident leads to the development of DIC?

A. Thromboembolism resulting from bedrest and micro emboli formation
B. Activation of the clotting mechanism by placental and fetal tissue
C. Hemolysis of red blood cells (RBCs) resulting from fetal enzyme release
D. Thrombocytopenic state, which normally occurs during pregnancy

16. Which statement does not support the rationale for heparin administration in the treatment of DIC?

A. The antithrombin activity of heparin neutralizes free-circulating thrombin
B. Heparin permits normalization of clotting test results
C. Heparin prevents fibrinogenesis
D. Heparin increases hemorrhagic manifestations

17. Which laboratory finding would indicate successful treatment of this patient?

A. Platelet count of 40,000/mm^3
B. PTT of 76 seconds
C. Fibrin degradation products of 10 ug/ml
D. Hemoglobin level of 7

18. Hemophilia A and hemophilia B are bleeding disorders that can be distinguished only by laboratory studies. Which statement about these disorders is true?

A. Hemophilia B is caused by a deficiency of Factor VIII
B. Hemophilia A is caused by a deficiency of Factor IX
C. Hemophilia A is more common than hemophilia B
D. Almost all of the individuals with hemophilia A are female

19. Hemarthrosis, especially of the knees, elbows, and ankles, is a common assessment finding in hemophilia. The nurse understands that the other common assessment findings would include:

A. Bruising and bleeding gums
B. Neuropathy and paresthesia
C. Pain and hematuria
D. All of the above

20. The most common cause of death in a patient with hemophilia occurs from bleeding of the:

A. GI tract
B. Heart
C. Cranium
D. Larynx

21. Diagnosis is typically based on a patient's bleeding pattern, family history, and physical examination. Confirming diagnostic studies indicate:

A. Factor VIII or Factor IX deficiency
B. Prolonged PT and PTT
C. Increased fibrinogen level
D. Decreased platelet count

22. A 17-year-old girl is admitted to the ED 10 days after an abortion. She continues to have heavy bleeding and lower abdominal pain. The physician suspects retained products of conception. While the patient is in the ED, her laboratory studies reveal a prolonged PT and PTT. The physician diagnoses disseminated intravascular coagulation (DIC). Priority nursing care of this patient would include all of the following except:

A. Immobilizing the right leg
B. Stopping local bleeding
C. Preventing deformity
D. Assisting with immediate aspiration of hemarthroses

23. A 40-year-old man with a history of alcohol abuse is admitted to the ED with hematemesis. His blood pressure is 88/56 mmHg, temperature 99 F, hemoglobin 8.4 g/dL, and hematocrit 24%. The patient's blood is typed and cross-matched for transfusion; his blood type is designated, as group AB. Which statement about group AB is true?

A. The plasma contains both A and B antibodies
B. The plasma contains both A and B antigens
C. The red cell membrane contains both A and B antigens
D. This blood group possesses neither A nor B antigens

24. Packed RBCs are recommended for transfusion. Which statement regarding packed RBCs and whole blood is true?

A. Both packed cells and whole blood cause the hemoglobin and hematocrit to increase at the same rate
B. Fresh packed cells provide all of the necessary blood components, including platelets and coagulation factors
C. Packed cells decrease the risk of anaphylactic reaction
D. All of the above statements are correct

25. The nurse who administers the transfusion of packed RBCs to a patient must be cognizant of standard transfusion practices. Which statement about blood transfusions is true?

A. Lactated Ringer's and normal saline are the only solutions used when administering blood products
B. During a blood transfusion, the nurse must assess the patient's vital signs before and after the transfusion only
C. When using a blood warmer, the temperature should not exceed 103.1°F (38.5°C)
D. An 18G or 20G catheter may be used during a blood transfusion

26. One hour after the transfusion has been initiated, the patient complains of chills and headache. The nurse checks his vital signs and notes that his temperature has increased to 103.1°F (39.5°C). Based on these findings, the nurse determines that the patient is probably experiencing a:

A. Febrile, nonhemolytic transfusion reaction
B. Hemolytic transfusion reaction
C. Delayed hemolytic transfusion reaction
D. Bacterial transfusion reaction

27. A 60-year-old man with thrombocytopenia is admitted to the ED because of rectal bleeding. The nurse knows that thrombocytopenia does not result from:

A. Chlorothiazide (Diuril) therapy
B. Zidovudine (AZT) therapy
C. Splenectomy
D. Viral infection

28. The nurse would expect a thrombocytopenic patient's platelet count to return to normal levels within what time after discontinuation of quinidine therapy:

A. 24 hours
B. 72 hours
C. 1 week
D. 2 weeks

29. A 28-year-old African-American man with a history of sickle cell disease is admitted to the ED. During assessment, the nurse notes the following symptoms: severe abdominal and back pain, aching joint pain, fever, vomiting, and dyspnea. The nurse understands that all of the following are forms of sickle-cell crisis except:

A. Aplastic crisis
B. Sequestration crisis
C. Painful crisis
D. Anemic crisis

30. Which nursing diagnosis would be inappropriate for a patient with sickle cell anemia?

A. Altered tissue perfusion related to increased blood viscosity
B. Pain related to ischemia from impaired blood flow
C. Impaired gas exchange related to dysfunctional RBCs
D. Decreased cardiac output related to impaired myocardial contractility

31. A 28-year-old African-American man with a history of sickle cell disease is admitted to the ED. During assessment, the nurse notes the following symptoms: severe abdominal and back pain, aching joint pain, fever, vomiting, and dyspnea. While obtaining the patient history, the nurse would question the patient about all of the following factors that may precipitate a crisis except:

A. Cigarette smoking
B. Infection
C. Increased fluid intake
D. A strenuous game of tennis

32. One of the treatments for a patient vomiting and in sickle-cell crisis involves hydration, which may be achieved by:

A. Inserting the smallest-possible-gauge IV catheter and infusing $D_5\frac{1}{2}$ NS solution at 100 mL/hour
B. Inserting a large-gauge IV catheter and infusing normal saline solution at 150 mL/hour
C. Inserting a large-gauge IV catheter and infusing Lactated Ringer's solution at 300 mL/hour
D. Having the patient drink 4 to 6 quarts (about 4 to 6 liters) of liquid within the following 24 hours

33. The nurse understands which analgesic would be contraindicated in a patient with sickle cell crisis?

A. Meperidine hydrochloride (Demerol).
B. Morphine sulfate IV
C. Aspirin or NSAIDs
D. Hydroxyurea

34. A 33-year-old man with a positive history of human immunodeficiency virus (HIV) is brought to the ED complaining of dyspnea and a productive cough. He has been taking zidovudine, also known as azidothymidine or AZT (Retrovir), for the past year. Which assessment finding is characteristic of a patient with acquired immunodeficiency syndrome (AIDS)?

A. Rapid weight loss and night sweats
B. Hairy leukoplakia and swollen lymph nodes
C. Purplish skin lesions and prolonged diarrhea
D. All of the above

35. Which laboratory finding would the nurse expect for a patient with a depressed immune system resulting from AIDS?

A. Hemoglobin of 8
B. High T_4:T_8 lymphocyte ratio
C. Platelet count of 40,000/mm^3
D. T lymphocyte count of 150/mm^3

36. The nurse knows that zidovudine is classified as an:

A. Antiviral agent used to decrease the replication of HIV
B. Antibiotic used to treat Pneumocystis carinii pneumonia
C. Antitubercular agent
D. Antifungal used to treat oral candidiasis

37. The physician orders aerosolized pentamidine isethionate (NebuPent) for a patient with HIV. Which statement about pentamidine therapy is false?

A. Pentamidine should be administered in a well-ventilated room
B. Respiratory precaution measures should be used during the administration of pentamidine
C. Pregnant nurses or those who are trying to become pregnant should avoid administering pentamidine
D. Pentamidine should be administered only via intermittent positive-pressure breathing

38. A 5-year-old boy is transferred to the ED by ambulance from his pediatrician's office with a suspected diagnosis of Reye's syndrome. When obtaining the nursing history from the child's mother, the nurse should inquire about a recent history of:

A. Chicken pox
B. Diarrhea
C. Measles
D. Insect bites

39. Which laboratory finding supports a diagnosis of Reyes syndrome?

A. Elevated serum glucose level
B. Elevated serum potassium level
C. Low WBC count
D. Elevated serum ammonia level

40. The physician is having difficulty establishing a peripheral IV line and considers inserting an intraosseous catheter. When the mother asks which bone will be used, the nurse responds appropriately that the most common insertion site is the:

A. Iliac crest
B. Sternum
C. Tibia `
D. Femur

41. A 17-year-old female model arrives at the ED complaining of generalized cramps and numbness in her fingers. When asked about her medical history, she informs the nurse that she has been on a high-protein diet for about 6 weeks. The nurse establishes an IV line and draws blood for laboratory studies. The patient's serum calcium level is 5.5 mg/dL. When assessing a patient for hypocalcemia, the nurse attempts to elicit Chvostek's sign by:

A. Applying a blood pressure (BP) cuff to the upper arm, inflating the cuff, and observing for carpopedal spasm
B. Tapping a finger on the skin above the supramandibular portion of the parotid gland and observing for twitching of the upper lip on the side opposite the stimulation
C. Tapping a finger on the skin above the supramandibular portion of the parotid gland and observing for twitching of the upper lip on the same side as the stimulation
D. Having the patient hyperventilate (expelling more than 30 breaths/minute) to produce carpopedal spasm caused by respiratory alkalosis

42. The nurse would assess a patient with hypocalcemia for which of the following electrocardiogram (EKG) changes?

A. Shortened PR intervals
B. Prolonged PR intervals
C. Prolonged QT intervals
D. Appearance of U waves

43. The nurse would assess a hypocalcemic patient for all of the following potential complications except:

A. Seizures
B. Oliguria
C. Laryngeal stridor
D. Bleeding abnormalities

44. A 71-year-old woman is brought to the ED because of fatigue and a change in mental status. Assessment findings reveal a rectal temperature of 96.8°F (36°C), a BP of 110/74 mmHg, a pulse rate of 48 beats/minute, a respiratory rate of 12 breaths/minute, periorbital edema, and yellowish skin pigmentation. The patient's daughter relates a history of thyroid problems and noncompliance with medical therapy. The physician diagnoses myxedema coma. The nurse would assess a patient admitted with myxedema coma (hypothyroid crisis) for which electrolyte abnormality?

A. Hyponatremia
B. Hypernatremia
C. Hyperglycemia
D. Hypocalcemia

45. Which acid-base imbalance would the nurse expect a patient with myxedema to have?

A. Respiratory acidosis
B. Respiratory alkalosis without compensation
C. Metabolic alkalosis
D. Respiratory alkalosis with compensation

46. Which signs would the nurse expect to note during the assessment of a patient with myxedema coma?

A. Increased urine output and hyperactive bowel sounds
B. Oliguria and abdominal distention
C. Diarrhea and hyperglycemia
D. Polycythemia and hypothermia

47. Which IV fluid is most likely to be used in the treatment of a patient with myxedema coma?

A. Dextrose 5% in water
B. Dextrose 10% in water
C. Dextrose 5% in normal saline solution
D. 0.3% sodium chloride

48. A 78-year-old woman arrives at the ED complaining of abdominal cramping. She states that she has had diarrhea and has felt tired for about 1 week. She has a history of diabetes mellitus and chronic renal failure. The nurse establishes an IV line and draws blood for laboratory studies. The serum potassium level is 6 mEq/L. The physician diagnoses hyperkalemia. The nurse would anticipate pharmacologic management of hyperkalemia to include administration of all of the following except:

A. Lactulose enemas
B. Dextrose 50% and regular insulin
C. Sodium bicarbonate
D. Calcium chloride

49. The nurse would assess a patient with hyperkalemia for which EKG changes?

A. Prolonged QT intervals
B. Peaked T waves
C. Prominent U waves
D. Shortened PR intervals

50. Which signs would the nurse expect to note during the physical assessment of a patient with hyperkalemia?

A. Apathy and absent bowel sounds
B. Ascending muscle weakness and bradycardia
C. Descending muscle weakness and tachycardia
D. Hyperactive bowel sounds and polyuria

51. Which acid-base imbalance is characteristic of a hyperkalemic patient?

A. Respiratory acidosis
B. Metabolic alkalosis
C. Respiratory alkalosis
D. Metabolic acidosis

52. A 52-year-old man with newly diagnosed multiple myeloma is admitted to the ED with back pain. He informs the nurse that he fell against a bookcase at home. X-rays reveal a rib fracture; electrolyte studies reveal a serum calcium level of 12.7. The physician diagnoses hypercalcemia. The nurse is aware that hypercalcemia occurs in multiple myeloma as a result of:

A. Mobilization of calcium from the bones
B. Release of calcium from lesions into the plasma
C. Increased tubular reabsorption of calcium
D. Increased intestinal reabsorption of calcium secondary to excessive vitamin D intake

53. The nurse assesses the patient for signs of hypercalcemia, which include:

A. Flank or thigh pain and polyuria
B. Anuria or oliguria and constipation
C. Diarrhea and metabolic alkalosis
D. Constipation and metabolic acidosis

54. The nurse understands which EKG change is characteristic of a patient with hypercalcemia?

A. Prolonged PR intervals
B. Prolonged QT intervals
C. Shortened ST segments
D. Appearance of U waves

55. A 52-year-old man with newly diagnosed multiple myeloma is admitted to the ED with back pain. He informs the nurse that he fell against a bookcase at home. X-rays reveal a rib fracture; electrolyte studies reveal a serum calcium level of 12.7. The physician diagnoses hypercalcemia. The nurse would expect the treatment for this patient to include the administration of:

A. Normal saline solution and loop diuretics
B. Normal saline solution and thiazide diuretics
C. Sodium polystyrene sulfonate (Kayexalate) enemas
D. Hemodialysis, glucose, and insulin

56. A 64-year-old man is admitted to the ED with altered mental status, jaundice, and increased abdominal girth. He has a medical history of cirrhosis. The nurse establishes an IV line and draws blood for laboratory studies. Liver enzyme levels (serum aspartate aminotransferase, serum alanine aminotransferase, and bilirubin) are elevated. The physician diagnoses hepatic encephalopathy. The nurse would assess a patient with hepatic failure for signs of:

A. Hypercalcemia
B. Hyperproteinemia
C. Hypokalemia
D. Free-water depletion

57. The nurse knows that respiratory alkalosis, a common acid-base imbalance in patients with hepatic failure, is a result of:

A. A high blood ammonia level, which acts as a respiratory stimulant
B. Hypocalcemia, which causes neuromuscular irritability
C. Hypokalemia, which causes hyperventilation
D. Hypomagnesemia, which causes hypoventilation

58. Aldosterone-blocking agents, such as spironolactone (Aldactone), may be administered to a patient with hepatic failure. The nurse would evaluate the effectiveness of these agents by assessing for:

A. Increased serum sodium levels and decreased serum potassium levels
B. Decreased serum sodium levels and increased serum potassium levels
C. Decreased serum sodium levels and increased serum magnesium levels
D. Decreased serum sodium and potassium levels

59. The nurse would anticipate the physician to order all of the following measures to treat hepatic failure except:

A. Administration of sodium polystyrene sulfonate enemas to remove excess potassium
B. Limiting the administration of hypotonic solutions
C. Decreasing or eliminating the patient's dietary protein intake
D. Decreasing the patient's dietary sodium intake

60. A 28-year-old woman is admitted to the ED after a house fire. She has second- and third-degree burns over approximately 30% of her body-surface area, including her face. Endotracheal intubation is performed, and IV lines are established. The goals of IV therapy for this patient would be based on all of the following except:

A. Gender and medical history
B. Depth and percentage of the burns
C. Urine output and urine specific gravity measurements
D. Hemoglobin and hematocrit values

61. During the initial treatment phase, fluid replacement at 4 mL/kg/percent of burns is given over the first 24 hours. The calculated amount of solution is divided so that:

A. One-third of the solution is given every 8 hours
B. One-half of the solution is given in the initial 8 hours, one-half in the next 16 hours
C. One-half of the solution is given in the first 12 hours, one-half in the next 12 hours
D. One-half of the solution is given in the first 16 hours, one-half in the next 8 hours

62. During the initial stages (first 3 days) of a burn injury, the nurse would expect the patient to show signs of:

A. Jugular venous distention and hypernatremia
B. Edema and hyperkalemia
C. Jugular venous distention and hyponatremia
D. Jugular venous distention and hypokalemia

63. During the later stages (after the first 3 days) of a burn injury, the nurse would expect the patient to show signs of:

A. Jugular venous distention and hypokalemia
B. Edema and hypokalemia
C. Oliguria and hypokalemia
D. Edema and hyponatremia

64. A 40-year-old man is admitted to the ED with lethargy and tachypnea. His skin is dry and flushed, and he has a fruity breath odor. An IV line is started and blood is drawn for laboratory studies. His blood glucose level is 840 mg/dL, and his urinalysis reveals +3 glucose, and +3 ketones. The physician diagnoses diabetic ketoacidosis. The nurse would expect to note all of the following physiologic abnormality during the assessment of this patient except:

A. Hyperkalemia
B. Hyperventilation
C. Poor skin turgor
D. Jugular venous distention

65. A 40-year-old man is admitted to the ED with lethargy and tachypnea. His skin is dry and flushed, and he has a fruity breath odor. An IV line is started and blood is drawn for laboratory studies. His blood glucose level is 840 mg/dL, and his urinalysis reveals +3 glucose, +3 ketones. The physician diagnoses diabetic ketoacidosis. The nurse's first priority in caring for this patient would be to:

A. Administer insulin IV
B. Administer insulin SC
C. Administer volume replacement fluids and insulin IV
D. Establish an airway and monitor its patency

66. A 40-year-old man is admitted to the ED with lethargy and tachypnea. His skin is dry and flushed, and he has a fruity breath odor. An IV line is started and blood is drawn for laboratory studies. His blood glucose level is 840 mg/dL, and his urinalysis reveals +3 glucose, +3 ketones. The physician diagnoses diabetic ketoacidosis. Which IV solution would the nurse expect to use in the initial treatment of this patient?

A. Isotonic saline solution
B. Hypotonic saline solution
C. Hypertonic saline solution
D. Hypotonic dextrose solution

67. A 40-year-old man is admitted to the ED with lethargy and tachypnea. His skin is dry and flushed, and he has a fruity breath odor. An IV line is started and blood is drawn for laboratory studies. His blood glucose level is 840 mg/dL, and his urinalysis reveals +3 glucose, +3 ketones. The physician diagnoses diabetic ketoacidosis. During therapy, the nurse's evaluation of this patient's serum potassium level is likely to demonstrate which pattern?

A. An initially elevated level, followed by gradually decreasing levels
B. An initially decreased level, followed by gradually increasing levels
C. An increased level that remains generally elevated
D. A decreased level that remains generally low

68. A 12-year-old boy arrives at the ED complaining of difficulty breathing. His parents inform the nurse that the family has a long history of asthma and that the child has suffered previous wheezing episodes but none this severe. Arterial blood gas (ABG) studies performed, while the patient is breathing room air (21% oxygen), reveal: pH 7.21, PO_2 65 mmHg, PCO_2 62 mmHg, and HCO_3^- 24 mEq/L. The nurse would interpret this patient's ABG result as:

A. Metabolic acidosis
B. Metabolic alkalosis
C. Respiratory acidosis
D. Respiratory alkalosis

69. A 12-year-old boy arrives at the ED complaining of difficulty breathing. His parents inform the nurse that the family has a long history of asthma and that the child has suffered previous wheezing episodes but none this severe. Arterial blood gas (ABG) studies performed while the patient is breathing room air (21% oxygen) reveal a of pH 7.21, PO_2 65 mmHg, PCO_2 62 mmHg, and HCO_3^- 24 mEq/L. Which action would be the nurse's lowest priority when caring for this patient?

A. Oxygen therapy
B. Inhaled bronchodilator therapy
C. Continuous cardiac monitoring
D. Preparation for possible tracheotomy

70. A 12-year-old boy arrives at the ED complaining of difficulty breathing. His parents inform the nurse that the family has a long history of asthma and that the child has suffered previous wheezing episodes but none this severe. Arterial blood gas (ABG) studies performed, while the patient is breathing room air (21% oxygen), reveal: pH 7.21, PO_2 65 mmHg, PCO_2 62 mmHg, and HCO_3^- 24 mEq/L. The nurse knows that, if therapy is not implemented immediately, this patient could suffer:

A. Respiratory arrest
B. Gastric aspiration
C. Adult respiratory distress syndrome
D. Acute renal failure

71. The patient stops breathing shortly after the nurse institutes inhaled bronchodilator therapy, as ordered. After initial ventilation with a bag-valve-mask device, the patient achieves good bilateral chest rising. He is then intubated with an orotracheal tube, and ventilation is continued. A repeat ABG analysis indicates pH, 7.12, PCO_2 55 mmHg, PO_2 33 mmHg, and HCO_3^- 25 mEq/L. No loss of vital signs is noted. The patient is then given 100 mEq of sodium bicarbonate. Ten minutes later, ABG analysis indicates pH, 7.55, PCO_2 35 mmHg, PO_2 425 mmHg, and HCO_3^- 36.5 mEq/L. Based on the latest ABG results, the nurse knows that the patient is exhibiting signs of:

A. Metabolic acidosis
B. Metabolic alkalosis
C. Respiratory acidosis
D. Respiratory alkalosis

72. The patient stops breathing shortly after the nurse institutes inhaled bronchodilator therapy, as ordered. After initial ventilation with a bag-valve-mask device, the patient achieves good bilateral chest rising. He is then intubated with an orotracheal tube, and ventilation is continued. A repeat ABG analysis indicates pH 7.12, PCO_2 55 mmHg, PO_2 33 mmHg, and HCO_3^- 25 mEq/L. No loss of vital signs is noted. The patient is then given 100 mEq of sodium bicarbonate. Ten minutes later, ABG analysis indicates: pH 7.55, PCO_2 35 mmHg, PO_2 425 mmHg, and HCO_3^- 36.5 mEq/L. The nurse should have anticipated the correct treatment after the patient stopped breathing to include:

A. Hyperventilation with a bag-valve-mask device
B. Administration of 1 mEq/kg of sodium bicarbonate IV push
C. Administration of 40% oxygen via a high flow oxygen (Venturi) mask
D. Administration of 1 mg of epinephrine IV

73. A 37-year-old woman arrives at the ED after having ingested ten 5 mg methamphetamine hydrochloride (Desoxyn) tablets about 2 hours ago. She appears excited and nervous. Her blood pressure is 145/70 mmHg, pulse rate 124 beats/minute, respiratory rate 44 breaths/minute, and temperature, 99.5°F (37.5°C). She complains of circumoral tingling and numbness as well as tingling in her hands and feet. An ABG analysis, which is taken while the patient is receiving 28% oxygen by facemask, indicates pH 7.60, PCO_2 15 mmHg, PO_2 140 mmHg, and HCO_3^- 22 mEq/L. This patient's ABG results may be interpreted as:

A. Metabolic acidosis
B. Metabolic alkalosis
C. Respiratory acidosis
D. Respiratory alkalosis

74. A 37-year-old woman arrives at the ED after having ingested ten 5 mg methamphetamine hydrochloride (Desoxyn) tablets about 2 hours ago. She appears excited and nervous. Her blood pressure is 145/70 mmHg, pulse rate 124 beats/minute, respiratory rate 44 breaths/minute, and temperature, 99.5°F (37.5°C). She complains of circumoral tingling and numbness as well as tingling in her hands and feet. An ABG analysis, which is taken while the patient is receiving 28% oxygen by facemask, indicates pH 7.60, PCO_2 15 mmHg, PO_2 140 mmHg, and HCO_3^- 22 mEq/L. The goal of treatment for this patient would be to increase:

A. Oxygenation
B. Ventilation
C. HCO_3^- level
D. CO_2 retention

75. An anxious 24-year-old presents to the emergency department (ED). An ABG analysis, which is taken while the patient is receiving 28% oxygen by facemask, indicates pH 7.60, PCO_2 15 mmHg, PO_2 140 mmHg, and HCO_3^- 22 mEq/L. All of the following statements about this patient are correct except:

A. After treatment in the ED, the patient will require follow-up care
B. The patient is having an anxiety attack
C. Emergency treatment for this patient should include rebreathing exhaled CO_2,
D. Emergency treatment for this patient should include the administration of sodium bicarbonate IV

76. An anxious 24-year-old complains of circumoral tingling and numbness as well as tingling in her hands and feet. An ABG analysis, which is taken while the patient is receiving 28% oxygen by facemask, indicates pH 7.58, PCO_2 17 mmHg, PO_2 240 mmHg, and HCO_3^- 23 mEq/L. The nurse suspects that the patient is experiencing numbness and tingling because:

A. Alkalosis causes vasodilation and paresthesia
B. Hypocapnia causes vasoconstriction and decreases calcium levels
C. Diazepam causes these symptoms
D. None of the above

77. A 43-year-old male is brought to the emergency department (ED). He has labored respirations and tachycardia. ABG analysis reveals pH, 7.03, PO_2 135 mmHg (28% O_2), PCO_2 43 mmHg, and HCO_3^- 11 mEq/L. The nurse would correctly interpret the patient's ABG results as an indication of:

A. Metabolic acidosis
B. Metabolic alkalosis
C. Respiratory acidosis
D. Respiratory alkalosis

78. A 78-year-old, 155-lb (70-kg) man was transported from a nursing home to the ED about 4 hours ago, complaining of difficulty voiding. His temperature upon arrival was 104.5° F (40.3°C). He is now demonstrating labored respirations and tachycardia. ABG analysis reveals pH 7.01, PO_2 125 mmHg (28% O_2), PCO_2 42 mmHg, and HCO_3^- 10 mEq/L. The bicarbonate deficit in this situation would be:

A. 10 mEq/L
B. 14 mEq/L
C. 24 mEq/L
D. 30 mEq/L

79. The nurse correctly calculates that the amount of sodium bicarbonate required for a 70-kg patient, with ABG results as pH 7.01, PO_2 125 mmHg (28% O_2), PCO_2 42 mmHg, and HCO_3^- 10 mEq/L, to correct the abnormality to be:

A. 44 mEq
B. 88 mEq
C. 100 mEq
D. 245 mEq

80. A 78-year-old, 155-lb (70-kg) man was transported from a nursing home to the ED about 4 hours ago, complaining of difficulty voiding. His temperature upon arrival was 104.5° F (40.3°C). He is now demonstrating labored respirations and tachycardia. ABG analysis reveals pH 7.01, PO_2 125 mmHg (28% O_2), PCO_2 42 mmHg, and HCO_3^- 10 mEq/L. ABG analysis reveals pH 7.01, PO_2 125 mmHg (28% O_2), PCO_2 42 mmHg, and HCO_3^- 10 mEq/L. Which laboratory studies are likely to provide essential information necessary for the treatment of this patient's acid-base imbalance?

A. Complete blood count and reticulocyte count
B. Creatine phosphokinase isoenzyme and serum amylase levels
C. Lactate level and anion gap
D. Electrolyte studies and acetone level

81. The nurse is in the process of resuscitating a 45-year-old man in the ED. ABG measurements (obtained 5 minutes ago) indicate pH 7.15, PO_2 50 mmHg, PCO_2 68 mmHg, and HCO_3^- 18 mEq/L. The nurse correctly interprets the ABG results to mean that the patient has:

A. Fully compensated respiratory acidosis
B. Fully compensated metabolic acidosis
C. Partially compensated respiratory alkalosis
D. Mixed metabolic and respiratory acidosis

82. The nurse is in the process of resuscitating a 45-year-old man in the ED. ABG measurements (obtained 5 minutes ago) indicate pH 7.15, PO_2 50 mmHg, PCO_2 68 mmHg, and HCO_3^- 18 mEq/L. The nurse anticipates that the best initial therapy for this patient would be to:

A. Improve oxygenation and ventilation
B. Defibrillate immediately
C. Administer sodium bicarbonate
D. Administer epinephrine

83. The nurse is in the process of resuscitating a 45-year-old man in the ED. ABG measurements (obtained 5 minutes ago) indicate pH 7.15, PO_2 50 mmHg, PCO_2 68 mmHg, and HCO_3^- 18 mEq/L. Which blood gas abnormalities, if not reversed, can seriously compromise this patient's myocardial function:

A. Hypoxemia and a low bicarbonate level
B. Acidosis and hypoxemia
C. Acidosis and a low bicarbonate level
D. Acidosis and hypercapnia

84. A family of five arrives at a small, rural ED complaining of headaches, malaise, nausea, and vomiting. This occurs during the winter, and toxic ingestion or inhalation is suspected. The father's ABG analysis indicates pH 7.25, PCO_2 47 mmHg, PO_2 97 mmHg, O_2 saturation 75%, and HCO_3^- 15 mEq/L. Other family members have similar results. This family's symptoms suggest:

A. Viral syndrome
B. CO_2 narcosis
C. Carbon monoxide poisoning
D. Radon poisoning

85. A family of five arrives at a small, rural ED complaining of headaches, malaise, nausea, and vomiting. This occurs during the winter, and toxic ingestion or inhalation is suspected. The father's ABG analysis indicates pH 7.25, PCO_2 47 mmHg, PO_2 97 mmHg, O_2 saturation 75%, and HCO_3^- 15 mEq/L. The nurse anticipates the initial treatment for this family to include:

A. Breathing into a paper bag
B. Administration of 100% O_2 via a non-rebreather mask
C. Acetylcysteine (Mucomyst) inhalant therapy
D. IV bronchodilator therapy

86. A family of five arrives at a small, rural ED complaining of headaches, malaise, nausea, and vomiting. This occurs during the winter, and toxic ingestion or inhalation is suspected. The father's ABG analysis indicates pH 7.25, PCO_2 47 mmHg, PO_2 97 mmHg, O_2 saturation 75%, and HCO_3^- 15 mEq/L. If initial treatment were unsuccessful, the nurse would prepare each patient for:

A. Hyperbaric therapy
B. Exploratory laparotomy
C. Cardiopulmonary bypass surgery
D. Hemodialysis

87. A family of five arrives at a small, rural ED complaining of headaches, malaise, nausea, and vomiting. This occurs during the winter, and toxic ingestion or inhalation is suspected. The father's ABG analysis indicates pH 7.25, PCO_2 47 mmHg, PO_2 97 mmHg, O_2 saturation 75%, and HCO_3^- 15 mEq/L. After appropriate treatment, when all family members are stabilized, the nurse formulates a nursing diagnosis of:

A. Ineffective family coping related to guilt
B. Noncompliance related to financial status
C. Powerlessness related to current health
D. Knowledge deficit related to the medical diagnosis of carbon monoxide poisoning

88. A 22-year-old man is unconscious when brought to the ED. The nurse notes that he is breathing rapidly and deeply. Although his skin is warm and dry, his pulse is 130 beats/minute and weak, and his blood pressure is 92/60 mmHg. The nurse draws blood for ABG and electrolyte studies and sends the specimens to the laboratory. The nurse would expect the physician to order the administration of which drugs at this time:

A. Dextrose 50% and naloxone (Narcan)
B. Regular insulin and sodium bicarbonate
C. NPH insulin and potassium
D. Activated charcoal and naloxone

89. A 22-year-old man is unconscious when brought to the ED. The nurse notes that he is breathing rapidly and deeply. Although his skin is warm and dry, his pulse is 130 beats/minute and weak, and his blood pressure is 92/60 mmHg. The nurse draws blood for ABG and electrolyte studies and sends the specimens to the laboratory. While awaiting the laboratory findings, the nurse learns from the patient's parents that the patient has a 10-year history of Type I diabetes mellitus. The ABG results reveal pH 7.03, PO_2 98 mmHg, PCO_2 28 mmHg, and HCO_3^- 12 mEq/L. Other laboratory studies indicate the following serum levels: sodium 140 mEq/L, potassium 5 mEq/L, chloride 104 mEq/L, CO_2 18 mEq/L, blood urea nitrogen (BUN), 40 mg/dL, and glucose 592 mg/dL. The physician gives a diagnosis of diabetic ketoacidosis (DKA). Which treatment would the nurse expect the physician to order next?

A. Dextrose 50% and naloxone
B. Regular insulin and sodium bicarbonate
C. NPH insulin and potassium
D. Activated charcoal and naloxone

90. Which IV fluid would be most appropriate for a patient with DKA?

A. 0.45% saline solution
B. 0.9% (normal) saline solution
C. Dextrose 5% in 0.45% saline (D_5 ½NS) solution
D. Dextrose 5% in normal saline solution

91. The nurse anticipates that the physician will order the preferred initial insulin treatment for a DKA patient by preparing to administer:

A. IV boluses of regular insulin 10 to 20 units/hour
B. An IV bolus of 20 units regular insulin followed by a continuous infusion of 4 to 8 units/hour
C. 10 units of regular insulin IV and 20 units of NPH insulin SC
D. 10 units of regular insulin IV and 10 units of regular insulin SC

92. Which history finding is considered a precipitating factor in the development of DKA?

A. Omission of or resistance to insulin in a patient with diabetes mellitus
B. Surgery or trauma in a patient with diabetes mellitus
C. Pancreatitis
D. All of the above

93. Which patient with insulin-dependent diabetes mellitus would the nurse determine is most at risk for DKA?

A. A child with otitis media
B. A child who participates in a gym class
C. A child who requires insulin twice a day
D. A child who self-administers insulin

94. The nurse knows that signs and symptoms of DKA may also occur in a child with:

A. Hypoglycemia
B. Appendicitis
C. Seizures
D. Upper respiratory tract infection

95. Which EKG abnormality may be assessed initially in a patient with DKA?

A. Sinus bradycardia
B. Appearance of U waves
C. ST-segment depression
D. Tall T waves

96. The nurse should assess for which electrolyte abnormality in a patient with DKA:

A. Hypomagnesemia
B. Hypophosphatemia
C. Hyperchloremia
D. Hypercalcemia

97. All of the following physical findings are characteristic of a patient with DKA except:

A. Acetone breath and slow respirations
B. Altered level of consciousness and Kussmaul's respirations
C. Polyuria and signs of dehydration
D. Tachycardia and possible hypotension

98. Which assessment findings would not support a diagnosis of DKA?

A. Decreased PCO_2, pH, and HCO_3^-
B. Elevated urine specific gravity and elevated BUN level
C. Elevated serum potassium level and decreased bicarbonate level
D. Decreased serum potassium level and decreased hematocrit

99. Which assessment finding is considered the most obvious sign of DKA?

A. Elevated serum potassium level
B. Elevated blood pH
C. Hypertension
D. Polyuria

100. The priority nursing diagnostic category for a patient with DKA would be:

A. Altered nutrition, less than body requirements
B. Ineffective breathing pattern
C. Impaired gas exchange
D. Fluid volume deficit

101. After instituting the appropriate treatment, the nurse should assess the patient for which potential treatment-related complication:

A. Hyperosmolar nonketotic hyperglycemic coma (HHNK)
B. Acute renal failure
C. Cerebral edema
D. Respiratory acidosis

102. Which other potential complication may occur in a patient treated for DKA:

A. Shock
B. Oliguria
C. Hypercalcemia
D. Hypokalemia

103. Which diabetic patient is considered at highest risk for hypovolemic shock from DKA?

A. A child
B. An adolescent
C. An elderly patient
D. A cardiac patient

104. Six hours after admission, the patient's serum glucose level decreases to 243 mg/dL. Which fluid therapy would the nurse expect the physician to order now?

A. 0.45% saline solution
B. Normal saline solution
C. D_5W NS solution
D. Lactated Ringers

105. Which parameter is most appropriate for determining a DKA patient's response to insulin therapy in the ED?

A. Laboratory studies of serum glucose levels
B. Laboratory studies of serum ketone levels
C. Bedside urine glucose measurements
D. Bedside capillary glucose measurements with a glucometer

106. All of the following treatments are appropriate for a patient with DKA except:

A. Continuous administration of NPH insulin at 4 to 8 units/hour
B. Rapid administration of fluids, initially 1,000 mL/hour
C. Infusion of $D_5\frac{1}{2}$ NS solution when serum glucose levels decrease to 250 mg/dL
D. Infusion of potassium as ketosis decreases and insulin therapy is begun

107. A 68-year-old woman is brought to the ED by her son, who informs the nurse that his mother has been experiencing weakness, polydipsia, and polyuria for the past few days. Initial laboratory studies reveal a serum glucose level of 2,000 mg/dL no ketones are detected in the urine. The physician diagnoses HHNK. Which assessment finding would result in a change in the level of consciousness in a patient with HHNK?

A. Serum osmolarity of 380 mOsm/L
B. BUN level of 50 mg/dL
C. Serum sodium level of 125 mEq/L
D. Nonketotic state

108. Which nursing action is not a priority during the initial management of a patient with HHNK?

A. Administering insulin
B. Administering hypotonic saline solution
C. Monitoring the patient's rectal temperature and notifying the physician if the temperature rises above 101°F (38.3°C)
D. Assessing the patient's neurologic status

109. The nurse would expect the management of a patient with HHNK to differ from that of a patient with DKA because the patient with HHNK requires:

A. Hypertonic fluid replacement and less insulin and potassium than that needed for a patient with DKA
B. Hypotonic fluid replacement and less insulin and potassium than that needed for a patient with DKA
C. Hypotonic fluid replacement and no insulin or potassium
D. Isotonic replacement fluid and more insulin and potassium than that needed for a patient with DKA

110. All of the following nursing diagnoses would be appropriate for a patient with HHNK except:

A. Fluid volume deficit related to osmotic diuresis
B. Potential for injury related to altered level of consciousness
C. Altered peripheral tissue perfusion related to decreased cardiac output
D. Ineffective breathing pattern related to hyperventilation

111. A 47-year-old man is brought to the ED. His family reports that he had become confused over the past 72 hours and suffered a seizure while on the way to the hospital. Upon arrival, the patient is minimally responsive. His respiratory rate is 32 breaths/minute, pulse rate 110 beats/minute, and blood pressure 120/90 mmHg. Immediate laboratory work reveals an abnormal sodium level of 117 mEq/L. The patient's chest X-ray reveals a mass in the right mid-lung field. The nurse suspects that the underlying factor responsible for this patient's change in mental status is related to:

A. Lung cancer with cerebral metastasis
B. Syndrome of inappropriate antidiuretic hormone (SIADH) secretion
C. Seizures associated with meningitis
D. Possible subarachnoid hemorrhage

112. Which patient would not be considered at risk for developing SIADH?

A. A 20-year-old patient who is transferred from a skilled nursing facility where he received prolonged positive-pressure ventilation
B. A 36-year-old patient receiving phenytoin sodium (Dilantin)
C. A 64-year-old patient with chronic obstructive pulmonary disease complicated by pneumonia
D. A 70-year-old patient with a lung carcinoma

113. The nurse knows that an increase in antidiuretic hormone (ADH) secretion may result from:

A. Chlorpropamide (Diabinese) therapy
B. Head trauma
C. Viral respiratory infection
D. All of the above

114. A 47-year-old man is brought to the ED. His family reports that he had become confused over the past 72 hours and suffered a seizure while on the way to the hospital. Upon arrival, the patient is minimally responsive. His respiratory rate is 32 breaths/minute, pulse rate 110 beats/minute, and blood pressure 120/90 mmHg. Immediate laboratory work reveals an abnormal sodium level of 117 mEq/L. The patient's chest X-ray reveals a mass in the right mid-lung field. Which laboratory finding is characteristic of a patient with SIADH?

A. Serum sodium level of 120 mEq/L
B. Serum potassium level of 6 mEq/L
C. Serum osmolarity of 350 mOsm/L
D. Urine specific gravity of 1.003

115. The nurse would expect the initial treatment of this patient to include all of the following except:

A. Administration of furosemide (Lasix)
B. Administration of 3% hypertonic saline solution
C. Fluid restriction
D. Administration of demeclocycline hydrochloride (Declomycin) 300 mg PO

116. Prevention of which potential complication is the goal of nursing care for a patient with SIADH:

A. Tetany
B. Seizures
C. Hypotension
D. All of the above

117. A 16-year-old boy is brought to the ED by his parents because he has been experiencing polydipsia and polyuria. His medical history reveals no significant findings. Immediate laboratory studies indicate a serum sodium concentration of 160 mEq/L and a urine osmolarity of 250 mOs/L. The physician diagnoses diabetes insipidus. Vasopressin tannate therapy is initiated. Which patient is most likely to develop diabetes insipidus?

A. An elderly man receiving thiazides and clofibrate (Atromid-S)
B. A young woman with severe pneumonia
C. A middle-aged man receiving vasopressin tannate for esophageal varices
D. A young man with a skull fracture resulting from a head trauma

118. Which laboratory finding would support a diagnosis of diabetes insipidus?

A. Decreased serum sodium level
B. Decreased serum osmolarity
C. Increased urine osmolarity
D. Urine specific gravity of 1.001

119. A 16-year-old boy is brought to the ED by his parents because he has been experiencing polydipsia and polyuria. His medical history reveals no significant findings. Immediate laboratory studies indicate a serum sodium concentration of 160 mEq/L and a urine osmolarity of 250 mOs/L. The physician diagnoses diabetes insipidus. The priority nursing intervention in this situation would be to:

A. Assess for signs and symptoms of hypovolemic shock
B. Initiate seizure precautions
C. Auscultate lung fields for crackles
D. Monitor the patient for cardiac arrhythmias

120. The nurse notes that a patient is not responding to vasopressin tannate (Pitressin tannate) therapy. This may be caused by:

A. Administration of vasopressin with calcium channel blockers
B. Mixing vasopressin with normal saline solution
C. Inadequate warming or agitation of the medication vial
D. Failure to keep medication refrigerated

121. The nurse would question administering vasopressin tannate to a patient who has:

A. Liver dysfunction
B. Brain tumor
C. Angina pectoris
D. Undergone kidney transplantation

122. A friend brings a 25-year-old man to the ED. The patient had been complaining of blurred vision, headache, slurred speech, and weakness. He is now comatose. Earlier in the morning, he had been playing tennis. Immediate laboratory studies indicate a serum glucose level of 34 mg/dL. The nurse suspects that this patient's symptoms resulted from:

A. Neuroglycopenia
B. Glycopenia
C. Decreased liver glycogenolysis
D. Decreased response of the sympathetic nervous system

123. The nurse knows that emergency management of a comatose patient with hypoglycemia includes:

A. Measurement of fasting blood sugar levels and administration of sweetened orange juice via a nasogastric tube
B. Measurement of fasting blood sugar levels and administration of 50 mL of dextrose 5% in water (D_5W) IV
C. Infusion of 1 liter of dextrose 5% in water followed by measurement of blood glucose levels
D. Administration of 50 mL of dextrose 50% IV

124. Which statement regarding myxedema coma is true:

A. It is an extremely advanced form of hypothyroidism
B. It does not occur in all patients with hypothyroidism
C. All patients who have myxedema coma are in a hypothyroid state
D. All of the above

125. Which electrolyte imbalance would the nurse expect a patient to have in myxedema coma?

A. Hyponatremia
B. Hypernatremia
C. Hypokalemia
D. Hyperkalemia

126. Paramedics bring a 66-year-old woman to the ED. Her blood pressure is 104/58 mmHg, pulse rate 44 beats/minute, respiratory rate 14 breaths/minute, and temperature 92.4°F (33.6°C). No medical history is available, except for the patient's statement of not feeling well for the past month. Physical examination reveals a lethargic, thin woman with dry skin and periorbital and facial edema. Bilateral pulmonary congestion is noted. EKG monitoring shows sinus bradycardia. The physician diagnoses impending myxedema coma. The patient remains hypothermic, with a temperature of 95°F (35°C). An appropriate nursing intervention would be to:

A. Apply a hypothermia blanket
B. Rewarm the patient with blankets
C. Administer a glycerin suppository every 4 hours as needed
D. All of the above

127. Paramedics bring a 66-year-old woman to the ED. Her blood pressure is 104/58 mmHg, pulse rate 44 beats/minute, respiratory rate 14 breaths/minute, and temperature 92.4°F (33.6°C). No medical history is available, except for the patient's statement of not feeling well for the past month. Physical examination reveals a lethargic, thin woman with dry skin and periorbital and facial edema. Bilateral pulmonary congestion is noted. EKG monitoring shows sinus bradycardia. The physician diagnoses impending myxedema coma. The patient remains hypothermic, with a temperature of 95°F (35°C). The nurse would anticipate the treatment for this patient to include all of the following except:

A. Fluid restriction
B. Thyroid hormone replacement
C. Electrolyte replacement
D. Diuretic administration

128. The nurse draws blood for arterial blood gas analysis. Measurements reveal pH, 7.28: PO_2, 50 mmHg, PCO_2, 64 mmHg, and HCO_3^- 20 mEq/L. Based on these findings, the nurse would expect to:

A. Administer dextrose 5% in Lactated Ringer's solution IV at 150 mL/hour
B. Administer 35% oxygen via a high flow oxygen (Venturi) mask
C. Measure the patient's serum electrolyte levels immediately
D. Prepare for endotracheal intubation

129. An obese patient with Addison's disease is admitted to the ED after ambulatory surgery. The paramedics report that the patient has a fever, pallor, rapid weak pulse, signs of dehydration, headache, confusion, restlessness, and a blood pressure of 90/50 mmHg. Laboratory findings reveal a serum potassium level of 6.5 mEq/L, white blood cell count, 15,000/mm^3 serum glucose level 55 mg/dL, and serum sodium level 124 mEq/L. The physician diagnoses adrenal crisis. The nurse suspects that this patient's adrenal crisis probably resulted from:

A. Obesity
B. Decreased exercise
C. Increased appetite
D. Fasting status before surgery

130. Nursing care of a patient with adrenal crisis should focus on the prevention of which life-threatening aspect of adrenal crisis:

A. Hypokalemia
B. Hyperglycemia
C. Vascular collapse
D. Hypernatremia

131. Which diagnostic test is the best indicator for a patient with adrenal crisis?

A. Plasma carcinoembryonic antigen level
B. 24-hour urine 17-hydroxycorticosteroid level
C. Plasma cortisol level
D. Adrenocorticotropic hormone (ACTH) infusion test

132. Which fluid replacement method would the nurse expect to administer to a patient with adrenal crisis?

A. Dextrose 5% in Lactated Ringer's solution at 100 mL/hour
B. 1 liter of dextrose 5% in normal saline in 2 hours
C. D$_5$W at 200 mL/hour
D. 1 liter of 0.45% saline solution in 6 hours

133. Which medication should the nurse prepare for immediate administration got a patient with adrenal crisis?

A. 0.1 mg of levothyroxine sodium (Synthroid)
B. 200 mg of dexamethasone (Decadron)
C. 200 mg of hydrocortisone (Cortef)
D. 0.1 mg of fludrocortisone acetate (Florinef)

134. The nurse would assess for hyperkalemia by observing for which EKG change:

A. T-wave depression with prolonged QT intervals
B. Peaked T waves, wide QRS complexes, and prolonged PR intervals
C. Q-wave inversion and shortened PR intervals
D. Bradycardia and bundle branch block

135. The clinical signs and symptoms of acute adrenal crisis are caused by:

A. Decreased aldosterone and cortisol levels
B. Decreased ADH and cortisol levels
C. Increased ADH and cortisol levels
D. Increased aldosterone and cortisol levels

136. A 55-year-old woman is admitted to the ED with a temperature of 105°F (40.5°C), blood pressure 180/110 mmHg, pulse rate 120 beats/minute, and respiratory rate 36 breaths/minute. She shows signs of dehydration and states that she has been experiencing muscle weakness and bone pain for the past week. She has a history of Grave's disease. The physician diagnoses thyroid crisis. The nurse would assess this patient for signs of:

A. Hypocalcemia and hypoglycemia
B. Hyperglycemia and hyponatremia
C. Hypernatremia and hypokalemia
D. Metabolic alkalosis

137. The nurse learns that a patient is iodine-sensitive and is in thyroid crisis. Based on this information, which drug would the nurse expect to be included in the treatment plan?

A. ACTH
B. Levothyroxine sodium (Synthroid)
C. Lithium carbonate (Lithobid)
D. Phenytoin (Dilantin)

138. A 55-year-old woman is admitted to the ED with a temperature of 105°F (40.5°C), blood pressure 180/110 mmHg, pulse rate 120 beats/minute, and respiratory rate 36 breaths/minute. She shows signs of dehydration and states that she has been experiencing muscle weakness and bone pain for the past week. She has a history of Grave's disease. The physician diagnoses thyroid crisis. Which nursing measure would be inappropriate in controlling a patient's pyrexia that is in thyroid crisis?

A. Administration of aspirin
B. Administration of muscle relaxants to control shivering
C. Application of ice packs to the axillae and groin
D. Use of a hypothermia blanket with a rectal probe

139. Which of the following would not be useful in assessing a patient's thyroid function:

A. Serum protein-bound iodine
B. Radioactive iodine uptake
C. Thyroid-stimulating hormone
D. Urine 17-ketosteroids

140. A 55-year-old woman is admitted to the ED with a temperature of 105°F (40.5°C), blood pressure 180/110 mmHg, pulse rate 120 beats/minute, and respiratory rate 36 breaths/minute. She shows signs of dehydration and states that she has been experiencing muscle weakness and bone pain for the past week. She has a history of Grave's disease. The physician diagnoses thyroid crisis. The patient begins to complain of bone pain and thirst. The nurse notes a decreased level of consciousness and hypotonicity of muscles. Which laboratory findings should be monitored in this situation?

A. Blood urea nitrogen
B. Serum potassium
C. Serum sodium
D. Serum calcium

141. A 65-year-old woman is brought to the ED by ambulance after fainting. Physical examination reveals central-type obesity with a fatty buffalo hump in the neck, hirsutism, thin and fragile extremities with ecchymotic areas, hypertension, and mild congestive heart failure. She informs the nurse that she has experienced extreme weakness and fatigue during the past month and that her sleep patterns have become altered. The nurse realizes that the patient's signs and symptoms are characteristic of:

A. Conn's syndrome
B. Cushing's syndrome
C. Diabetes insipidus
D. Myxedema coma

142. A 65-year-old woman is brought to the ED by ambulance after fainting. Physical examination reveals central-type obesity with a fatty buffalo hump in the neck, hirsutism, thin and fragile extremities with ecchymotic areas, hypertension, and mild congestive heart failure. She informs the nurse that she has experienced extreme weakness and fatigue during the past month and that her sleep patterns have become altered. Which statement regarding the pathophysiology of the patient's condition is true?

A. It is caused by removal of the pituitary gland
B. It is a disorder of the posterior lobe of the pituitary gland and caused by vasopressin deficiency
C. The clinical manifestations reflect excessive adrenocortical activity
D. The clinical manifestations reflect deficient adrenocortical activity

143. A 65-year-old woman is brought to the ED by ambulance after fainting. Physical examination reveals central-type obesity with a fatty buffalo hump in the neck, hirsutism, thin and fragile extremities with ecchymotic areas, hypertension, and mild congestive heart failure. She informs the nurse that she has experienced extreme weakness and fatigue during the past month and that her sleep patterns have become altered. The nurse would expect to assess this patient for signs of:

A. Hypernatremia
B. Hypokalemia
C. Hyperglycemia
D. All of the above

144. A 65-year-old woman is brought to the ED by ambulance after fainting. Physical examination reveals central-type obesity with a fatty buffalo hump in the neck, hirsutism, thin and fragile extremities with ecchymotic areas, hypertension, and mild congestive heart failure. She informs the nurse that she has experienced extreme weakness and fatigue during the past month and that her sleep patterns have become altered. The patient's condition produces anti-inflammatory effects. Which nursing diagnosis best reflects this assessment?

A. Potential for injury related to decreased protein catabolism
B. Potential for infection related to altered metabolism
C. Altered body image related to physical appearance
D. Sleep pattern disturbance related to anxiety

145. Which assessment finding would a patient with increased mineralocorticoid and glucocorticoid levels exhibit:

A. Increased heart rate with atrial premature complexes
B. Decreased serum osmolarity
C. Elevated calcitonin levels
D. Chvostek's sign

146. During the later stages (after the first 3 days) of a burn injury, the nurse would expect the patient to show signs of:

A. Jugular venous distention and hypokalemia
B. Edema and hypokalemia
C. Oliguria and hypokalemia
D. Edema and hyponatremia

147. What condition could be the cause of the following symptoms seen together in the same patient: chronic nighttime cough, earache, dysphagia, hoarseness, and epigastric pain?

A. Peptic ulcer
B. Cholecystitis
C. Pancreatitis
D. Gastro esophageal reflux disease (GERD)

148. A young woman is brought into the ED after a motor vehicle accident. She is complaining of severe pain in her abdomen and left shoulder. Upon exam, you note ecchymosis around her navel. You should be most concerned about:

A. Intestinal perforation
B. Pancreatic contusion
C. Splenic rupture
D. GI hemorrhage

149. A patient presents to the emergency department with sudden onset of confusion, angioedema, and bronchospasm while having lunch in a restaurant. The patient is hypotensive. What medication should not be administered?

A. Albuterol
B. Methylprednisolone
C. Atropine
D. Diphenhydramine

150. What phase of a tonic-clonic, often referred to as gran mal, seizure is a patient having if she is having violent and severe muscle body contractions accompanied by a loss of continence?

A. Tonic period
B. Clonic period
C. Aversive
D. Absence

GENERAL MEDICAL EMERGENCIES: RATIONALE

1. **B** In this situation, the nurse should be particularly alert for signs and symptoms of anticoagulant overdose, including petechiae, tachycardia, hypotension, hematuria, epistaxis, bleeding gums, ecchymoses, tarry stools, and coffee-ground vomitus. Pruritus and facial flushing are clinical signs of an allergic drug reaction.

2. **A** A patient on long-term anticoagulant therapy is at risk for serious hemorrhagic complications, most commonly involving the intracranial compartment and GI tract. GI hemorrhage is typically associated with underlying lesions, such as ulcers. Minor bleeding, as evidenced by epistaxis or hematuria, may occur because of capillary rupture. Bleeding of the genitourinary or respiratory tract rarely occurs in patients on long-term anticoagulant therapy but may result from instrumentation.

3. **B** The nurse would expect the physician to order administration of vitamin K, the treatment of choice for warfarin overdose. Because the patient ingested a large amount of warfarin, which has a half-life of 48 to 72 hours, the physician would need to reverse the effects rather than allow them to wear off gradually, as gradual wearing off may prolong the bleeding. Administering vitamin K, either orally or parenterally, antagonizes warfarin, thereby reversing its effects. Peritoneal dialysis, ethylenediaminetetraacetic acid (EDTA) chelation therapy, and plasmapheresis are not indicated in this situation because warfarin's effects can be easily reversed with vitamin K. Additional orders could include transfusion of PRBCs (if the patient's hemoglobin/hematocrit is low) and fresh frozen plasma (FFP).

4. **D** Administration of protamine sulfate would be inappropriate for a patient with hemorrhagic complications from oral anticoagulant therapy. Protamine sulfate neutralizes the effects of parenterally administered heparin and is therefore used to treat heparin overdose. Therapy for hemorrhagic complications from oral anticoagulants includes fluid volume replacement, clotting factor replacement, administration of vitamin K, and infusion of fresh frozen plasma and whole blood.

5. **A** A patient receiving anticoagulant therapy should be instructed to avoid excessive alcohol intake because prolonged usage destroys liver cells, causing impaired coagulation from lack of clotting factors. Such a patient should also be cautioned to wear gloves while gardening, to use an electric shaver rather than one with a straight-edged blade, to use a soft-bristled toothbrush, and to avoid trimming corns and calluses, as these measures help prevent trauma and decrease the risk of bleeding.

A medical-alert bracelet or necklace is recommended for all patients receiving anticoagulant therapy.

6. **C** An appropriate nursing intervention for a patient receiving heparin therapy would be to test the patient's urine and stool for blood. The nurse also should observe for other signs and symptoms of GI hemorrhage, including tachycardia, hypotension, and hematemesis. The partial thromboplastin time (PTT), not the prothrombin time (PT), is normally monitored to maintain therapeutic anticoagulation in heparin therapy; the therapeutic range should be 1.5 to 2.5 times the patient's control. PT is normally monitored during warfarin therapy. A patient receiving anticoagulant therapy should avoid aspirin because it aggravates bleeding tendencies.

7. **C** Massaging an area before or after a subcutaneous injection of heparin is inappropriate because it increases the risk of trauma and hematoma formation at the injection site. Appropriate nursing actions would include changing the injection site with each dose to prevent massive hematoma formation; using the iliac crest or abdominal fat layer because injecting these sites produces minimal trauma to subcutaneous tissues; and observing the site for prolonged bleeding.

8. **D** To prevent overdosage and the risk of prolonged bleeding during continuous administration, the drip rate must be accurately calculated and controlled. The PTT must be checked just before the next scheduled dose to ensure that clotting times are not dangerously prolonged. Larger doses and frequent injections are required during intermittent infusion to maintain therapeutic prolonged clotting times. Major bleeding episodes occur more commonly with intermittent IV infusion than with continuous IV infusion because larger doses must be given.

9. **A** Acute lymphocytic leukemia, a malignant disease of the bone marrow and lymphatic system that affects the hematologic cells and causes a proliferation of nonfunctional white blood cells and possibly the destruction of red blood cells and platelets, primarily affects young children; it is uncommon after age 20. Approximately 80% of all patients with this disease are between ages 2 and 5.

10. **C** An appropriate nursing diagnosis for a patient with acute lymphocytic leukemia would be Potential for infection related to immunosuppression because infection uncontrolled by dysfunctional white blood cells is a serious complication and a leading cause of death in acute cases. Other major causes of death include chemotherapeutic side effects, bleeding resulting from anemia, and thrombocytopenia. Infection is commonly caused by gram-negative sepsis. Frequent cultures are necessary, and treatment with appropriate antibiotics is required. The patient may require placement in a protected environment, because anemia and thrombocytopenia occur. Altered tissue perfusion related to enhanced coagulation from thrombocytosis and altered tissue perfusion related to increased blood viscosity from polycythemia vera would be inappropriate diagnoses. Seizures rarely occur in this disease; therefore, potential for injury related to seizures would be an inappropriate diagnosis.

11. **B** The nurse would expect to treat a leukemic patient with an elevated temperature with acetaminophen. Fever is perhaps the most important sign of infection in such a patient; judicious use of analgesic and antipyretic medications is appropriate. Granulocytosis and inflammation are commonly absent; therefore the presence of a fever is an important indicator of the onset of infection. Frequent use of analgesics or antipruritics may mask fever. Bleeding is another major complication;

therefore, aspirin must be used cautiously because of its antiplatelet activity and the risk of Reye's syndrome. Azathioprine and antibiotics are inappropriate for treating fever.

12. **A** Chemotherapy destroys abnormal leukemic cells, causes bone marrow depression, and depresses the patient's immunologic defense mechanisms. Chemotherapy produces granulocytopenia, so the patient must be observed for the first signs of infection.

13. **C** The most significant clinical finding in a patient with disseminated intravascular coagulation (DIC) is abnormal bleeding—such as hemoptysis, petechiae, or hematuria—without a history of a serious bleeding disorder. Other signs and symptoms include a prolonged PT and PTT, decreased fibrinogen levels, decreased platelet count, increased fibrin degradation products, and an elevated blood urea nitrogen level. Leukopenia, maculopapular rash, and severe hypertension are not symptoms of DIC.

14. **D** Bleeding may occur from mucous membranes, venipuncture sites, and the GI and genitourinary tracts. In DIC, widespread clotting occurs in small blood vessels, leading to the consumption of clotting factors and platelets and the development of a bleeding disorder.

15. **B** Activation of the clotting mechanism via fetal and placental tissue may lead to the development of DIC. In pregnancy, a normally hypercoagulable (not thrombocytopenic) state, amniotic fluid causes clot-promoting activities. However, because dead fetal and placental tissues also cause clot-promoting activities, such conditions as retained dead fetus and abruptio placentae may release clots into the maternal circulation that can lead to DIC. Under these conditions, the

incidence of DIC approaches 50%. Treatment involves blood factor replacements and removal of fetal material. Hemolysis of red blood cells does not occur from fetal enzyme release. Although thromboembolism may occur in a postpartum patient, it does not cause DIC.

16. **D** Because heparin therapy retards the coagulation process, it decreases hemorrhagic manifestations and permits normalization of clotting test results. Its antithrombin activity neutralizes free-circulating thrombin, thus preventing proliferation of thrombin (which leads to the formation of fibrin) and further blood clotting.

17. **C** A fibrin degradation products result of 10 ug/mL is considered normal and therefore reflects a successful treatment outcome. A platelet count of 40,000/mm^3 is still quite low, and a PTT of 76 seconds is still prolonged; both indicate a state of impaired coagulation. A hemoglobin level of 7 g/dL is low, reflecting blood loss.

18. **C** Hemophilia A (a deficiency of Factor VIII) is five times more common than hemophilia B (a deficiency of Factor IX). Both types are inherited as X-linked traits; therefore, almost all affected individuals are male. The mothers and some sisters of hemophiliacs may be asymptomatic carriers of the disorder.

19. **D** Bleeding near peripheral nerves causes neuropathy, pain, paresthesia, and muscle atrophy. Bleeding gums and hematuria, unrelated to trauma, are common. Abnormal bleeding occurs through the absence or deficiency of a specific clotting factor. About one-half of all hemophiliacs have severe, spontaneous bleeding into joints, which can lead to crippling and deformity.

20. **C** The most common cause of death in a patient with hemophilia occurs from bleeding of the cranium. Intracerebral hemorrhage may also lead to shock and death. Other less common bleeding sites include the GI and genitourinary tracts, pharynx, and heart.

21. **A** Confirming diagnostic studies in hemophilia indicate a Factor VIII or Factor IX deficiency, a prolonged PTT and normal PT, a normal fibrinogen level, and a normal platelet count.

22. **D** Assisting with immediate aspiration of hemarthroses would be inappropriate in this situation, as hemarthroses should not be aspirated unless the patient is feeling acute pain and pressure; aspiration may cause infection and additional bleeding. Treatment should focus on preventing crippling deformities and prolonging life expectancy. Joint bleeding is initially managed by immobilizing the affected limb and applying ice packs to diminish swelling and reduce pain. Because the plasma level of the deficient factor must be raised, an immediate infusion of cryoprecipitate (Factors VIII, XIII, and fibrinogen) may be necessary. Hemarthroses are not associated with von Willebrand's disease.

23. **C** In the four main blood groups of the ABO system A, B, AB, and O, the antigens are located on the red cell membrane and match the blood group designation. Therefore, in a patient with group AB, the red cell membrane contains both A and B antigens; in group A, the red cell membrane contains A antigens; in group B, the red cell membrane contains B antigens and in group O, there are no antigens present. The antibodies of the ABO system are located in the serum; they do not correspond to the antigens on the red cell membrane because antibodies cannot be produced against antigens present.

24. **C** Packed red blood cells (RBCs) decrease the risk of anaphylactic reaction. A unit of whole blood, which contains all the necessary blood components, including platelets and coagulation factors, is centrifuged to separate the RBCs from the plasma. Packed cells consist of the same RBC mass as whole blood with only small amounts of plasma, leukocytes, and platelets. Because only a small amount of plasma is present, the risk of plasma protein reaction, which may cause an anaphylactic reaction, decreases. A transfusion of packed RBCs causes the hemoglobin and hematocrit levels to rise faster than a whole blood transfusion does. In the average patient, the hemoglobin raises 1 g/dL, and the hematocrit rises 2% to 3%. With a whole blood transfusion: a similar increase will be seen; however, it typically occurs 24 hours after administration. Packed RBCs restore or maintain oxygen-carrying capacity and are indicated in anemia or surgical blood loss or to increase RBC mass. Whole blood is indicated when massive hemorrhage occurs.

25. **D** When administering a blood transfusion, an 18 or 20G catheter may be used. To prevent hemolysis, 18G catheters are recommended for most blood transfusions. However, 20G catheters are acceptable for average transfusion rates. Only normal saline solution may be used when administering blood products. Lactated Ringer's solution causes agglutination, and dextrose 5% in water (D_5W) causes hemolysis. During a blood transfusion, the patient's vital signs should be assessed before initiating the transfusion, 15 minutes after initiation, and after the transfusion is completed. Assessing the vital signs at these times enables the nurse to detect any adverse effects. It is particularly important to assess the vital signs 15 minutes after the initiation of the transfusion, because this is when most severe reactions occur. When using a blood warmer, the

temperature should not exceed 98.6°F (37°C); RBCs heated above this temperature may hemolyze.

26. **A** Based on these signs and symptoms, the nurse would determine that the patient is experiencing a febrile, non-hemolytic transfusion reaction, and the most common of the immediate reactions. This type of reaction, which typically occurs in patients who have received multiple transfusions, is characterized by fever, chills, headache, hypotension, lumbar pain, palpitations, and malaise. The fever typically occurs 1 to 6 hours after the transfusion has been initiated. A hemolytic transfusion reaction, the most acute and most dreaded adverse effect of a transfusion, occurs because of ABO blood group incompatibility. It is characterized by the immediate onset of a fever that may exceed 104.9°F (40.5°C), facial flushing, chills, lumbar pain, hypotension, headache, chest pain, dyspnea, oliguria, and shock. A delayed hemolytic transfusion reaction, which typically occurs 2 or more days after a transfusion, most commonly occurs in patients who have received previous transfusions. It is characterized by continued anemia, decreased hemoglobin level, hemoglobinuria, and bilirubinuria. A bacterial transfusion reaction, a rare occurrence, is caused by bacterial contamination of the blood product. It is characterized by high fever, severe hypotension, dry flushed skin, pain in the abdomen and extremities, vomiting, and bloody diarrhea.

27. **C** The nurse knows that thrombocytopenia (a decreased number of thrombocytes) does not result from a splenectomy, which would cause the platelet count to increase. The spleen collects one-third of all the platelets, and its removal eliminates the site of platelet antibody production, thus decreasing platelet destruction. Chlorothiazide may cause thrombocytopenia because of platelet antibody formation. Both chlorothiazide and zidovudine (AZT) suppress thrombocyte production because of

bone marrow depression. A viral infection may cause thrombocytopenia because the virus can destroy circulating platelets or impair platelet production.

28. **C** The nurse would expect the platelet count to return to normal levels within 1 week after discontinuation of quinidine therapy. Thrombocytopenia, which occurs in only 1 in 100,000 persons taking quinidine, develops as a result of an idiosyncratic reaction to platelet antibody formation. It may develop within 12 hours after quinidine therapy is started and typically recedes within 24 hours after discontinuation of the drug. A normal platelet count and even mild thrombocytosis should occur within 1 week.

29. **D** Anemic crisis is not a form of sickle-cell crisis. Sickle-cell crisis, the initiation of sickling of red blood cells leading to severe hemolytic anemia, may take on one of three forms: aplastic, sequestration, or painful. In aplastic crisis, the bone marrow stops producing RBCs and the hemoglobin level drops. In sequestration crisis, which is caused by splenic blockage, the patient has a sudden, large pooling of blood in the spleen. In painful crisis, the most common form of sickle-cell crisis, sickled cells occlude the blood vessels, decreasing blood flow and producing ischemia and infarction.

30. **D** Sickle cell anemia usually does not result in impaired myocardial contractility; therefore a diagnosis of decreased cardiac output related to impaired myocardial contractility would be inappropriate. The other nursing diagnoses are appropriate for a patient with sickle-cell anemia. Increased blood viscosity (from clumping of sickled cells) may decrease the blood flow to the organs and extremities. Impaired blood flow causes tissue ischemia and pain. Because sickled cells are

dysfunctional, and occluded peripheral vessels prevent oxygen delivery to tissues, impaired gas exchange occurs.

31. **C** Increased fluid intake will prevent sickle-cell crisis by preventing dehydration; therefore, it would not be considered a precipitating factor. Cigarette smoking, infection, and such physically demanding activities as tennis may precipitate a painful episode of sickle-cell crisis. Cigarette smoking contributes to sickle-cell crisis by interfering with oxygen exchange. Although infection is considered a precipitating factor, the precise relationship between infection and sickle-cell crisis has not been identified; researchers are uncertain whether the decreased oxygen state is caused by infection or whether the crisis encourages infection. Physically demanding activities, such as tennis, lead to overexertion and dehydration. The dehydration potentiates the sickling process, thereby causing a crisis.

32. **A** Inserting the smallest-possible-gauge IV catheter and infusing D 5 ½% saline solution at 100 mL/hour would be the best way to maintain hydration in this patient. Inserting a small-gauge IV catheter, such as a 21G or 23G catheter, will minimize trauma and reduce tissue scarring. Patients with sickle-cell anemia have a lifelong illness in which venous access must be preserved. To avoid fluid overload and congestive heart failure, the recommended rate of infusion is 100 to 150 mL/hour. Patients with sickle-cell anemia should normally consume 4 to 6 quarts (about 4 to 6 liters) of liquid every 24 hours. In sickle-cell crisis, adequate hydration is critical because it assists in halting the sickle cycle by decreasing blood viscosity. In this situation, however, the patient has been vomiting and probably would not be able to tolerate oral fluids.

33. **A** The analgesic used varies with the severity of the crisis; typically, oral analgesics are ordered before IM or IV agents are given. Meperidine (Demerol) is contraindicated for routine analgesia. Morphine, acetaminophen, aspirin and NSAIDs may be given. Hydroxyurea is the only drug currently approved by the FDA for the treatment of sickle cell disease. For frequent and severe pain, long-term hydroxyurea is currently the accepted treatment. Hydroxyurea increases total hemoglobin in sickle cell disease. The increase in hemoglobin retards the sickling of RBCs.

34. **C** The signs and symptoms of HIV and AIDS vary depending on the phase of infection. Some assessment findings and symptoms include: rapid weight loss, night sweats, hairy leukoplakia, swollen lymph nodes, purplish skin lesions and prolonged diarrhea.

35. **D** A T lymphocyte count of $150/mm^3$ reflects a depressed immune system; normal counts range from 600 to 1,000. Because T_4 cells are the lymphocytes affected in AIDS, the nurse would expect a low $T_4 : T_8$ ratio. Platelets and hemoglobin levels are not reflective of a person's immune status.

36. **A** Zidovudine (AZT), classified as an antiviral agent used to decrease the replication of human immunodeficiency virus (HIV), is the only FDA-approved medication for AIDS. It may be given to those with a positive HIV status to prevent the development of AIDS. Sulfamethoxazole trimethoprim (Bactrim) is the antibiotic most useful in treating Pneumocystis carinii pneumonia. Rifampin and isoniazid are antitubercular agents. Clotrimazole (Mycelex) is an antifungal agent effective against oral candidiasis.

37. **D** Pentamidine is administered via a nebulizer. Because it is unknown whether the patient has tuberculosis, which is contagious, or Pneumocystis carinii pneumonia, which is not considered a threat to someone with an intact immune system, and because aerosolized pentamidine stimulates coughing, pentamidine should be administered in a well-ventilated room, using acid fast bacilli (AFB) respiratory measures. Such measures include placing the patient in a closed room with special ventilation to prevent the spread of tuberculosis. Administering this drug in a well-ventilated room while wearing a mask reduces the nurse's exposure to the drug, which may cause irritation to the eyes and throat. Because researchers do not know whether pentamidine causes fetal damage, pregnant nurses and those who are trying to become pregnant should avoid administering the drug.

38. **A** The nurse should inquire about a recent history of chicken pox, influenza, and salicylate (aspirin) ingestion, which have been associated with the development of Reyes syndrome. Diarrhea, measles, and insect bites have no bearing in this situation.

39. **D** Because liver dysfunction occurs with Reyes syndrome, an elevated serum ammonia level is considered indicative of this disease. Other common findings include increased aspartate aminotransferase, alanine aminotransferase, and lactic dehydrogenase (LDH) levels. Hypoglycemia (decreased glucose levels) may also occur as glucose stores become depleted because of the stress, anorexia, and vomiting associated with this disease.

40. **C** The anterior aspect of the tibia below the knee is the most common site for insertion of an intraosseous catheter. Although the iliac crest may sometimes be used, it is a difficult site to

maintain for catheterization; it also decreases the patient's mobility. The sternum and femur are not used for intraosseous catheterization.

41. **C** A positive Chvostek's sign is indicative of hypocalcemia because a decrease in ionized calcium causes an increase in neuromuscular excitability. To elicit Chvostek's sign, the nurse would tap a finger on the skin above the supramandibular portion of the parotid gland and observe for twitching of the upper lip on the same side as the stimulation. Applying and inflating a blood pressure cuff to the patient's upper arm and having the patient hyperventilate are two methods of eliciting carpopedal spasm (Trousseau's sign). A positive Trousseau's sign also is indicative of hypocalcemia.

42. **C** When assessing a patient for hypocalcemia, the nurse would observe for a prolonged QT interval on electrocardiogram (EKG), an indication of impaired cardiac contractility resulting from hypocalcemia. A prolonged QT interval predisposes the patient to a polymorphous ventricular tachycardia (torsades de pointes).

43. **B** Oliguria is not one of the potential complications of hypocalcemia. Bleeding abnormalities occur in hypocalcemia because calcium assists in converting prothrombin to thrombin in the coagulation cascade. Bronchospasm can lead to laryngeal stridor and seizures because of neuromuscular irritability caused by reduced calcium levels.

44. **A** A patient with myxedema coma typically suffers from hyponatremia, which results from the interstitial accumulation of a mucopolysaccharide substance that attracts water and produces water retention. Therefore, the hyponatremia is caused by dilution from water retention. Another common finding in

myxedema coma is hypoglycemia, which results from the patient's hypometabolic state. Because the thyroid gland produces the calcium-lowering hormone calcitonin, calcium levels may rise in hypothyroidism.

45. **A** The nurse would expect a patient with myxedema coma to have respiratory acidosis and CO_2 narcosis as a result of lowered thyroxine (T_4) and triiodothyronine (T_3) levels. These hormones increase metabolic functions, such as respiration. Thus, a decrease in T_3, and T_4 levels depresses respiratory function, thereby causing hypoventilation. Metabolic acidosis also may develop as hypoxia increases serum lactate levels.

46. **B** The nurse would expect to note oliguria and abdominal distention during the assessment of a patient with myxedema coma since this condition causes dilutional hyponatremia and a decreased cardiac output. Decreased cardiac output leads to a decreased renal perfusion and glomerular filtration rate (GFR), which results in oliguria. Dilutional hyponatremia may cause decreased intestinal peristalsis, resulting in abdominal distention and, possibly, paralytic ileus. The patient also may exhibit hypothermia, hypoventilation, seizures, hypoglycemia, and anemia.

47. **C** Because myxedema coma is associated with dilutional hyponatremia, treatment usually consists of fluid restriction initially, followed by the administration of a hypertonic solution, such as dextrose 5% in normal saline (D_5NS). Since fluid therapy aims at correcting imbalances, an infusion of D_5NS would provide necessary calories, prevent hypoglycemia, and correct the underlying hyponatremia. Administering a hypotonic solution, such as D_5W or 0.3% sodium chloride, would worsen the patient's hyponatremic state. Although $D_{10}W$

would correct the hypoglycemia, it would be of no value in treating hyponatremia.

48. **A** The nurse would anticipate the treatment of a patient with hyperkalemia to include of the administration of dextrose 50%, regular insulin, sodium bicarbonate, and calcium chloride, but not lactulose enemas; lactulose is used to treat hepatic failure. The dextrose converts to glucose, which drives potassium into the cells, as does the administration of IV insulin. Sodium bicarbonate corrects the accompanying metabolic acidosis, causing potassium to move out of the cell. IV calcium stimulates cardiac contractility, thereby counteracting the depressant effects of excess potassium on the heart.

49. **B** During the initial stages of hyperkalemia, the nurse would expect to see peaked T waves on EKG. The impaired neuromuscular transmission that occurs in hyperkalemia produces intraventricular conduction disturbances, which manifest as repolarization changes (reflected as peaked T waves). As potassium levels increase, other changes occur, including prolongation of PR intervals, absence of P waves, and widening of QRS complexes.

50. **B** During the physical assessment of a patient with hyperkalemia, the nurse would expect to note ascending muscle weakness and bradycardia. Ascending muscle weakness typically originates in the legs and travels to the trunk; because the diaphragm and intercostal muscles are usually spared, the respiratory function remains unimpaired. Because peristalsis is increased in a patient with hyperkalemia, diarrhea is common and hyperactive bowel sounds may be heard. Apathy is common to both hypokalemia and hyperkalemia. Polyuria is not a sign of hyperkalemia.

51. **D** Hyperkalemia is commonly associated with metabolic acidosis. In an acidotic state, hydrogen shifts from the extracellular compartment into the cell to reduce the acidosis. As potassium is the major intracellular electrolyte, it shifts from the cell into the extracellular compartment in exchange. Thus, metabolic acidosis produces a relative increase in serum potassium levels.

52. **B** In multiple myeloma, hypercalcemia results from the release of calcium from lesions into the extracellular compartment (plasma). Other causes of hypercalcemia unrelated to multiple myeloma include increased mobilization of calcium from the bone in primary hyperparathyroidism, altered renal tubular reabsorption of calcium, and increased intestinal reabsorption of calcium secondary to a large dietary intake or an excessive administration or intake of vitamin D.

53. **A** Signs of hypercalcemia include flank or thigh pain, and polyuria, and constipation. Flank and thigh pain, which result from renal calculi, occur in approximately two-thirds of all hypercalcemic patients. Polyuria results from the inhibition of ADH by calcium in the distal tubules. Anuria or oliguria, diarrhea, and metabolic acidosis or alkalosis are not signs of hypercalcemia.

54. **C** The increased extracellular levels of calcium predispose the patient to repolarization changes (as reflected in shortening of the ST segment) and ultimately cardiac arrest. If a patient is receiving digitalis therapy, hypercalcemia may cause an enhanced digitalis effect, which can contribute to arrhythmias or cardiac arrest.

55. **A** Treatment for this patient would include the administration of normal saline solution and loop diuretics.

Normal saline solution is administered to increase the patient's GFR and calcium excretion. Loop diuretics are used to prevent tubular reabsorption of calcium. Thiazide diuretics should be avoided, as they decrease calcium excretion. Other treatments for hypercalcemia include the administration of corticosteroids to decrease the GI absorption of calcium, plicamycin (mithramycin) to stimulate bone uptake of calcium, and oral phosphates to bind calcium. Sodium polystyrene sulfonate enemas, glucose, insulin, and hemodialysis are used to treat hyperkalemia.

56. **C** The nurse would assess the patient for signs of hypokalemia. In hepatic failure, this occurs because of elevated aldosterone levels; aldosterone reabsorbs sodium and causes the kidneys to excrete potassium. Other signs of hepatic failure include decreased plasma protein level (hypoproteinemia)— which results from hypoalbuminemia, decreased calcium levels (hypocalcemia)—which results from inadequate storage of vitamin D, and free-water excess—as dilutional hyponatremia may result from increased ADH secretion.

57. **A** Respiratory alkalosis results from increased ammonia levels, which act to stimulate the respiratory drive and lead to hyperventilation. Hypermagnesemia produces hypoventilation. Hypokalemia can result from metabolic alkalosis because, in this state, potassium shifts into the cell. Hypocalcemia usually is not associated with acid-base imbalances, except in the case of chronic renal failure, which produces metabolic acidosis.

58. **B** Aldosterone causes the body to retain both sodium and water and to excrete potassium. Spironolactone is an aldosterone-blocking agent that is used to enhance sodium excretion and potassium retention; therefore, the nurse would assess for a decrease in serum sodium levels and an increase in

serum potassium levels. It is important to prevent hypokalemia in the patient with liver dysfunction because decreased serum potassium levels can contribute to the development of hepatic encephalopathy. Magnesium levels should not be affected significantly by spironolactone.

59. **A** The nurse would not expect the physician to order Kayexalate enemas in this situation, as they decrease potassium levels and the patient's levels are already decreased. Lactulose enemas are used to eliminate intestinal ammonia. Limiting the administration of hypotonic solutions restricts free-water intake, a necessary measure to prevent further dilution of intravascular sodium, as plasma hyponatremia is present in those with hepatic failure. Both dietary protein and sodium are restricted in patients with hepatic failure.

60. **A** The goals of IV therapy for the patient in this situation would not be based on gender and medical history. Fluid replacement is a lifesaving step in the initial treatment of burns. Hemoconcentration (as determined by hemoglobin and hematocrit values), increased urine specific gravity, and oliguria are common sequelae in the early stages of burn injury. These result from intravascular depletion, as body fluids shift into the intracellular and interstitial compartments. Careful monitoring of urine specific gravity and urine output for signs of impending renal failure is necessary. The depth and percentage of burn injury (using the Rule of Nines) serve as the basis for determining the amount of fluid required.

61. **B** During the initial treatment phase of a burn injury, one-half of the solution is given in the first 8 hours, during which time the patient undergoes generalized dehydration and decreased circulating volume peak, and the remaining fluid is administered over the next 16 hours. Nurses should keep in

mind that this fluid replacement formula is only a guide; the patient's individual response to fluid therapy is the determining factor in replacement therapy. The patient's response is determined by hourly vital sign assessments, hourly urine output assessments, and monitoring of urine specific gravity every 8 hours.

62. **B** During the initial stages of burn injury, the nurse would expect the patient to show signs of edema and hyperkalemia. At this time, the patient experiences a plasma-to-interstitial fluid shift, causing a leakage through the capillaries, resulting in tissue edema. Because of cellular trauma, potassium is released to the extracellular space, resulting in hyperkalemia. After the initial stage, usually after 36 hours, the body begins to mobilize burn edema; fluid shifts back into the intravascular space, thereby predisposing the patient to circulatory overload. Also at this time, potassium is excreted in large amounts in the urine because of an increase in intravascular volume. Aldosterone, which reabsorbs sodium and excretes potassium, is released in large quantities in response to the dilutional hyponatremia that develops as intracellular and interstitial fluid shifts back into the intravascular compartment.

63. **A** During the later stages of burn injury, the nurse would expect the patient to show signs of jugular venous distention and hypokalemia. At this time, the patient experiences and interstitial to plasma fluid shift into the intravascular compartment, resulting in circulatory overload (as evidenced by jugular venous distention) and dilutional hyponatremia. Aldosterone is released in response to hyponatremia, resulting in the reabsorption of sodium and excretion of potassium from the kidneys. Hypokalemia is further perpetuated as the expanding intravascular volume fosters an increasing urine output with resultant potassium loss.

64. **D** The nurse would not expect to note jugular venous distention, a sign of fluid overload, in a patient with diabetic ketoacidosis (DKA). Instead, the nurse would expect to note signs of severe intravascular dehydration, such as poor skin turgor. The nurse would also expect the patient to have hyperkalemia, an initial response to metabolic acidosis, as well as hyperventilation, as the body attempts to compensate for the metabolic acidosis by eliminating carbon dioxide.

65. **D** The first priority in caring for any patient is to establish and maintain a patent airway. The patient with DKA typically displays Kussmaul's respirations (slow, deep, regular breathing) in response to the acidotic state. Frequent patient assessment and arterial blood gas (ABG) studies are vital. Administration of volume replacement fluids and IV insulin are secondary interventions in this situation.

66. **A** Because a patient with DKA typically exhibits severe intravascular depletion and cellular dehydration, the nurse would expect the initial treatment to focus on stabilizing hemodynamic status by infusing isotonic saline solution to promote intravascular rehydration. If the circulatory system is stable but cellular dehydration is present, body fluid repletion can be achieved with a hypotonic solution, such as half normal saline solution. Because the circulatory system is unstable in DKA, hypotonic saline solution should be avoided. After fluid therapy and insulin administration have been initiated, careful monitoring of electrolyte and glucose levels is crucial. When the serum glucose level falls between 250 and 300, insulin is discontinued and fluid therapy is changed to a hypertonic solution containing glucose, such as $D_5\frac{1}{2}$ NS, thereby preventing the development of hypoglycemia, hypokalemia, and cerebral edema.

67. **A** During DKA therapy, the patient typically follows a pattern of initially elevated serum potassium levels followed by gradually decreasing levels. In DKA, serum potassium levels initially are elevated in response to the body's acidotic state, which causes shifting of cellular potassium into the intravascular space. However, in time, renal loss of potassium occurs from polyuria. Serum potassium is further depleted as potassium shifts into the intracellular compartment in response to insulin therapy and correction of acidosis.

68. **C** Respiratory acidosis is an emergency in an asthmatic patient. During the early stages of an asthma attack, ABG measurements reveal respiratory alkalosis from hyperventilation. However, as airway obstruction progresses, respiratory acidosis results, as reflected in this patient's ABG measurements. The rationale for determining respiratory acidosis is that the PCO_2 is greater than 40 mmHg (the respiratory component) and the pH is less than 7.35 (acidosis); the bicarbonate buffer remains unchanged.

69. **D** Preparing for a possible tracheotomy is not a priority action in this situation. However, the nurse may need to prepare for oral intubation if initial therapy is unsuccessful. Initial management includes oxygen therapy, continuous cardiac monitoring, establishment of an IV line, and the delivery of inhaled bronchodilator therapy, as ordered.

70. **A** If this patient is not treated, respiratory arrest will occur as a result of airway obstruction, acidosis, and hypoxemia.

71. **B** Metabolic alkalosis is indicated by a pH greater than 7.45, an HCO_3^- level greater than 26 mEq/L, and a normal PCO_2 (respiratory component). In this situation, the patient's metabolic alkalosis could only have been caused by overzealous

administration of sodium bicarbonate. Respiratory arrest would have caused the patient to experience respiratory acidosis followed by metabolic acidosis. Hyperventilation would cause respiratory alkalosis. Excessive oxygen administration can cause O_2 toxicity and, in patients with obstructive lung disease, respiratory acidosis.

72. **A** The correct treatment in this situation should have been limited to hyperventilation with a bag-valve-mask device. The patient's initial ABG measurements showed a respiratory acidosis secondary to ineffective ventilation. Hyperventilating this patient with a bag-valve-mask device would have blown off CO_2, thus correcting the acidosis. Sodium bicarbonate is unnecessary because the HCO_3^- level is normal. The patient's acid-base imbalance is unrelated to oxygen therapy. Epinephrine is not indicated because the patient did not lose pulse or blood pressure.

73. **D** This patient is hyperventilating and, as a result, is in respiratory alkalosis. The pH is elevated above 7.45, and the PCO_2, (respiratory component) is low. The metabolic component of HCO_3^- is normal.

74. **D** The goal of therapy for this patient is to increase CO_2, retention by helping the patient gain control of her respirations, which are presently uncontrolled because of hyperventilation. That can be accomplished by using a paper bag to induce rebreathing of exhaled air, which will lead to CO_2, retention, breaking the cycle and slowing the respiratory rate. The patient's oxygen and bicarbonate levels are already normal.

75. **D** The patient does not require sodium bicarbonate administration, which is indicated for metabolic acidosis. The patient had an anxiety attack and took an overdose of

medication; therefore, she requires either inpatient or outpatient follow-up.

76. **B** This patient is experiencing numbness and tingling because hypocapnia causes vasoconstriction and decreased calcium levels. Carbon dioxide is a potent vasoactive agent. Hypocapnia leads to vasoconstriction of cerebral and peripheral vessels, resulting in the paresthesias associated with hyperventilation. Alkalosis also decreases serum calcium levels, resulting in numbness, tingling, and paresthesias. Diazepam does not cause numbness or tingling.

77. **A** The correct interpretation is metabolic acidosis. The pH is below 7.35, indicating acidosis; the respiratory component (PCO_2) is normal, but the metabolic component (HCO_3^-) is extremely low (normal is 22 to 26 mEq/L), indicating acid excess.

78. **B** The bicarbonate deficit is the amount of bicarbonate anion that would theoretically be necessary to fully correct the acid-base imbalance. It can be calculated by subtracting the measured bicarbonate (10) from the desired bicarbonate (average, 24). Therefore, the bicarbonate deficit in this situation would be 14 mEq/L.

79. **D** A total of 245 mEq of sodium bicarbonate would be necessary to correct this acid-base imbalance. The patient may require a continuous infusion to receive this large amount of bicarbonate. The calculation to correct acidosis is as follows: bicarbonate deficit x weight (kg) x 0.25 (a conversion factor accounting for the bicarbonate space in the body) = dose of sodium bicarbonate (mEq). Therefore: 14 x 70 x 0.25 = 245 mEq of sodium bicarbonate.

80. **C** A lactate level and anion gap would provide essential information for the treatment of this patient because they give diagnostic clues to the source of the acid-base imbalance. An elevated lactate level (above 16 mg/dL) indicates lactic acidosis, usually a result of cardiogenic or septic shock or severe hypoxemia. An anion gap (normal is 12 mEq/L) may be calculated by subtracting the total serum anions from the total serum cations. The calculation is as follows: anion gap is $(Na^+ + K^+) - (Cl^- + HCO_3^-)$. A metabolic acidosis with a normal anion gap results from a loss of HCO_3^-, such as occurs in diarrhea or acute tubular necrosis or in chloride excess following the administration of calcium chloride or hydrochloric acid. A metabolic acidosis with an increased anion gap occurs in patients with lactic acidosis, DKA, or uremia. Complete blood count (CBC) and electrolyte studies would also be performed to provide information about infection and electrolyte status. Creatine phosphokinase (CPK) isoenzyme levels are useful in diagnosing myocardial infarction. A reticulocyte count provides information about bone marrow function. Serum amylase levels aid in diagnosing pancreatitis, whereas acetone levels aid in diagnosing DKA.

81. **D** In this situation, the patient has mixed metabolic and respiratory acidosis, a result of cardiopulmonary arrest. The pH is low; the respiratory component (PCO_2) is elevated, indicating CO_2, retention; and the metabolic component (HCO_3^-) is low, indicating excess systemic acids.

82. **A** The initial therapy for this patient is to improve oxygenation and ventilation. If respiratory acidosis still exists after resuscitation measures have been instituted and the patient is intubated, some impediment to ventilation exits, such as pneumothorax, esophageal intubation, or pulmonary embolus. Improved oxygenation will prevent progression of metabolic

acidosis. Sodium bicarbonate may then be required to reverse the metabolic acidosis. The patient's cardiac rhythm was not stated, so it is unclear whether defibrillation or epinephrine is indicated.

83. **B** The two parameters that will cause a severe problem for this patient's myocardial function are acidosis and hypoxemia. Both depress contractility and reduce stroke volume. Myocardial contractility decreases dramatically as the pH falls below 7.25, a result of a dysfunction of calcium influx into the cell. Bicarbonate and carbon dioxide levels do not directly affect myocardial contractility.

84. **C** Based on the presenting symptoms, the family probably is suffering from carbon monoxide poisoning. An O_2 saturation of 75% with a PO_2, of 97 mmHg suggests that a molecule other than oxygen is occupying the hemoglobin molecule. Diagnosis is confirmed by a high arterial carboxyhemoglobin level (normal is 0% to 2% in nonsmokers, 2% to 5% in smokers).

85. **B** The nurse would anticipate the initial treatment for a patient with carbon monoxide poisoning to be the administration of 100% O_2 via a non-rebreather mask. This should clear the blood of carbon monoxide in approximately 80 minutes. Breathing into a paper bag is the usual treatment for respiratory alkalosis induced by an anxiety attack. Administering acetylcysteine and bronchodilators is the treatment for an asthma attack. Acetylcysteine also is used to treat acetaminophen overdose.

86. **A** Secondary treatment of carbon monoxide poisoning includes hyperbaric oxygen therapy. For carboxyhemoglobin levels above 20%, authorities recommend hyperbaric oxygen therapy. When carboxyhemoglobin levels approach critical

levels, permanent neurologic damage can occur if treatment is not begun.

87. **D** An appropriate nursing diagnosis after treatment has been instituted and the family is stabilized would be knowledge deficit related to the medical diagnosis of carbon monoxide poisoning. The nurse must instruct the family on the sources of carbon monoxide exposure, such as wood stoves, propane heaters, smoldering charcoal, and incomplete combustion of organic materials, as well as on the signs and symptoms of potential exposure, such as headache, dizziness, nausea, and vomiting. No information provided supports the formulation of the other nursing diagnoses listed.

88. **A** When an ED patient is unconscious and the cause is unknown, the appropriate treatment is to administer one ampule of dextrose 50% and 0.8 to 2 mg of naloxone. Dextrose is administered in case the patient is in insulin shock, a condition more dangerous than DKA. Naloxone is administered to reverse respiratory depression, in case an overdose of narcotics caused the unconsciousness. Administering insulin to an unconscious patient before establishing the cause of unconsciousness could be harmful because it may result in furthering hypoglycemia. Not enough information is provided to determine the appropriateness of administering sodium bicarbonate, potassium, or activated charcoal.

89. **B** Regular insulin and sodium bicarbonate should be administered to a patient whose serum glucose level is 592 mg/dL and pH is 7.03. Regular insulin is preferred over NPH insulin because of its rapid onset of action; sodium bicarbonate should be administered to a patient with DKA if the pH falls below 7.10. Naloxone, dextrose, and activated charcoal are not

indicated in the treatment of DKA. Potassium therapy normally is instituted after correction of the acid-base imbalance.

90. **B** The patient has tachycardia and hypotension, indicating intravascular volume depletion. Therefore, the most appropriate solution in this situation would be 0.9% (normal) saline solution. Usually, therapy involves the infusion of 1 liter of normal saline solution every hour for 2 to 3 hours, until the blood pressure returns to normal or urine output improves. Hypertonic solutions, such as dextrose 5% in 0.45% normal saline (D_5 ½NS) and dextrose 5% in normal saline, and hypotonic solutions, such as 0.45% saline, are inappropriate initially. Hypertonic solutions would cause further cellular depletion, and hypotonic solutions would cause further intravascular volume loss as fluid shifts into the cell.

91. **B** The preferred initial insulin treatment would be an IV bolus of 20 units of regular insulin, followed by a continuous infusion of 4 to 8 units/hour. The insulin should be diluted in a glass bottle, because it will bind to plastic containers. The subcutaneous route should be avoided in hypotensive patients because absorption is variable. Continuous infusion maintains a steady blood insulin level. Use of NPH insulin should be avoided initially because of its delayed action.

92. **D** Precipitating factors in the development of DKA include omission of or resistance to insulin in a patient with diabetes, surgery or trauma in a patient with diabetes, and pancreatitis, which interferes with insulin production and release. These conditions produce stress, thereby increasing glucocorticoid release, which results in elevated blood glucose levels.

93. **A** Children at risk for DKA include those who have infections, who are under emotional stress, or who do not

comply with insulin therapy. Younger children are more prone to infections, whereas adolescents tend to suffer more from emotional stress and to not comply with therapy. An increase in activity, such as participation in a gym class, may precipitate hypoglycemia by lowering insulin requirements. A child requiring two injections of insulin per day or who self-administers insulin is at no greater risk of developing DKA.

94. **B** Signs and symptoms of DKA may also occur in a child with appendicitis or urinary tract infection; in fact, the symptoms are similar enough that misdiagnosis is possible. For example, the abdominal pain associated with DKA is so severe that it mimics an acute surgical abdomen or sickle-cell crisis; polyuria may cause DKA to be mistaken for a urinary tract infection.

95. **D** During the initial stages of DKA, the nurse may note tall T waves on EKG. The appearance of tall T waves and wide QRS complexes, along with absence of P waves, signals hyperkalemia, a common initial finding in a patient with DKA. Hyperkalemia is caused by the shifting of potassium out of the cell as a result of metabolic acidosis. As the acidosis is reversed, potassium returns to the cell; this may result in hypokalemia caused by osmotic diuresis. EKG findings indicative of hypokalemia include ST-segment depression and the appearance of U waves. The patient with DKA typically experiences sinus tachycardia, not sinus bradycardia, from hypovolemia.

96. **B** Hypophosphatemia, manifested by muscle weakness, may occur in DKA as a result of total body phosphate depletion resulting from diuresis and acidosis. Initial phosphate measurements may be normal or high, as seen with potassium measurements, but may drop after therapy. Both phosphate and

potassium may be replaced by administration of potassium phosphate IV. Hypomagnesemia, hyperchloremia, and hypercalcemia do not typically occur in DKA.

97. **A** Slow respirations are not indicative of a patient with DKA. Clinical manifestations of this condition include altered level of consciousness, poor skin turgor, hypotension, and tachycardia, which are the result of dehydration. Hyperglycemia promotes osmotic diuresis, resulting in polyuria, polydipsia, and cellular and intravascular fluid depletion. The breakdown of body fats releases excessive ketones, resulting in metabolic acidosis and acetone breath odor. An increase in the rate and depth of respirations compensates for the acidosis by blowing off carbon dioxide; this is known as Kussmaul's respirations.

98. **D** A decreased serum potassium level and decreased hematocrit would not support a diagnosis of DKA. Initial diagnostic studies typically reveal decreased arterial pH, HCO_3, and CO_2, levels caused by metabolic acidosis with respiratory compensation. The patient's blood urea nitrogen (BUN) and hematocrit levels and urine specific gravity increase as a result of dehydration. Potassium shifts from the cells into the intravascular fluid, with a corresponding hydrogen shift into cells. This compensatory mechanism is an attempt to buffer the acidosis, which produces an elevated potassium level.

99. **D** Polyuria, the most obvious sign of DKA, initially results from the osmotic diuretic effect of hyperglycemia. Although the ketone-induced metabolic acidosis causes a shift of potassium into the serum, the resulting elevated serum potassium level is not so obvious. Metabolic acidosis decreases blood pH; Kussmaul's respirations compensate for this. A patient with

DKA is typically hypotensive because of the associated fluid loss.

100. **D** The priority nursing diagnostic category for a patient with DKA would be Fluid volume deficit, as an elevated serum glucose level results in intracellular dehydration and intravascular depletion. Hyperglycemia increases the serum osmolarity, thereby causing a shift of intracellular fluid into the intravascular space, producing intracellular dehydration. An increased serum osmolarity produces osmotic diuresis and poly uria (excessive urination). Although a patient with DKA has altered nutrition, this is not a priority at this time. The other categories are inappropriate because the respiratory alkalosis that results from Kussmaul's respirations is a beneficial compensatory mechanism to combat metabolic acidosis.

101. **C** Cerebral edema can result from overzealous fluid replacement and administration of sodium bicarbonate. Although a rare complication, it most commonly occurs in children and adolescents during the first day of treatment. Mannitol (Osmitrol), an osmotic diuretic, is the treatment of choice. Acute renal failure may occur if treatment is not instituted and dehydration continues. HHNK and respiratory acidosis are not treatment-related complications.

102. **D** After initiation of therapy, hypokalemia may result from the correction of acidosis or from insulin therapy. Once intravascular fluid depletion has been reversed, 20 to 40 mEq of potassium should be added to each liter of IV fluid.

103. **A** A child is at highest risk for hypovolemic shock from DKA because, compared to an adolescent or adult, a child has less body fluid and therefore less to lose before becoming dehydrated. A child with DKA can lose up to 10% of his body

weight through dehydration. Children and adolescents also have a higher risk of developing cerebral edema during fluid replacement. Elderly and cardiac patients are at increased risk of developing pulmonary edema.

104. **C** Once the patient's serum glucose level has fallen between 250 and 300 mg/dL, the nurse would expect the physician to order D_5W NS to prevent hypoglycemia and cerebral edema. The other solutions do not contain dextrose, which the patient now requires in small doses since his serum glucose level has fallen.

105. **D** In the ED, the most effective parameter for determining a DKA patient's response to insulin therapy is taking bedside capillary measurements with a glucometer. This provides instantaneous results; sending serum specimens to the laboratory may take 1 to 2 hours for results. Urine measurements are inconsistent because urine glucose thresholds are variable, and glycosuria usually occurs when the serum glucose level is above 180 mg/dL.

106. **A** Continuous administration of NPH insulin at 4 to 8 units/hour is inappropriate for a patient with DKA. NPH insulin is an intermediate-acting insulin and should never be administered IV specific treatments for such a patient aim to restore fluid balance; restore normal carbohydrate, fat, and protein metabolism; and maintain electrolyte balance and function of related systems. During restoration of fluid balance, rapid administration of fluid (up to 1,000 mL/hour) may be ordered initially. When the patient's serum glucose level falls to 250 mg/dL, the initial infusions of 0.45% saline or normal saline solution should be changed to $D_5\frac{1}{2}$ NS with potassium to prevent hypoglycemia, hypokalemia, and cerebral edema. To restore normal carbohydrate, fat, and protein metabolism, rapid-

acting insulin (regular) should be administered, preferably as a continuous infusion of 4 to 8 units/hour (alternatives include IM or IV loading doses) or as an IV bolus of 10 to 25 units/hour. During treatment, electrolyte levels, especially potassium, should be monitored.

107. **A** Hyperglycemia results in an elevated plasma osmolarity (normal serum osmolarity is 275 to 295 mOsm/L). This hyperosmolar state causes the brain cells to become dehydrated, thereby producing a change in level of consciousness. A BUN level of 50 mg/dL would not alter the patient's level of consciousness. A serum sodium level of 125 mEq/L could cause a change in mental status, but serum sodium levels are typically elevated (not lowered) in HHNK. A nonketotic state would not cause a change in mental status.

108. **C** Monitoring the patient's rectal temperature and notifying the physician if the temperature rises above 101°F (38.3°C) is not a priority nursing action during the initial management of HHNK. Although, HHNK may be precipitated by prolonged total parenteral nutrition administration, pneumonia, burns, cerebrovascular accident, or recent surgery, and temperature assessment is an important component of managing these states, monitoring temperature is not a priority concern in the initial management. Initially, the patient should be rehydrated with a hypotonic solution, such as 0.45% saline solution if the blood pressure is stable, or normal saline solution if intravascular depletion occurs. Frequent neurologic assessments are necessary because cerebral intracellular dehydration results in mental status changes. The serum glucose level should be normalized by insulin administration.

109. **B** The nurse would expect the patient with HHNK to require hypotonic fluid replacement and less insulin and

potassium than that needed for a patient with DKA. Hypotonic (0.45% saline) solution is preferred to isotonic (0.9% saline) solution because of the marked hyperosmolarity associated with HHNK. Because of this severely dehydrated state, as much as 4 to 6 liters may be required in the first 10 hours. In the absence of acidosis, potassium loss in the urine is greatly decreased during the initial stages of glycosuria. Less insulin usually is required to reduce the hyperglycemia in a patient with HHNK as compared with a patient with DKA.

110. **D** Ineffective breathing pattern related to hyperventilation would be inappropriate because compensatory hyperventilation resulting from metabolic acidosis does not develop in HHNK. Appropriate nursing diagnoses for a patient with this condition would include Fluid volume deficit related to osmotic diuresis, which is induced by the hyperglycemic state; Potential for injury related to altered level of consciousness because of the possibility of confusion, obtundation, and seizures secondary to severe intracerebral dehydration; and Altered peripheral tissue perfusion related to a decreased cardiac output, which may result from fluid volume loss.

111. **B** Based on the assessment findings, the nurse would suspect that the patient's change in level of consciousness resulted from syndrome of inappropriate antidiuretic hormone (SIADH) secretion. Dilutional hyponatremia and altered mental status are indications of this disorder; a mass in the right lung field may reflect oat-cell carcinomas, which produce antidiuretic hormone (ADH). Cerebral metastasis typically produces neurologic dysfunction of one area or one side of the body rather than a generalized state of confusion or stupor. Acute purulent meningitis could cause an altered mental status without such dysfunction, but the lack of a fever or an elevated white blood cell count makes meningitis a less likely diagnosis.

A subarachnoid hemorrhage presents with a more abrupt onset of severe headache and photophobia.

112. **B** Phenytoin has not been associated with SIADH; therefore, a 36-year old patient receiving phenytoin sodium is not considered at risk for developing SIADH. Patients at risk include those with lung carcinomas, as in oat-cell carcinoma that synthesizes, stores, and releases ADH from the tumor tissue. Those who have received prolonged positive-pressure ventilation, as a reduction in left atrial filling may stimulate central ADH release. Also, those with pneumonia, tuberculosis, lung abscesses, or empyema, as inflamed pulmonary tissue may lead to ADH secretion.

113. **D** SIADH is caused by increased secretion of ADH by the posterior pituitary gland. Precipitating factors include tuberculous meningitis; extracranial malignant tumors, especially bronchogenic and pancreatic tumors; head traumas, such as skull fractures; medications, such as chlorpropamide, clofibrate, and thiazides; and viral respiratory infections.

114. **A** A serum sodium level of 120 mEq/L is characteristic of a patient with SIADH. An increase in ADH secretion promotes excessive water retention by the kidneys. This lowers the serum sodium level and produces a marked decrease in serum osmolarity (the normal range for serum osmolarity is between 275 and 295 mOsm/L). Dilutional hypokalemia also results (normal potassium levels range from 3.5 to 5 mEq/L). Urine output decreases as a result of increased reabsorption of water. The concentrated urine that is produced has high specific gravity and osmolarity (urine specific gravity ranges from 1.001 to 1.030, depending on its concentration).

115. **D** Use of demeclocycline and other drugs that block the effect of ADH on the renal tubules are inappropriate for the acute treatment of SIADH but may be appropriate for long-term therapy. Hyponatremia and its resultant decreased osmolarity are responsible for the patient's seizures. The goal of initial treatment is to raise the serum sodium level to at least 125 mEq/L to avoid neurologic symptoms. At this level, the patient's mental status should improve. Administering furosemide should produce diuresis; administering a 3% hypertonic saline solution and restricting fluids should raise the serum sodium level.

116. **B** Preventing seizures is the primary goal of nursing care in a patient with SIADH. The clinical manifestations of SIADH result from excessive water retention, which leads to overhydration and water intoxication. Water intoxication dilutes serum sodium levels, producing hyponatremia, which results in neurologic changes. Signs and symptoms of hyponatremia and water intoxication vary from a mild headache to seizures, coma, and death. The patient is probably hypertensive because of the fluid overload. Tetany is a sign of hypocalcemia.

117. **D** Diabetes insipidus may develop from various causes, one of which is head trauma, especially involving a basal skull fracture. It most commonly develops in neurosurgical patients. Other precipitating factors include inflammatory or degenerative conditions, such as tubercular meningitis, syphilis, sarcoidosis, Hodgkin's disease, and tumors. Severe pneumonia and therapy with thiazides and vasopressin predispose the patient to SIADH.

118. **D** Laboratory findings for a patient with diabetes insipidus typically show a urine specific gravity between 1.001 and 1.005. Diabetes insipidus results from a defect in the release or

synthesis of ADH within the pituitary or a defect in renal tubular response to ADH. In diabetes insipidus, the patient has impaired renal conservation of water; therefore, little water reabsorption occurs. As water is lost from the body, the serum sodium level rises, resulting in an increased serum osmolarity. As the kidneys fail to conserve water, the urine remains dilute, resulting in a decreased urine osmolarity and a specific gravity between 1.001 and 1.005.

119. **A** Diabetes insipidus can be complicated by severe volume depletion and dehydration, resulting in hypovolemic shock. The appropriate nursing intervention would be to assess for signs and symptoms of rapidly developing hypovolemic shock. Meticulous recording of fluid intake and output, monitoring of vital signs, and daily weight monitoring are mandatory. Instituting seizure precautions and auscultating lung fields for crackles are appropriate interventions for a patient with SIADH. Although arrhythmias are possible in diabetes insipidus, they are uncommon and monitoring for them is not a priority.

120. **C** The mainstay of management in diabetes insipidus is the administration of vasopressin tannate because the patient is deficient in ADH, or vasopressin. If Pitressin tannate is prescribed, the vial must be warmed under hot water for several minutes and vigorously shaken. In this situation, inadequate warming or agitation of the medication vial may have caused the patient's unresponsiveness to therapy. The other choices have no bearing on the effectiveness of vasopressin.

121. **C** The nurse would question administering vasopressin to a patient with angina pectoris. Vasopressin must be used cautiously in patients with heart disease because its vasoconstrictive properties may precipitate myocardial ischemia. It increases water reabsorption by the renal tubules

and constriction of the smooth muscle of the arterioles. Vasopressin may be safely administered in a patient with liver dysfunction, a brain tumor, or a transplanted kidney.

122. **A** In this situation, the patient has symptoms of hypoglycemia that probably resulted from a neurologic response. During hypoglycemia, insulin-antagonist hormones, such as epinephrine, are released, causing the patient to experience the characteristic symptoms of neuroglycopenia (tachycardia, diaphoresis, tremors, and nervousness).

123. **D** Emergency management of a patient in hypoglycemic coma includes the administration of 50 mL of dextrose 50% IV. If there is any doubt about whether a comatose patient is hypoglycemic or hyperglycemic, the nurse should obtain a serum glucose measurement by finger stick. A fasting blood sugar level measurement is not feasible in this situation because the nurse would not know whether the patient had fasted before the measurement was obtained.

124. **D** Myxedema occurs in patients with moderate to severe hypothyroidism. If the hypothyroidism is allowed to progress, the patient's condition will deteriorate and coma will eventually ensue. Myxedema coma is extremely advanced hypothyroidism; all persons who develop myxedema coma are in a hypothyroid state, but not all patients with hypothyroidism have myxedema coma.

125. **A** The nurse would expect a patient with myxedema coma to have hyponatremia. Low sodium levels are caused by impaired water excretion, which can be due to dilution in nature. Potassium levels are typically normal in myxedema, unless the patient has another underlying condition.

126. **B** Rewarming should take place gradually, using blankets or sheets only. The use of a hypothermia blanket is strongly contraindicated because rapid rewarming can precipitate vasodilation, which can cause cardiac arrhythmias, circulatory collapse, or death. Once thyroid replacement has begun, the body will begin to compensate and slowly return to a normal temperature. No benefit occurs from glycerin suppositories in this condition.

127. **D** Diuretic therapy may result in sodium loss, thereby lowering sodium levels further; it is therefore contraindicated in patients with myxedema coma. Fluid restriction may be indicated in myxedema coma to correct hyponatremia. If the hyponatremia is severe (levels less than 115 mEq/L), infusion of normal saline solution (electrolyte replacement) may be necessary to elevate the serum sodium level. Thyroid hormone replacement is essential to correct the decreased secretion of thyroid hormone.

128. **D** The patient's PCO_2, level is 64 mmHg, indicating acute respiratory acidosis; therefore, the appropriate nursing intervention at this time would be to prepare for endotracheal intubation. Myxedema coma causes changes in the thoracic ventilatory capacity and respiratory center. The initial assessment indicated bilateral pulmonary congestion. The patient also may have pleural effusion and ascites. The nurse must assess the respiratory system carefully to determine the need for ventilatory assistance. Arterial blood gas measurements usually demonstrate respiratory acidosis with PCO_2, narcosis.

129. **D** The patient has a history of Addison's disease, which can be controlled by corticosteroids. However, because he had been fasting and did not take his medication, the blood level of

corticosteroids decreased. Abrupt discontinuation of steroid therapy precipitated the adrenal crisis.

130. **C** The most serious threat in adrenal crisis is peripheral vascular collapse. A patient may lose as much as 20% of extracellular fluid volume. Therefore, the first goal of emergency treatment is fluid replacement. Secondary interventions are aimed at achieving electrolyte balance and a normal glucose state. A patient with Addison's disease typically has hypoglycemia, hyperkalemia, and hyponatremia.

131. **C** The most definitive diagnostic test for adrenal crisis is measurement of plasma cortisol levels. Abnormally low levels indicate adrenocortical insufficiency. Adrenocorticotropic hormone (ACTH) and 24-hour urine 17-hydroxycorticosteroid level measurements are used to help diagnose adrenal disorders; however, they are contraindicated for a patient with adrenal crisis because of the potentially life-threatening delay associated with the tests. Plasma carcinoembryonic antigen levels help diagnose cancer or abnormal cells in the body.

132. **B** To combat the patient's fluid deficit, the nurse would expect to infuse 1 liter of dextrose 5% in normal saline. The infusion rate should be extremely rapid (1 to 2 hours), barring such complications as cardiac or renal disease. Fluid replacement should raise the blood pressure by volume expansion and contribute needed glucose and sodium. After the first liter, the patient may require additional fluids at a rate of 1 liter every 3 to 4 hours. A 0.45% saline solution, D_5W, and dextrose 5% in Lactated Ringer's solution are inappropriate because they do not contain enough sodium, which is needed to correct the hyponatremia associated with adrenal crisis.

133. **C** Hydrocortisone, a soluble cortisol replacement for lost glucocorticoids, is commonly used to treat adrenal crisis. The usual dosage is 100 to 200 mg IV immediately, then every 6 hours. Sodium levothyroxine is used to treat thyroid disease. Dexamethasone and fludrocortisone, mineralocorticoid replacements, may be used to treat adrenal crisis; however, they are not urgently required because saline solution and hydrocortisone adequately compensate for lost mineralocorticoids.

134. **B** When adrenal crisis is complicated by hyperkalemia, the EKG will show peaked T waves, wide QRS complexes, and prolonged PR intervals. Hyperkalemia may cause bradycardia; it is not associated with bundle branch block or T-wave depression.

135. **A** Adrenal crisis, or acute adrenocortical insufficiency, is caused by decreased cortisol and aldosterone secretion by the adrenal cortex. ADH is secreted by the posterior pituitary and has no significance in adrenal crisis.

136. **B** In this situation, the nurse would assess for signs and symptoms of hyperglycemia and hyponatremia. Excessive thyroid hormone levels appear to produce an increase in glycogenolysis and rapid intestinal glucose absorption. Also, increased adrenergic activity may cause insulin resistance and impair insulin secretion, resulting in hyperglycemia. Diaphoresis in a patient with a high fever, who consumes large quantities of water without adequate salt intake, may induce water toxicity or dilutional hyponatremia.

137. **C** For patients who are iodine-sensitive, lithium carbonate is used to inhibit thyroid hormone release. Levothyroxine sodium is used for thyroid hormone replacement. ACTH is used

mainly in treating adrenal diseases. Phenytoin is an antiepileptic agent.

138. **A** Aspirin would be inappropriate in this situation because salicylates are thought to interfere with the binding of triiodothyronine (T_3 and thyroxine (T_4) to circulating thyroid-binding protein. The increase of free T_3 and T_4 may exacerbate the existing hyperthyroidism. Non-aspirin antipyretics should be used in thyroid storm. Administering muscle relaxants to control shivering, applying ice packs to the axillae and groin, and using a hypothermia blanket with a rectal probe are acceptable methods of treating fever.

139. **D** Measurement of 24-hour urine 17-ketosteroids is used to assess adrenal, not thyroid function. Serum protein-bound iodine, radioactive iodine uptake, and thyroid-stimulating hormone measurements help assess thyroid function.

140. **D** In this situation, the patient's serum calcium level should be monitored because bone pain, muscle weakness, and hypotonic muscles are symptoms of hypercalcemia, which is caused by hypermetabolism of the bone. Hypercalcemia also causes thirst, lethargy, and drowsiness, which may progress to stupor and coma.

141. **B** The patient's signs and symptoms are the classic manifestations of Cushing's syndrome and constitute the associated protein catabolic, gluconeogenic, mineralocorticoid, androgenic, and behavioral effects that are characteristic of this disorder.

142. **C** Cushing's syndrome, the opposite of Addison's disease, presents with clinical manifestations of excessive rather than deficient adrenocortical activity. The syndrome may result from

excessive administration of cortisone or ACTH or from hyperplasia of the adrenal cortex. Removal of the pituitary gland may cause vasopressin deficiency, resulting in diabetes insipidus.

143. **D** A patient with Cushing's syndrome should be monitored for mineralocorticoid effects, including increased serum sodium levels (hypernatremia), decreased serum potassium levels (hypokalemia), hypertension, and edema. Increased blood glucose levels (hyperglycemia) are a gluconeogenic effect manifested by glucose intolerance.

144. **B** Potential for infection related to altered metabolism best reflects the anti-inflammatory effects of excessive glucocorticoid levels seen in a patient with Cushing's syndrome. Such effects produce increased susceptibility to infection and mask infections that do occur. Potential for injury related to decreased protein catabolism is incorrect because the patient with Cushing's syndrome experiences excessive, not decreased, protein catabolism, resulting in muscle weakness and an increased risk for soft tissue injuries and fractures from progressive osteoporosis. Altered body image related to physical appearance and Sleep pattern disturbance related to anxiety may be relevant diagnoses; however, they are not associated with the anti-inflammatory effects of this disease.

145. **A** The hypokalemia associated with Cushing's syndrome produces an increased heart rate, frequently with atrial premature complexes. Also, increased serum aldosterone levels result in an increased serum osmolarity and hypernatremia. Elevated calcitonin levels may be seen in hyperthyroidism. Chvostek's sign occurs in hypocalcemia.

146. **A** During the later stages of a burn injury, the nurse would expect the patient to show signs of jugular venous distention and hypokalemia. At this time, the patient experiences an interstitial-to-plasma fluid shift into the intravascular compartment, resulting in circulatory overload, as evidenced by jugular venous distention and a dilutional hyponatremia. Aldosterone is released in response to hyponatremia, resulting in the re-absorption of sodium and excretion of potassium for the kidney. Hypokalemia is further perpetuated as the expanding intravascular volume fosters an increase in the urine output with resultant potassium loss.

147. **D** GERD is the chronic regurgitation of stomach acids into the esophagus, causing cellular and tissue damage over the long-term, including Barrett esophagus and esophageal cancer. Symptoms of a peptic ulcer include bloody/tarry stools, nausea, vomiting, and abdominal pain, and occur when an overproduction of stomach acid irritates the lining of the GI tract. Cholecystitis is the inflammation and obstruction of the bile duct, and most commonly occurs in women who are overweight and between 20 to 40 years of age. Severe upper right quadrant pain, sometimes radiating to the back, and nausea/vomiting are the most common symptoms. Patients with pancreatitis also present with abdominal pain and nausea/vomiting. Their pain is often in the left upper quadrant.

148. **C** Bruising around the umbilicus, Cullen sign is the most common signs of splenic rupture. Left shoulder pain, or Kehr sign, is frequently seen in patients with intra-abdominal bleeding. Splenic injuries occur frequently in blunt abdominal trauma simply because the spleen is not as well protected by the ribs as other organs. In contrast, pancreatic injuries are less common from blunt trauma because the pancreas is so well protected. Patients with pancreatic injuries may also vomit bile,

in addition to having diffuse abdominal pain. Intestinal perforation is significantly more likely to occur with penetrating trauma, such as a gunshot or knife wound, than with blunt trauma from a motor vehicle accident. Symptoms include acute abdominal pain, distention and rigidity, tachycardia, and nausea/vomiting.

149. **C** The most likely cause of the patient's symptoms is an anaphylactic reaction in response to something eaten at lunch. Albuterol should be given to relieve the bronchospasm. Oxygen and fluids should also be administered for hypotension. Diphenhydramine should be administered to treat the underlying allergy, and methylprednisolone can be given after initial treatment with Benadryl and albuterol as its therapeutic onset is more delayed. Frequent monitoring is necessary because of the potential for airway loss if the allergic reaction progresses.

150. **B** In a tonic-clonic seizure a patient initially has stiffening of the muscles throughout the entire body. The patient's eyes may roll back and loss of consciousness can occur. This is called the tonic period and lasts approximately 10 to 30 seconds. Following the tonic period is the clonic period of the seizure, lasting around 30 to 90 seconds. The patient suffers violent and rhythmic contractions over her whole body. The patient may be incontinent of both urine and stool.

GENITOURINARY AND GYNECOLOGIC EMERGENCIES

1. The most appropriate nursing action for an uncircumcised male patient with a zipper injury would be to:

A. Delicately unzip the zipper after the physician administers a local anesthetic
B. Delicately unzip the zipper using no anesthesia
C. Cut the zipper around the injury, allowing the tracks to separate
D. Prepare the patient for circumcision to remove the injured foreskin

2. Which statement regarding urethral trauma is true:

A. Urethral trauma is most common in women
B. Urethral trauma commonly occurs when the bladder is full
C. Urethral trauma is diagnosed by intravenous pyelography (IVP)
D. The patient with urethral trauma should be instructed not to void

3. Which statement regarding the assessment or treatment of urethral trauma is true?

A. Urethral trauma is difficult to diagnose because it is painless
B. An indwelling urinary catheter should be inserted as soon as possible to maintain urethral patency
C. A suprapubic catheter may be inserted to divert urine
D. The patient typically suffers urinary incontinence as a result of sphincter damage

4. The nurse is assessing a patient with a hard scrotal mass that cannot be transilluminated. This finding most likely indicates:

A. Hydrocele
B. Spermatocele
C. Testicular tumor
D. Epididymitis

5. The nurse understands that IVP usually is not indicated for a patient with acute renal failure because:

A. It would be of no diagnostic value
B. It places the patient at increased risk for an allergic reaction to the contrast media
C. It may cause a fluid volume deficit because of the osmotic effect of the contrast media
D. The contrast media would have a nephrotoxic effect

6. Which finding differentiates decreased renal perfusion from acute tubular necrosis (ATN):

A. Serum creatinine level of 4 mg/dL
B. Urine sodium level of 15 mEq/L
C. Urine output of 350 mL/24 hours
D. Urine specific gravity of 1.010

7. Anuria is a common symptom of:

A. Urethral injury
B. Bladder injury
C. Postrenal acute renal failure ARF
D. All of the above

8. The nurse would expect a patient with ureteral trauma to be best managed by:

A. Surgical repair
B. Insertion of an indwelling urinary catheter
C. Insertion of a suprapubic catheter
D. Bed rest and monitoring of urine output

9. The nurse would anticipate a penile fracture to be treated by:

A. Insertion of a suprapubic catheter
B. Surgical repair
C. Splinting
D. Casting

10. Which common assessment finding is considered a nonspecific sign of genitourinary trauma?

A. Flank pain
B. Hypotension
C. Urine retention
D. Hematuria

11. Signs and symptoms of epididymitis may be confused with those of:

A. Testicular torsion
B. Priapism
C. Urinary tract infection (UTI)
D. Pyelonephritis

12. A 24-year-old man is brought to the emergency department (ED), after having sustained blunt trauma to the left kidney during a boxing match. He is awake and alert. His chief complaint is flank tenderness. Urinalysis reveals microscopic hematuria. All other laboratory values are within normal limits. Vital signs are blood pressure 130/70 mmHg, pulse rate 76 beats/minute, and respiratory rate 20 breaths/minute. He is scheduled for transfer to the medical-surgical unit as soon as a bed is available. Which assessment findings indicate renal trauma:

A. Severe, colicky flank pain, and diaphoresis
B. Hematuria and flank pain
C. Severe flank pain and urethral bleeding
D. Severe flank pain and no urine output

13. Which injury resulting from blunt renal trauma typically resolves without surgery?

A. Contusion
B. Rupture of a major renal artery
C. Renal pedicle injury
D. None of the above

14. A patient's assessment findings reveal ecchymosis around the left flank area. This would best be interpreted as:

A. Pulled muscles in the flank area
B. Fractured ilium
C. Retroperitoneal bleeding
D. All of the above

15. The physician determines that your patient has a renal contusion. Priority intervention would include:

A. Immediate surgery
B. Maintaining the patient on his affected side to apply pressure to the area
C. Percutaneous evacuation of blood from the abdominal cavity
D. No treatment other than observation for worsening of the injury

16. In a patient with renal contusion, if the patient's pain increases, the nurse's main priority would be to:

A. Administer narcotics, as ordered
B. Monitor the patient's serum electrolyte studies, blood urea nitrogen (BUN) level, and glucose level
C. Monitor the patient's serum hematocrit
D. Measure the patient's blood pressure

17. The nurse should suspect renal trauma in any patient with:

A. A positive Chvostek's sign
B. Oliguria
C. Hematoma in the flank area
D. Dysuria

18. Which injury would lead the nurse to suspect kidney trauma:

A. Chest trauma
B. Fractured pelvis
C. Deceleration injury
D. All of the above

19. Which test would confirm a diagnosis of renal trauma most conclusively?

A. Kidney-ureter-bladder (KUB) urethrography
B. Abdominal computed tomography (CT) scan
C. IVP
D. Peritoneal tap

20. A 62-year-old man arrives at the ED after being unable to urinate for the past 2 days. He appears slightly confused and complains of nausea, vomiting, and swollen ankles. His history reveals no renal dysfunction but a history of benign prostatic hypertrophy. Laboratory findings indicate a serum BUN level of 38 mg/dL and a serum creatinine level of 4 mg/dL. The nurse suspects that this patient is exhibiting signs and symptoms of:

A. Acute renal failure (ARF)
B. Congestive heart failure (CHF)
C. Pyelonephritis
D. Chronic renal failure

21. Which symptom is considered the hallmark assessment finding in a patient with acute renal failure (ARF)?

A. Edema
B. Rising BUN and creatinine levels
C. Anuria
D. Confusion

22. A 62-year-old man arrives at the ED after being unable to urinate for the past 2 days. He appears slightly confused and complains of nausea, vomiting, and swollen ankles. His history reveals no renal dysfunction but a history of benign prostatic hypertrophy. Laboratory findings indicate a serum BUN level of 38 mg/dL and a serum creatinine level of 4 mg/dL. Which test would the nurse expect the physician to order initially when diagnosing this patient's condition:

A. KUB urethrography
B. Abdominal CT scan
C. IVP
D. Peritoneal tap

23. A 58-year-old male has arrived at the ED complaining that he has not been able to urinate for 3 days. After inserting an indwelling urinary catheter and draining 2,500 mL of urine from the patient's bladder, the nurse formulates a nursing diagnosis of:

A. Fluid volume excess related to kidney dysfunction
B. Fluid volume deficit related to restoration of urine flow
C. Potential for injury related to potassium excess
D. Potential for injury related to metabolic acidosis

24. After inserting a urinary catheter on a 58-year-old male, who complained of not being able to urinate for 3 days, and draining 2,500 mL of urine, the most important nursing intervention at this time would involve:

A. Clamping the catheter
B. Requesting an order for fluid replacement
C. Requesting an order for a diuretic
D. Preparing the patient for emergency surgery

25. A 62-year-old man arrives at the ED after being unable to urinate for the past 2 days. He appears slightly confused and complains of nausea, vomiting, and swollen ankles. His history reveals no renal dysfunction but a history of benign prostatic hypertrophy. Laboratory findings indicate a serum BUN level of 38 mg/dL and a serum creatinine level of 4 mg/dL. After establishing an IV line, the nurse would expect to administer:

A. Dextrose 5% in water at a keep-vein-open rate
B. 3% saline solution at 20 mL/hour
C. Normal saline solution and potassium chloride at 30 mL/hour
D. Dextrose 5% in 0.45% saline solution and potassium chloride at 160 mL/hour

26. A 35-year-old woman arrives at the ED complaining of nausea, vomiting, malaise, and a decreased urine output. She recently completed a 2-week course of cephradine (Velosef) for a UTI. Urinalysis reveals a sodium level of 40 mEq/L with a urine specific gravity of 1.0. Urine sediment includes casts, with few red blood cells (RBCs) or white blood cells (WBCs). Other laboratory findings include a serum BUN level of 40 mg/dL and a serum creatinine level of 4 mg/dL. Which condition is suggestive of the patient's assessment findings?

A. Recurrence of UTI
B. Dehydration from vomiting
C. Allergic drug reaction
D. Acute tubular necrosis

27. A 48-year-old male arrives at the ED complaining of a decreased urine output. Which assessment finding is the most accurate indicator of this patient's renal function?

A. Serum creatinine level
B. Serum BUN level
C. Urine sodium level
D. Urine specific gravity

28. Which laboratory finding is an indirect measurement of a patient's glomerular filtration rate (GFR)?

A. Creatinine clearance
B. BUN level
C. Urine sodium level
D. Urine specific gravity

29. A 35-year-old woman arrives at the ED complaining of nausea, vomiting, malaise, and a decreased urine output. She recently completed a 2 week course of cephradine (Velosef) for a UTI. Urinalysis reveals a sodium level of 40 mEq/L with a urine specific gravity of 1.0. Urine sediment includes casts, with few red blood cells (RBCs) or white blood cells (WBCs). Other laboratory findings include a serum BUN level of 40 mg/dL and a serum creatinine level of 4 mg/dL. The nurse would expect treatment for this patient to include:

A. Antibiotic therapy with penicillin or an aminoglycoside
B. Fluid restriction
C. Furosemide (Lasix) administration
D. Electrolyte replacement

30. A 35-year-old woman arrives at the ED complaining of nausea, vomiting, malaise, and a decreased urine output. She recently completed a 2 week course of cephradine (Velosef) for a UTI. Urinalysis reveals a sodium level of 40 mEq/L with a urine specific gravity of 1.0. Urine sediment includes casts, with few red blood cells (RBCs) or white blood cells (WBCs). Other laboratory findings include a serum BUN level of 40 mg/dL and a serum creatinine level of 4 mg/dL. The nurse should also assess this patient for:

A. Hypernatremia
B. Metabolic alkalosis
C. Hyperkalemia
D. Hypercalcemia

31. A 35-year-old woman arrives at the ED complaining of nausea, vomiting, malaise, and a decreased urine output. She recently completed a 2 week course of cephradine (Velosef) for a UTI. Urinalysis reveals a sodium level of 40 mEq/L with a urine specific gravity of 1.0. Urine sediment includes casts, with few red blood cells (RBCs) or white blood cells (WBCs). Other laboratory findings include a serum BUN level of 40 mg/dL and a serum creatinine level of 4 mg/dL. Which finding would indicate that the patient's treatment has been effective?

A. Serum BUN level of 54 mg/dL
B. Serum creatinine level of 72 mg/dL
C. Creatinine clearance of 125 mL/min
D. Urine sodium level of 50 mEq/L

32. A male patient is admitted to the ED complaining of sudden onset of pain to the testicular area, especially upon elevation of the scrotum. The pain radiates to the flank area and is accompanied by nausea, vomiting, and testicular edema. The patient's signs and symptoms are characteristic of which condition:

A. Testicular tumor
B. Priapism
C. Acute epididymitis
D. Testicular torsion

33. A male patient is admitted to the ED complaining of sudden onset of pain to the testicular area, especially upon elevation of the scrotum. The pain radiates to the flank area and is accompanied by nausea, vomiting, and testicular edema. This condition is most common among which age group:

A. Children and adolescents
B. Young adults
C. Middle-age adults
D. Older adults

34. A male patient is admitted to the ED complaining of sudden onset of pain to the testicular area, especially upon elevation of the scrotum. The pain radiates to the flank area and is accompanied by nausea, vomiting, and testicular edema. The nurse would expect treatment of this problem to include:

A. Antibiotic therapy
B. Application of ice packs and manual manipulation
C. Immediate orchiectomy
D. Sedation

35. The nurse knows that end-stage renal disease (ESRD) develops when:

A. The serum creatinine level reaches 4 mg/dL
B. 90% of the nephrons are destroyed
C. The kidneys can no longer concentrate urine
D. The kidneys can no longer absorb sodium

36. A 52-year-old diabetic man with a 1-year history of chronic renal failure that is treated with continuous ambulatory peritoneal dialysis is unconscious when admitted to the ED. His blood pressure is 190/100 mmHg; serum potassium level, 7.8 mEq/L; serum BUN level, 200 mg/dL, and serum creatinine level, 10 mg/dL. Available medical records indicate that 2 years ago he had been receiving 28 units of NPH insulin daily. The nurse anticipates that the patient's hyperkalemia will be treated with:

A. Ion-exchange resin
B. Sodium bicarbonate
C. Calcium chloride
D. All of the above

37. An unconscious 32-year-old male has arrived at the ED. Available medical records indicate that 2 years ago he had been receiving 24 units of NPH insulin daily. Which statement best describes how ESRD has most likely affected the patient's diabetes over the course of 2 years?

A. Insulin requirements have decreased
B. Insulin requirements have increased
C. Hyperglycemic episodes have occurred more frequently
D. Symptoms of diabetic neuropathy have increased

38. An end-stage renal patient has pulmonary edema, and peritoneal dialysis is required. In preparing for the setup of dialysis for the patient, which clinical procedure would the novice nurse be expect to perform?

A. Call the nephrologist
B. Insert PD catheter
C. Setup of the PD machine
D. A rapid flush of the PD ports.

39. When administering PD dialysate solution, the nurse should assess for signs of:

A. Hypervolemia
B. Hyperkalemia
C. Hypercalcemia
D. Hyperglycemia

40. During peritoneal dialysis, the dialysate solution has difficulty draining from the abdomen. An appropriate nursing intervention to facilitate drainage would be to:

A. Aspirate drainage from the catheter using a syringe
B. Flush the catheter with a heparinized syringe
C. Instill another liter of dialysate
D. Reposition the patient from side to side

41. A 52-year-old diabetic man with a 1-year history of chronic renal failure that is treated with continuous ambulatory peritoneal dialysis and he is unconscious when admitted to the ED. Available medical records indicate that 2 years ago he had been receiving 28 units of NPH insulin daily. The nurse should also assess this patient for developing:

A. Coagulopathies
B. Heart block
C. Hypercalcemia
D. Metabolic alkalosis

42. A 58-year-old man arrives at the ED, diaphoretic and complaining of severe pain in the right side. He informs the nurse that he had been walking his dog when he suddenly felt a horrible pain. Assessment findings reveal that his blood pressure is 160/70 mmHg, pulse 124 beats/minute and regular, temperature 98.6°F (37°C), and respiratory rate 24 breaths/minute. His abdomen, when palpated, reveals tenderness in the right flank. Urinalysis indicates RBCs in the urine. The patient has a history of hypertension and no known allergies. The physician diagnoses renal calculi and requests a consultation with the urologist. The nurse would expect the history of a patient with renal calculi to reveal a previous diagnosis of:

A. Prostatic hypertrophy
B. Hypothyroidism
C. Hyperparathyroidism
D. Chronic renal failure

43. Which question typically elicits the most valuable information from a patient complaining of flank pain?

A. "When did the pain start?"
B. "Is the pain steady or does it increase and decrease in severity?"
C. "What helps to relieve your pain?"
D. "Does the pain radiate anywhere?"

44. Which action should be the nurse's priority when treating a patient with renal colic?

A. Straining the patient's urine
B. Encouraging the patient to drink fluids
C. Monitoring the patient's fluid intake and output
D. Relieving the patient's pain

45. Which procedure would the nurse most likely expect to see used to confirm a diagnosis of renal calculi?

A. CT scan with contrast
B. Non-contrast spiral CT
C. KUB
D. Abdominal ultrasonography

46. If a kidney were partially obstructed by a calculus, the nurse would expect the patient's urine output to:

A. Increase
B. Decrease
C. Remain the same
D. Stop completely

47. Which medication should be avoided if renal calculi are suspected?

A. Atropine sulfate
B. Furosemide
C. Antacids
D. Antibiotics

48. Which assessment data are characteristic of UTI?

A. Dysuria, fever, many bacteria in the urine, and urinary frequency
B. Dysuria, low WBC count, and acetone in the urine
C. Dysuria, many platelets, and glucose in the urine
D. Dysuria, acetone, and protein in the urine

49. Which information about a UTI should the nurse include in the discharge teaching for a patient:

A. UTI is not a serious illness; therefore, the patient does not need to be anxious
B. The patient must take the full course of antibiotic therapy ordered
C. The patient should avoid sexual intercourse for the next 6 weeks to avoid contaminating her partner
D. Now that the patient has a history of UTI, she should have a routine urinalysis every 3 months

50. Which diagnostic study would be necessary if a patient had hematuria?

A. A count of RBCs in the urine
B. A count of RBC casts in the urine
C. A count of leukocytes in the urine
D. A Gram stain of the urine

51. A 26-year-old woman arrives at the ED complaining of dysuria, fever of 101°F (38.3°C), and urinary frequency. She has had these symptoms for 36 hours. Physical examination reveals suprapubic tenderness but no flank pain. No history of UTI or urologic instrumentation is evident. She informs the nurse that she had sexual intercourse 12 hours before the onset of symptoms. She has no significant medical history and takes no medications. Her complete blood count, serum electrolyte, BUN, and glucose levels are normal. A tentative diagnosis of UTI is made, and urine specimens for analysis and culture are sent to the laboratory. When taking the health history, the nurse should remember to ask the patient about:

A. Previous surgeries or instrumentation of the genitourinary tract
B. A previous diagnosis of hypoparathyroidism
C. A history of sexually transmitted disease
D. Which birth control methods the patient uses

52. Which organism is the most common cause of UTI?

A. Staphylococcus saprophyticus
B. Klebsiella species
C. Proteus species
D. Escherichia coli

53. Which nursing action is most appropriate in the treatment of UTI?

A. Avoiding catheterizing the patient to obtain a urine specimen so that the infection does not spread
B. Requesting an order for phenazopyridine hydrochloride (Pyridium) if the patient complains of bladder discomfort
C. Encouraging the patient to drink coffee or tea to aid in diuresis
D. Telling the patient that cranberry juice should be avoided because it is a bladder irritant.

54. A 35-year-old man arrives at the ED with pain in the right flank that began 2 hours ago, spontaneously abated, and then suddenly recurred. The pain is severe, sharp, and radiates to the groin. Physical examination reveals tenderness in the right costovertebral angle. The patient's pulse rate is 110 beats/minute, blood pressure 150/94 mmHg, temperature 100°F (37.8°C), and respiratory rate 24 breaths/minute. Laboratory results indicate a WBC count of 10,000/mm^3, normal hemoglobin and hematocrit levels, and normal serum electrolyte, BUN, and glucose levels. Urinalysis reveals an RBC count greater than 100 cells via high-powered field. An indwelling urinary catheter is inserted, and 800 mL of urine is obtained. The patient is sent for an emergency IVP. The nurse knows that management of a patient with obstructive uropathy is directed primarily toward:

A. Preventing acute renal failure (ARF)
B. Correcting acidosis
C. Decompressing the urinary tract above the level of obstruction
D. Decompressing the urinary bladder to relieve pressure on the obstructed area

55. Which urinalysis finding is consistent with obstructive uropathy?

A. Normal urinalysis
B. Proteinuria of 3.5 g/day
C. Acetone 2+
D. Glycosuria 2%

56. The nurse notes that no urine has drained from a patient's catheter for 2 hours. Which is the most appropriate nursing action to take?

A. Change the patient's position
B. Check the catheter for patency
C. Reinsert a new catheter
D. Assume that the obstruction has worsened and call the physician

57. The IVP reveals 100% obstruction of the right ureter with severe hydronephrosis in the right kidney. The physician determines the need for percutaneous nephrostomy. Which is the most appropriate explanation the nurse can offer the patient about this procedure:

A. The nephrostomy will cure the patient's uropathy
B. Urine will temporarily drain through a tube in the patient's side
C. The procedure is necessary to prevent bilateral renal failure
D. All of the above

58. The physician determines the need for a percutaneous nephrostomy. The initial goal in caring for this patient would be to:

A. Relieve the patient's pain
B. Reduce the patient's blood pressure
C. Prevent cardiac arrhythmias
D. Maintain normal fluid and electrolyte balance

59. The physician determines the need for percutaneous nephrostomy. Which test will provide the health care team with the most valuable diagnostic information in this situation?

A. Abdominal X-ray
B. Renal ultrasonography
C. Renal arteriography
D. IVP

60. Which nursing diagnosis would be appropriate for a patient who has undergone percutaneous nephrostomy:

A. Potential fluid volume deficit related to the creation of an additional source of urine flow
B. Potential for infection related to altered skin integrity
C. Potential for injury related to metabolic acidosis
D. Fluid volume excess related to decreased renal perfusion

61. The nurse knows that prerenal azotemia results from all of the following except:

A. Shifting of fluid volume from the intravascular space to the interstitial space
B. Hemorrhage
C. Lodging of calcium oxalate calculi in a ureter
D. Hypotension

62. If a patient with acute renal failure (ARF) exhibits a pericardial friction rub, the nurse should immediately:

A. Notify the physician because the patient requires hemodialysis
B. Assess for pulsus paradoxus
C. Administer oxygen
D. Request an order for furosemide

63. A 56-year-old man is admitted to the ED because of shortness of breath. He has a history of congestive heart failure, myocardial infarction, and hypertension. Assessment findings reveal the following: blood pressure 220/110 mmHg, pulse rate 100 beats/minute-full and bounding, and respiration rate 34 breaths/minute, deep, fast, and labored. Auscultation reveals pericardial friction rub and crackles in both lung bases. EKG monitoring reveals normal sinus rhythm with tall, tented T waves. The nurse notes that the patient has distended jugular veins and edema of the hands, feet, periorbital areas, and sacrum. Indwelling urinary catheterization yields 20 mL of dark amber urine. Arterial blood gas studies show PH 7.25, PO_2 60 mmHg, PCO_2 36 mmHg, and HCO_3^- 14 mEq/L. Laboratory results reveal a serum BUN level of 50 mg/dL and a serum creatinine level of 5.5 mg/dL. The physician diagnoses acute renal failure (ARF). The physician determines that hemodialysis is necessary for this patient. The nurse should explain to the patient that:

A. Because his kidneys no longer function, he is now in acute renal failure (ARF) and will need dialysis for the rest of his life
B. His kidneys do not function, but dialysis will repair them
C. His breathing will be easier once hemodialysis removes fluid and toxins that his kidneys cannot
D. Hemodialysis will not remove all toxins

64. The tall, tented T waves noted on a patient's EKG are indicative of:

A. Hypercalcemia
B. Hypochloremia
C. Hypophosphatemia
D. Hyperkalemia

65. A 24-year-old man who was involved in a head-on automobile accident is brought to the ED. Paramedics report that the dashboard and steering wheel were pinned against the patient's abdomen and legs for 1 hour before rescue workers were able to release him. The patient is conscious and in severe abdominal and pelvic pain. His vital signs are stable: blood pressure, 120/70 mmHg, pulse rate 86 beats/minute, and respiratory rate 22 breaths/minute. The nurse notes that the patient's penis and testes are swollen and painful and that blood is oozing from his urethra. The physician diagnoses a pelvic fracture with genitourinary trauma, and then calls the urologist. Which history finding would lead the nurse to suspect that the patient has a ruptured bladder?

A. The bladder was full when injury occurred
B. The patient is male
C. The patient suffered a straddle-type injury
D. The patient received injuries to the lower chest

66. A patient with a ruptured bladder should also be assessed for:

A. Ruptured spleen
B. Pancreatitis
C. Rectal injury
D. Spinal cord injury

67. The nurse would expect a patient with a ruptured bladder to exhibit which signs and symptoms:

A. Pyuria, fever, and distended bladder
B. Hematuria and fever
C. Pyuria and severe pelvic pain
D. Hematuria, pelvic discomfort, and difficulty voiding

68. Besides providing pain relief, which nursing action should be included in the plan of care for a patient who has sustained testicular trauma?

A. Application of ice packs and testicular elevation
B. Application of heat packs and testicular elevation
C. Application of heat packs and leaving the testes in their natural position to avoid further trauma
D. Application of ice packs and leaving the testes in their natural position to avoid further trauma

69. Which symptom is present when the urethra is completely transected?

A. Hematuria
B. Abdominal distention from urine extravasation
C. Urethral bleeding
D. Severe colicky pain

70. A 29-year-old woman is admitted to the ED with suspected pelvic inflammatory disease (PID). She is complaining of bilateral lower abdominal pain and a slight, whitish-yellow, odorless vaginal discharge. Her blood pressure is 100/70 mmHg, pulse rate 96 beats/minute, respiratory rate 24 breaths/minute, and temperature 100.6°F (38.1°C). The patient informs the nurse that she has had the discharge for 3 days and that the lower abdominal pain began 2 days ago and has become increasingly worse. Her fever has persisted since yesterday. She also mentions that she has an intrauterine device (IUD) in place. The physician orders a complete blood count, blood culture, and cervical culture as well as a urinalysis and ultrasound studies. Which organism causes PID?

A. Neisseria gonorrhoeae
B. Mycobacterium tuberculosis
C. Chlamydia trachomatis
D. All of the above

71. The nurse knows that the signs and symptoms of PID may be confused with those of:

A. Pregnancy
B. Gallbladder disease
C. Acute pancreatitis
D. Appendicitis

72. Which condition is a potential complication of PID?

A. Peritonitis
B. Ectopic pregnancy
C. Infertility
D. All of the above

73. Which history finding places a patient at increased risk for PID?

A. Abnormal menstrual cycles
B. Stress
C. IUD use
D. Continued use of antibiotics

74. Which statement indicates that a patient with PID who has been placed on continuing antibiotic therapy understands discharge instructions?

A. "I need to be on bed rest while taking the antibiotics"
B. "I need to take all of the medication"
C. "I can stop the medication when the discharge disappears"
D. "My partner does not need to be treated"

75. Discharge planning for a patient with PID should include:

A. Genetic counseling for future pregnancies
B. Education and treatment of sexual contacts
C. Education for stress reduction
D. Follow-up ultrasound studies every 6 months

76. A 27-year-old woman is admitted to the ED after losing consciousness at home. Now fully alert, she complains of achiness, nausea, vomiting, and fever, which began yesterday morning. The patient has no medical or gynecologic history. She is 3 days into her menstrual period. She informs the nurse that she uses super-absorbent tampons and, occasionally, contraceptive sponges. The patient's vital signs are blood pressure 86/48 mmHg, temperature 103°F (39.4°C), pulse rate 124 beats/minute, and respiratory rate 28 breaths/minute. Based on the above symptoms, the nurse would suspect that the patient has:

A. Ectopic pregnancy
B. Vaginitis
C. Toxic shock syndrome
D. Ovarian cyst

77. A 27-year-old woman is admitted to the ED after losing consciousness at home. Now fully alert, she complains of achiness, nausea, vomiting, and fever, which began yesterday morning. The patient has no medical or gynecologic history. She is 3 days into her menstrual period. She informs the nurse that she uses super-absorbent tampons and, occasionally, contraceptive sponges. The patient's vital signs are blood pressure 86/48 mmHg, temperature 103°F (39.4°C), pulse rate 124 beats/minute, and respiratory rate 28 breaths/minute. What additional symptoms would the nurse assess for in this patient:

A. Cutaneous petechiae over the trunk
B. Diffuse macular erythroderma
C. Mucous membrane lesions
D. Vesicular rash over the palms and soles

78. The nurse would suspect that the bacteria that causes toxic shock syndrome is caused by:

A. Staphylococcus aureus
B. Chlamydia trachomatis
C. Escherichia coli
D. Treponema pallidum

79. Which factors place a patient at high risk for toxic shock syndrome?

A. Poor personal hygiene, deodorant tampon use, and IUD use
B. Prolonged use of super-absorbent tampons, contraceptive sponges, or a diaphragm
C. Prolonged use of tampons and frequent use of commercial douche preparations
D. Prolonged oral antibiotic therapy and alternating use of tampons and vaginal pads during menses

80. A 27-year-old woman is admitted to the ED after losing consciousness at home. Now fully alert, she complains of achiness, nausea, vomiting, and fever, which began yesterday morning. The patient has no medical or gynecologic history. She is 3 days into her menstrual period. She informs the nurse that she uses super-absorbent tampons and, occasionally, contraceptive sponges. The patient's vital signs are blood pressure 86/48 mmHg, temperature 103°F (39.4°C), pulse rate 124 beats/minute, and respiratory rate 28 breaths/minute. An appropriate nursing diagnosis for this patient would be:

A. Decreased cardiac output related to vasodilation and decreased myocardial contractility
B. Potential for infection related to fever and achiness
C. Fluid volume deficit related to vaginal hemorrhage and fever
D. Potential for injury related to seizures

81. Which nursing interventions would be the main priority in managing toxic shock syndrome?

A. Rapidly infuse IV fluid, as ordered, and closely monitor the patient's vital signs and urine output
B. Administer antipyretic medications, as ordered, and administer tepid sponge bath to reduce fever
C. Draw blood for cultures, as ordered, and monitor the patient's vital signs
D. Prepare for a spinal tap and monitor the patient's temperature

82. The nurse should observe the patient for which condition associated with untreated toxic shock syndrome:

A. Adult respiratory distress syndrome
B. Disseminated intravascular coagulation
C. Severe metabolic acidosis
D. All of the above

83. A 21-year-old woman is admitted to the ED, complaining of a vaginal discharge and painful, frequent urination. An enzyme-linked immunosorbent assay of vaginal discharge reveals gonorrhea. The nurse knows that anyone infected with gonorrhea also should be tested for:

A. Chlamydia
B. Human immunodeficiency virus (HIV)
C. Syphilis
D. Herpes

84. Which question asked during the nursing history should elicit important information about the sexually transmitted infections and possible treatment?

A. "When did you become sexually active?"
B. "Which birth control method do you use?"
C. "What kind of sexual practices do you engage in?"
D. "Have you ever had a sexually transmitted disease?"

85. The nurse explains that recurrence of sexually transmitted diseases places the patient at increased risk for all of the following conditions except:

A. Ectopic pregnancy
B. Renal disease
C. HIV
D. PID

86. The nurse initiates a discussion about sexually transmitted diseases and the use of contraceptives. The patient's decision to use which contraceptive method indicates the need for further teaching:

A. Oral contraceptives
B. Diaphragm
C. Condoms
D. Contraceptive sponges

87. In a patient diagnosed with a UTI, the nurse practitioner writes prescriptions for Bactrim and Pyridium. Which statement best reflects that the patient needs further discharge instructions?

A. "I will take and finish all medications as prescribed"
B. "I should use a form or barrier birth control while on antibiotics."
C. "I should return to the ER if I notice a change in the color of my urine."
D. "I should be drinking enough fluids to urinate at least every 2 to 3 hours."

88. The receiving nurse knows that the most important message to convey initially to any victim of sexual assault is that:

A. All medical tests will be handled confidentially
B. The examination will be done quickly
C. The patient is now in a safe, secure environment
D. Medications are available to prevent pregnancy

89. A 20-year-old woman walks into the ED and states, "I was raped." Her clothes are torn and her face is severely bruised. Trembling and withdrawn, she avoids eye contact with immediate personnel and is escorted by the nurse to a private room. When obtaining the nursing history, the nurse should determine whether the patient has done which activity since the assault:

A. Urinated or defecated
B. Changed clothes
C. Rinsed her mouth
D. All of the above

90. Which nursing action would be most appropriate when collecting a raped patient's clothing?

A. Have the victim place all of her clothing together in a plastic bag
B. Have the victim fold each piece of clothing inward and place each article in a separate paper bag
C. Shake each piece of clothing separately, then place all articles together in a paper bag
D. Not collect the clothing of the victim who had been totally undressed before the assault.

91. A patient who has been raped should be instructed to return to her physician for a repeat serologic test for syphilis (Venereal Disease Research Laboratory test) within how many weeks:

A. 1 to 2
B. 3 to 4
C. 5 to 6
D. 7 to 8

92. A 20-year-old woman walks into the ED and states, "I was raped." Her clothes are torn and her face is severely bruised. Trembling and withdrawn, she avoids eye contact with immediate personnel and is escorted by the nurse to a private room. Upon discharge, the nurse should provide the patient with:

A. Written discharge instructions
B. Suitable clothing, if the clothing has been retained for evidence
C. A list of referral telephone numbers
D. All of the above

93. Your patient has been given the diagnosis of anemia due to dysfunctional uterine bleeding. Which of the following would not be a good source of iron for her diet?

White fish
Spinach
Chicken
Baked potato

94. Which of the following laboratory tests would best indicate the patient may have renal insufficiency?

A. Elevated creatinine
B. Elevated alkaline phosphatase
C. Decreased chloride
D. Decreased calcium

95. Which of the following would not be commonly seen in a patient suffering from kidney stones?

A. Diaphoresis
B. Fever
C. Hematuria
D. Abdominal, flank or pelvic pain

96. Which of the following is not seen in a patient with prostatitis?

A. Lower back pain
B. Dysuria or urinary frequency
C. Fever
D. Incontinence

97. In caring for a patient with an indwelling urinary catheter, strategies to reduce the risk of infection would include all except:

A. Performing regular bladder irrigation
B. Using a closed drainage system
C. Using proper aseptic technique when inserting or caring for catheter
D. Gently clean around the urinary meatus daily

98. A critically high potassium value was just received on a patient with end state renal failure. Of the following medications, which would be most useful to temporarily decrease the potassium level?

A. Furosemide
B. Sodium polystyrene sulfonate
C. Hydrochlorothiazide
D. Amiodarone

99. Your patient, with known acute renal failure, has a potassium level of 6.0 mEq/dl. What EKG findings would commonly be seen with hyperkalemia?

A. Peaked T-waves
B. New-onset Q-waves
C. Bradycardia
D. Bundle branch block

100. A female patient is in the (emergency department) ED with a fever and toxic shock syndrome due to Staphylococcus aureus. What is the most common cause of this condition?

A. Aspirin use
B. Tampon use
C. Vibratory tool use
D. Cocaine use

GENITOURINARY & GYNECOLOGIC: RATIONALE

1. **C** The most appropriate nursing action in this situation would be to cut the zipper around the injury, allowing the zipper tracks to separate. No further tissue trauma should ensue. Another effective method would be to delicately unzip the zipper, using petrolatum as a lubricant. Local anesthetics should be avoided because edema will result. Cutting the skin or performing a circumcision may cause extensive scarring or may damage the urethra if the patient has epispadias (a condition in which the urethra is located at the top of the glans) or hypospadias (a condition in which the urethra is located at the bottom of the glans).

2. **D** A patient with urethral trauma should be instructed not to void because urine may extravasate into the peritoneum, causing pain and inflammation. Urethral injuries, which are more common in men, are associated with straddle-type injuries. This type of trauma can be diagnosed by kidney-ureter-bladder (KUB) or retrograde urethrography. Bladder injuries commonly occur when the bladder is full.

3. **C** A suprapubic catheter may be inserted to divert urine in a patient with urethral trauma. The nurse should never catheterize a patient with this type of injury. The physician should request an emergency consultation with the urologist, who will insert either an indwelling urinary or a suprapubic catheter based on his own assessment. Urethral trauma is associated with localized dull or sharp acute pain in the suprapubic or perineal area. A patient with urethral trauma typically cannot void, although he may have the desire to do so, because sphincter damage may have occurred.

4. **C** A hard scrotal mass that does not transilluminate most likely indicates a testicular tumor. In transillumination, a light beam is shone through the scrotum, resulting in a red glow emanating through the skin. This glow is not present in masses resulting from blood or tissue. Therefore, a mass filled with fluid, as in hydrocele or spermatocele, will transilluminate. Epididymitis does not produce a mass, although the scrotum is edematous.

5. **D** Intravenous pyelography (IVP) is contraindicated in acute renal failure (ARF) because the contrast media has an osmotic and nephrotoxic effect and can further compromise renal function. Contrast medium has a high osmolarity, which may cause further fluid overload in a patient with acute renal failure. A patient with iodine sensitivity may have an allergic reaction but may be premedicated with steroids or antihistamines to counteract it. IVP may help diagnose acute renal failure from obstructive causes.

6. **B** A urine sodium level of 15 mEq/L helps the nurse to differentiate decreased renal perfusion from acute tubular necrosis (ATN). In decreased renal perfusion, the kidneys reabsorb sodium and water in an effort to increase intravascular volume. This is reflected in a urine sodium level below 20 mEq/L. The urine is concentrated, resulting in a urine specific gravity above 1.010. The serum creatinine level is typically normal. In ATN, the damaged kidney loses its ability to reabsorb sodium, as reflected by a urine sodium level greater than 40 mEq/L. The urine is typically plasma like, with a specific gravity of about 1.010. The serum creatinine level is typically elevated above 2 mg/dL. A low urine output, such as 350 mL/24 hours, is characteristic of both decreased renal perfusion and the early phase of ATN.

7. **D** Anuria, the inability to void, is a common symptom of urethral injury, bladder injury, and postrenal acute renal failure (ARF). Sphincter damage may have occurred from trauma to the urethra, resulting in urine retention. Extravasation of urine in the peritoneum typically occurs in bladder rupture and results in anuria. Urine outflow is obstructed in postrenal ARF, resulting in the patient's inability to void.

8. **A** Ureteral trauma is best treated by surgical repair. In this type of injury, disruption of the structural integrity of the ureters occurs, usually because of penetrating abdominal trauma. Surgical anastomosis is required. Indwelling urinary and suprapubic catheterization are of no value because the urine cannot reach the bladder; hence, urine cannot be measured.

9. **C** Penile fracture, which is commonly associated with straddle-type injuries or violent sexual intercourse, usually is treated by splinting and the application of ice packs. Surgical evacuation of a hematoma may be required if extravasation occurs. An indwelling urinary or suprapubic catheter may be inserted to divert urine if edema occurs; however, catheterization does not aid in treating the fracture. Casting is inappropriate in this situation.

10. **D** Hematuria, whether frank or microscopic, is a common, nonspecific sign of genitourinary trauma. However, it does not necessarily occur in all cases. Menstruation, anticoagulant overdose, and bleeding disorders must be ruled out before the bleeding can be attributed to genitourinary trauma. Flank pain may be indicative of renal hemorrhage or urinary calculi. Hypotension is not a sign of renal trauma except when massive hemorrhage occurs. Urine retention is common in bladder rupture and urethral trauma.

11. **A** Epididymitis and testicular torsion are commonly mistaken for one another. Similar signs and symptoms include unilateral testicular pain, swelling, and fever. Differentiation occurs upon elevation of the scrotum, which relieves the pain of epididymitis but increases the pain of testicular torsion.

12. **B** Hematuria and flank tenderness indicate renal trauma. Microscopic hematuria is associated with minor contusions, whereas gross blood in the urine is consistent with major renal damage. Flank pain may reflect hemorrhage or extravasation of urine. Colicky pain is associated with obstruction rather than trauma. Urethral bleeding is a manifestation of urethral trauma. Urine output does not initially change because of trauma but may become oliguric, if acute renal failure develops, or anuric, if complete obstruction occurs.

13. **A** Contusion of the kidney, disruption of the fornix, and lacerations that do not extend beyond the renal cortex are considered minor renal injuries. These typically resolve without surgical intervention. Deep cortical lacerations and injuries involving the renal pedicle or renal pelvis are considered life threatening and require surgery. Disruption of a major renal artery causes massive bleeding and also warrants surgery.

14. **C** When trauma causes rupture of the renal vasculature, bleeding into the retroperitoneal space occurs. The amount of bleeding depends on the degree of injury. This condition may be so severe that the patient succumbs to shock, resulting from hemorrhage. Pulled muscles and a fractured ilium do not directly result in ecchymoses.

15. **D** Renal contusions are minor injuries and require no immediate treatment other than observation for worsening of the injury.

16. **D** The nurse's main priority in this situation would be to measure the patient's blood pressure. If the patient is hypotensive, bleeding should be suspected. Expansion of a hematoma in the kidney may cause increased pain or tenderness. The nurse may administer narcotics, as ordered, to control pain; however, this is not the primary intervention for bleeding. In some instances, narcotics are withheld to avoid masking symptoms, such as increased pain. Although monitoring the patient's serum hematocrit level is important, the initial action should be to assess vital signs. Monitoring serum electrolyte, blood urea nitrogen (BUN), and glucose levels is of no value in this situation.

17. **C** Renal trauma should be suspected in any patient with a hematoma in the flank area. Other signs and symptoms of renal trauma include frank or microscopic hematuria, flank pain that increases with movement and possibly radiates to the groin, and abdominal rigidity. Hypotension and hypovolemic shock may result if significant blood loss occurs. Swelling or a mass in the flank area may be noted on palpation. Chvostek's sign, facial twitching that is elicited by tapping the facial nerve, indicates hypocalcemia. Oliguria is a common finding in acute prerenal and intrarenal failure. Dysuria, or painful urination, is a sign of urinary tract infection (UTI) and renal calculi.

18. **D** Kidney trauma should be suspected in any patient with chest trauma, a fractured pelvis, or a deceleration injury. Chest trauma can cause kidney injuries, especially if the lower ribs have been fractured. Deceleration injuries, such as those caused by motor vehicle accidents and contact sports, are the most common cause of renal trauma. Although most kidney injuries are from blunt trauma, penetrating trauma, such as gunshot or stab wounds, may also result in renal trauma.

19. **B** An abdominal computed tomography scan confirms renal trauma most conclusively because of its high accuracy, ease of performance, and ability to visualize all renal structures. KUB urethrography also may help determine renal injury; it is especially valuable in demonstrating the size, shape, and location of renal anatomy. IVP also may help to diagnose renal trauma that results in hematomas or lacerations; however, before this test, the patient should be checked for any allergy to contrast media or iodine. Hydrocortisone (Solu-Cortef) and diphenhydramine hydrochloride (Benadryl) should be available if the allergy history is unknown. Peritoneal tap is indicated if bowel trauma is suspected.

20. **A** The patient has signs and symptoms consistent with postrenal acute renal failure (ARF). Postrenal ARF occurs when urine flow becomes completely obstructed, most commonly from renal calculi, prostatic hypertrophy, or tumors of the bladder, pelvis, or prostate gland. Serum BUN and creatinine levels rise because metabolic waste products cannot be eliminated from the body. A patient with congestive heart failure typically has oliguria, not anuria. A patient with pyelonephritis has signs of infection and urine frequency. The fact that the patient has no history of renal dysfunction rules out chronic renal failure.

21. **C** The hallmark symptom of postrenal acute renal failure (ARF) is anuria, the absence of urine output. Prerenal and intrarenal ARF are characterized by oliguria, a urine output of less than 400 mL/day. Polyuria typically develops later in intrarenal ARF. Other signs and symptoms of postrenal ARF— edema, shortness of breath, nausea, vomiting, and confusion— result from hypervolemia and uremia.

22. **A** The nurse practitioner will probably order KUB urethrography to help diagnose the patient's condition. This procedure should demonstrate enlargement of the structures distended with urine from the obstruction. Ultrasonography also may be used to diagnose postrenal obstruction.

23. **B** In this situation, the nurse would formulate a diagnosis of fluid volume deficit related to restoration of urine flow. After the restoration of urine flow, the patient with postrenal acute renal failure (ARF) is at risk for fluid volume deficit because the urine is characteristically dilute and rich in electrolytes. More fluid is drawn in the urine, therapy diluting the high osmolarity of electrolytes. The other nursing diagnoses would be appropriate before the urine flow is reestablished. Acute renal failure from postrenal obstruction causes a fluid volume overload, potassium excess, and metabolic acidosis. This occurs because of the inability to rid the body of urine, which results in a rise in electrolyte levels and metabolic waste products.

24. **B** After the drainage of 2,500 mL of urine, the most important intervention would be to request an order for fluid replacement to restore fluid balance. Once the obstruction is removed, diuresis of dilute urine high in electrolytes results. If fluids are not replaced, dehydration and electrolyte imbalance may occur. The indwelling urinary catheter should be clamped after 800 mL of fluid drains. Emergency surgical consultation is not indicated because the obstruction has been temporarily relieved. Because the urine is already dilute, diuretics are not indicated.

25. **D** The nurse would expect to administer dextrose 5% in 0.45% saline solution and potassium chloride at 160 mL/hour. The most appropriate solution for fluid replacement is dextrose 5% in 0.45% saline solution. Sodium and potassium must be

replaced as per serum test results. A 0.45% saline solution is hypotonic and is used to replace intracellular volume. Standard fluid replacement calls for replacing two-thirds of lost urine over 24 hours, plus another 30 mL/hour for insensible water loss.

26. **D** This patient has the signs and symptoms of ATN (acute tubular necrosis), a form of ARF (acute renal failure) resulting from drug-induced nephrotoxicity. When intrarenal damage occurs, the kidneys can no longer reabsorb sodium and concentrate urine. The urine sodium level is characteristically above 40 mEq/L, and urine specific gravity is plasma like 0.01. Casts, or cellular debris, appear in the urine because the renal tubules have been damaged. BUN and creatinine levels rise as metabolic wastes accumulate, producing the symptoms of nausea, vomiting, and malaise. A recurrent UTI would produce more signs and symptoms of infection, such as fever and white blood cells in the urine. If the patient had been dehydrated only, the serum creatinine level would be normal. An allergic drug reaction typically occurs earlier in antibiotic therapy.

27. **A** The serum creatinine level is the most accurate indicator of a patient's renal function. Creatinine, the end product of muscle metabolism, is produced at a constant rate and excreted by the kidneys at a constant rate with no reabsorption. The normal serum creatinine level is 1 to 2 mg/dL. BUN, the end product of protein metabolism, is a less accurate indicator than serum creatinine, because BUN is not produced at a constant rate and is excreted as well as reabsorbed. BUN levels are typically elevated in those who consume high-protein diets and in those are dehydrated or have blood in the GI tract. The normal serum BUN level is 10 to 20 mg/dL. Urine sodium levels provide information about the kidney's ability to reabsorb

sodium. Urine specific gravity provides information about the kidney's ability to concentrate urine.

28. **A** Creatinine clearance is an indirect measurement of the patient's glomerular filtration rate (GFR). GFR, the amount of water filtered out of the plasma through the glomerular capillary walls per minute, cannot be measured directly but only inferred from the creatine clearance because creatinine is produced and excreted at a constant rate. The creatinine clearance test involves the collection of a 24-hour urine specimen and a serum creatinine specimen. Normal GFR (and creatinine clearance) is 125 mL/minute.

29. **B** The nurse would expect this patient's treatment to include fluid restriction to correct the hypervolemia and oliguria caused by impaired kidney function. Penicillin and aminoglycosides produce nephrotoxic effects and would not be indicated because the patient does not have signs of infection. Furosemide administration and electrolyte replacement are indicated in prerenal conditions; in this situation, such therapy could compound the patient's nephrotoxicity. Also, the patient is probably retaining electrolytes and would not require their replacement at this time.

30. **C** A patient with ATN should also be monitored for hyperkalemia because of decreased renal excretion. Hyperkalemia occurs when the serum potassium level rises above 5 mEq/L. It may be represented by tall T waves and cardiac arrhythmias on electrocardiogram. Symptoms of hyperkalemia include nausea, vomiting, and weakness. Other common electrolyte abnormalities associated with ATN include hyponatremia, which results from the kidney's inability to reabsorb sodium, and hypocalcaemia and hyperphosphatemia (after 1 week) from decreased vitamin D utilization. Metabolic

acidosis occurs because of the inability to excrete hydrogen ions.

31. **C** A creatinine clearance of 125 mL/min is a normal finding and indicates that interventions have been successful in restoring normal kidney function. The other findings (elevated serum BUN and creatinine levels and a high urine sodium level) are still indicative of acute renal failure and the kidney's inability to reabsorb sodium.

32. **D** This patient's signs and symptoms suggest testicular torsion, or twisting of the spermatic cord. If untreated for more than 4 hours, testicular ischemia may result. The pain is severe and increases upon elevation of the testes. Acute epididymitis, infection of the male reproductive system, can be confused with testicular torsion; however, elevating the scrotum relieves pain from epididymitis. Testicular tumor would be suspected if palpation reveals a hard, testicular mass; pain may or may not be present. Priapism, an involuntary, painful erection, is not associated with testicular torsion.

33. **A** Testicular torsion is most common in children and adolescents, but it also may occur in young adults. It may be caused by a congenital abnormality of the spermatic cord.

34. **B** Treatment of testicular torsion includes the application of ice packs to reduce edema and manual manipulation by a urologist to reduce the torsion. Surgery may be necessary if manipulation is unsuccessful. Antibiotic therapy is indicated for epididymitis. Testicular tumor requires orchiectomy. Analgesia, not sedation, is part of the therapy for testicular torsion.

35. **B** End-stage renal disease (ESRD) develops when 90% of the nephrons are destroyed. Functional nephrons hypertrophy to

maintain integrity of the renal system. The serum creatinine level is about 10 mg/dL when ESRD occurs. Inability to concentrate urine occurs during the recovery phase of acute tubular necrosis. Impaired sodium reabsorption occurs throughout all phases of acute and chronic renal failure.

36. **D** Hyperkalemia can be treated with the administration of ion-exchange resins, sodium bicarbonate, calcium chloride, and insulin and dextrose 50% solution. Ion-exchange resins, such as sodium polystyrene sulfonate (Kayexalate), exchange sodium for potassium ions in the intestine. Sodium bicarbonate temporarily shifts potassium back into the cells by creating alkalosis. Although calcium chloride and calcium gluconate do not decrease the serum potassium level, these agents protect the heart from the adverse effects of hyperkalemia and enhance contraction. Insulin and dextrose 50% solution also decrease the serum potassium level by temporarily shifting potassium into the cell. Potassium enters the cell along with glucose; insulin helps glucose enter the cell.

37. **A** This patient's insulin requirements most likely have decreased over the past 2 years; during the last year of ESRD, before dialysis is instituted, insulin requirements typically decrease by 40% to 50%. Peripheral tissues become resistant to insulin, resulting in an increased half-life. Institution of dialysis typically improves the use and excretion of insulin, thereby decreasing its half-life. As renal failure progresses, the catabolism of exogenous and endogenous insulin decreases, resulting in more frequent hypoglycemic, not hyperglycemic, episodes. Diabetic neuropathy is unaffected by ESRD.

38. **D** A rapid flush is an expected procedure for the nurse to perform. The nurse would not insert a PD catheter. The setup of the machine is likely outside of the competence of the novice

nurse (or experienced nurse). Calling the nephrologist is not a procedure.

39. **D** When administering the 4.25% dialysate solution, the nurse should assess for signs of hyperglycemia because of the solution's high glucose concentration. Careful monitoring is especially necessary in diabetic patients. If the glucose draws too much fluid, hypovolemia may occur. Dialysis may help correct hyperkalemia. A slight decrease in calcium levels may result from peritoneal dialysis because protein and calcium are drawn off.

40. **D** Repositioning the patient from side to side may facilitate drainage of the dialysate from the abdomen. Disconnecting the catheter to aspirate drainage and flushing the catheter with a heparinized syringe are contraindicated because of the high risk of contamination and peritonitis. Instilling another liter of dialysate might impair ventilation by pushing on the diaphragm.

41. **A** The nurse should also assess this patient with chronic renal failure for developing coagulopathies because of impaired platelet function and clotting mechanisms resulting from uremia. Capillary membranes become more fragile because of hypocalcemia. Anemia results from decreased erythropoiesis. All these problems place the patient at increased risk for hemorrhage. The patient with chronic renal failure also may have bradycardia and metabolic acidosis.

42. **C** The nurse would expect a patient with renal calculi to have a history of hyperparathyroidism. Hyperparathyroidism is characterized by excess parathyroid hormone (parathormone) in the serum. Excess levels of this hormone pull calcium from the bone into the blood and increase renal tubular reabsorption of calcium. Excess calcium in the urine contributes to calculus

formation. A patient with bone carcinoma is also at risk for renal calculus formation because bone lesions may release calcium into the blood. Prostatic hypertrophy, hypothyroidism, and chronic renal failure are not considered risk factors in the development of renal calculi.

43. **B** The nurse must determine whether the patient's pain is colicky or non colicky. To elicit this information, the nurse should ask whether the pain is steady or whether it increases or decreases in severity. Colicky pain is commonly associated with renal pelvis or ureter problems. Renal colic is characterized by severe, acute pain of a sudden onset. The patient typically experiences crescendo-decrescendo variations in the pain. Acute non-colicky pain is steady; its onset and severity vary from patient to patient. The other questions are helpful in understanding the patient's pain but are not helpful in establishing an association to renal calculi.

44. **D** The priority nursing action would be to relieve the patient's pain. Straining the patient's urine, encouraging fluids, and monitoring fluid intake and output are important measures to include in the care plan for this patient; however, they are not the nurse's highest priority in this situation.

45. **B** The non-contrast spiral CT is currently the best method for diagnosing stones in either the kidneys or the ureters. This test is fast, does not require instruments or foreign chemicals to enter the body, and provides detailed accurate images of even very small stones. If stones are not present, a spiral CT scan can often identify other causes of pain in the kidney area. It is better than X-rays, ultrasound, and IVP (intravenous pyelogram) - the previous standard test for detecting kidney stones. KUB may be able to detect a stone and identify its general location.

Abdominal ultrasonography would only be able to detect renal calculi that are located in the kidneys.

46. **C** When a kidney is partially obstructed, urine output remains virtually the same. Because urine output and urine constituents are unchanged, the diagnosis may be delayed unless other symptoms are present.

47. **A** Atropine sulfate causes urine retention and should be avoided if renal calculi are suspected. The patient with renal calculi probably is dehydrated from vomiting, fever, and diaphoresis. IV fluids are necessary to rehydrate the patient and to aid in the passage of calculi. Atropine would interfere with this process. Furosemide (Lasix), antacids, and antibiotics are not known to interfere with the passage of renal calculi.

48. **A** Dysuria, fever, many bacteria in the urine, and urinary frequency are characteristic of UTI. Dysuria results from decreased bladder compliance and inflammation of the genitourinary mucosa. Normally, the bladder-stretching reflex is stimulated at 350 to 400 mL, thereby producing the urge to urinate. Inflammation decreases bladder elasticity, producing pain with minimal distention. This decrease in bladder elasticity, along with irritation from inflamed tissues, produces urinary frequency. Fever is the body's normal response to infection. Urinalysis typically reveals many white blood cells (WBCs), which suggests bacteria in the urine, and must be followed up by a culture and sensitivity report.

49. **B** Antibiotic therapy is the only treatment for UTI. The nurse must ensure that the patient understands the significance of the treatment and that she needs to continue the full course of medication even when symptoms are relieved. The nurse should stress that UTI is a serious illness that, if untreated, can ascend

to the kidneys and cause severe complications. The patient should not be released from the ED without this information. The patient should avoid sexual intercourse during the course of antibiotic therapy to avoid reinfection. Routine urinalysis is not indicated.

50. **B** When a patient with suspected UTI has hematuria the physician should order a count of red blood cell (RBC) casts in the urine to help identify the source of bleeding and the appropriate treatment. Normally, no RBC casts are seen in UTI. The presence of casts indicates that the source of bleeding is glomerular. The presence of RBCs that are of normal contour indicates that the source of bleeding is the urinary tract. This differentiation is important, as the treatment plan differs significantly. A count of leukocytes in the urine and a Gram stain of urine would not help to identify the source of the patient's hematuria.

51. **A** History of surgery or instrumentation is associated with the development of UTI. A history of hypoparathyroidism, sexually transmitted disease, or birth control methods has no significance in UTI.

52. **D** Escherichia coli, the most common causative agent of UTI, ascends the urinary tract after being transported to the urethra from the anal area. Although other microbes, such as Staphylococcus saprophyticus and certain Klebsiella and Proteus species may cause UTI, but E. coli is by far the most common.

53. **B** Requesting an order for an antispasmodic agent, such as phenazopyridine hydrochloride, if the patient complains of bladder discomfort is the most appropriate nursing action in this situation. If the patient is menstruating, catheterization may be

necessary to obtain a true urine specimen. Encouraging the patient to drink coffee or tea to aid in diuresis is inappropriate because these substances are bladder irritants and may increase bladder discomfort. The nurse should instruct the patient to increase her fluid intake, especially that of cranberry juice, which helps to acidify the urine and prevent reinfection.

54. **C** Decompressing the urinary tract above the level of the obstruction is essential in a patient with obstructive uropathy, either through percutaneous nephrostomy or cystostomy. This should allow urine to flow out of the kidney, thereby relieving hydronephrosis, which results from obstruction. An obstruction causes urine to flow back up to the kidney, where it stagnates. The degree of damage depends on the duration and completeness of the blockage and on the presence or absence of infection. Treatment aims to drain the genitourinary tract of urine above the level of obstruction to prevent kidney damage. The type of procedure (cystostomy or nephrostomy) also depends on the location of the obstruction. Cystostomy and nephrostomy are temporary measures used to improve the general health of the patient until more definitive procedures, such as surgery, can be performed. A consequence of relieving hydronephrosis is the prevention of acute renal failure (ARF). The situation does not mention whether the patient is acidotic; therefore, correcting acidosis is not applicable. Besides, acidosis would not occur until ARF occurs. Decompressing the bladder would not necessarily relieve pressure on the obstructed area and would be of no value in restoring urine flow.

55. **A** If only one kidney is obstructed, the urinalysis should remain normal because an unobstructed kidney can function normally, releasing urine of normal composition into the bladder. An obstructed kidney, however, cannot release urine. Hematuria may be present because trauma from the obstruction

may cause some bleeding. Sediment is not usually found in the urine. If the urinalysis is normal, the patient should have no protein, acetone, or glucose in the urine.

56. **B** The most appropriate action in this situation would be to check the catheter for patency. Urine flow can stop when the catheter becomes obstructed from blood clots or kinks. Changing the patient's position would not be therapeutic. Reinserting a new catheter may be necessary if the present catheter is dislodged; however, this should be done only after the catheter's patency is checked. Assuming that the patient's condition has worsened is premature; this should not be done until after catheter placement is checked.

57. **B** Percutaneous nephrostomy involves the insertion of a catheter tube above the level of obstruction to allow urine to flow from the kidney's collecting system, through the nephrostomy tube, and into a drainage bag. Obstructed urine flows backs into the kidney. Over time, this hydronephrosis causes damage to the tubules, which allows greater reabsorption of tubular fluid, especially sodium and water. When the obstruction is chronic, tubular function diminishes until it becomes lost; the concentrating ability is the first to cease. The more severe and prolonged the obstruction, the worse the damage. Untreated chronic obstruction can lead to complete kidney failure, in this case, of the right kidney. A nephrostomy rarely cures the patient's uropathy; rather, it temporarily alleviates such symptoms as pain or acidosis and promotes a better state of health before more permanent and definitive procedures, such as surgery, can be performed. A nephrostomy can help prevent further damage, but it cannot reverse damage already incurred.

58. **A** The initial goal would be to relieve the patient's pain and distress, then decompress the urinary tract above the obstruction and improve the patient's condition to permit more definitive treatment. Pain relief measures will most probably help reduce the patient's blood pressure. Cardiac arrhythmias are not commonly associated with obstructive uropathy. Because this situation developed only recently, the patient's fluid and electrolyte status probably is still normal.

59. **D** IVP, the best technique to delineate the urinary tract, would most clearly identify the exact location of obstruction and degree of hydronephrosis. An abdominal X-ray, the easiest and most readily available test, would show only calcifications or masses as well as the position of the kidneys. Renal ultrasonography would not provide information about the patient's renal function; however, it would yield information about the size, shape, and location of the kidneys and the presence or absence of hydronephrosis. It is typically used to help guide the physician during percutaneous nephrostomy. Renal arteriography shows the condition and distribution of the renal vasculature, which is not the primary problem in obstruction.

60. **B** Since a percutaneous nephrostomy drains urine from the kidney through the abdominal wall and into a drainage bag, the patient is at risk for infection. Therefore, potential for infection related to altered skin integrity would be an appropriate nursing diagnosis. The patient is not at risk for fluid volume deficit from an additional source of urine flow because the kidney will continue to produce the same amount of urine. The patient also would not be at risk for metabolic acidosis or fluid volume excess because urine flow has been reestablished.

61. **C** Prerenal azotemia does not result from the lodging of calcium oxalate calculi in a ureter. It results from any condition that reduces perfusion of the kidneys, such as fluid shifting from the intravascular space to the interstitial space, hemorrhage, or hypotension. When the blood supply is reduced, the efferent arteriole will constrict in an attempt to maintain filtration. The filtrate will then remain in the glomerulus for a longer period. This allows for a backflow of urea into the blood, accounting for a disproportionate rise in BUN levels compared to creatinine levels. As poor oxygenation to the kidneys persists, ischemic changes occur and cellular debris obstructs the flow of filtrate into the tubules. If perfusion is restored, renal blood flow and oxygenation will improve, thereby restoring kidney function. If the cause is not corrected, ischemic changes persist, the patient remains oliguric, and recovery from acute renal failure (ARF) can take months. Obstruction in a ureter from calculi can cause postrenal failure.

62. **B** The nurse should immediately assess for pulsus paradoxus, an exaggerated decline in the pulse or blood pressure during inspiration. Pericardial friction rub is a manifestation of pericarditis that results from the accumulation of uremic toxins and fluid in the pericardial sac. Although pericarditis can be reversed by hemodialysis, the nurse's primary responsibility in this situation would be to assess for a pulsus paradoxus, which would indicate the extent of fluid accumulation in the pericardial sac. When the pericarditis progresses to pericardial effusion, a friction rub can no longer be heard. Although oxygen may be necessary, the nurse would not necessarily assume that it should be administered, as oxygen needs are determined on an individual basis. Furosemide (Lasix) is of no value in treating pericarditis.

63. **C** The nurse must remember that the patient is extremely ill and short of breath. Offering the simplest explanation that is truthful and that offers hope and support would be most appropriate in this situation. Therefore, the nurse should tell the patient that he would be able to breathe easier once hemodialysis removes fluid and toxins that the kidneys cannot. Hemodialysis does not repair kidney function but effectively removes metabolic waste products. The nurse in this situation would not know whether the patient requires only a short course of hemodialysis or ongoing therapy for the rest of his life.

64. **D** Tall, tented T waves and prolonged PR intervals are indicative of hyperkalemia, a common complication of acute renal failure (ARF). As hyperkalemia progresses, wide QRS complexes develop; if hyperkalemia is not treated promptly, asystole ensues. Chronic renal failure results in hypocalcemia and hyperphosphatemia. Calcium and phosphorus imbalances usually do not occur in ARF.

65. **A** A ruptured bladder is most likely to occur when the bladder is full. It occurs equally in both sexes and is commonly associated with blunt abdominal (not chest) trauma and fracture of the pelvis. The nurse would suspect urethral trauma in a patient with a straddle-type injury.

66. **C** A patient with a ruptured bladder should also be assessed for rectal injury, which significantly increases morbidity and mortality. Damage to the iliac vessels also may occur. Ruptured spleen, pancreatitis, and spinal cord injury usually are not associated with bladder ruptures.

67. **D** Signs and symptoms of bladder rupture include hematuria, pelvic discomfort, and difficulty voiding. Hematuria

and pelvic discomfort result from tissue trauma. The degree to which the patient experiences these symptoms depends on the extent of damage and the presence of other injuries. Difficulty voiding occurs because the muscles responsible for urination are unable to function. Pyuria and fever indicate infection. A ruptured bladder would not be capable of distention.

68. **A** Besides pain relief measures, the plan of care should include the application of ice packs and testicular elevation. Because the patient is in severe pain, pain relief is a priority for this patient. Applying ice packs will help to reduce swelling and pain. Trauma may cause bleeding into the penis and scrotal sac. The collection of extravasated blood typically produces pain. Immobilizing and elevating the testes will help minimize further bleeding, thereby minimizing the pain. Applying heat packs will contribute to further bleeding.

69. **C** Urethral bleeding is present when trauma to the urethra occurs. This must be distinguished from hematuria, which occurs from injury to other parts of the genitourinary system. Hematuria does not occur with urethral trauma because urine cannot travel down the transected urethra. When the posterior urethra is completely transected, urine extravasation typically does not occur because the bladder neck remains competent. Because an incomplete transection can become completely transected, catheterization is not recommended. The patient with urethral trauma may have acute dull or sharp pain; colicky pain is associated with renal calculi.

70. **D** Pelvic inflammatory disease (PID), an inflammation of the female reproductive organs, can result from various causes but most commonly from a sexually transmitted bacterial infection. Pathogens carrying sexually transmitted disease, such as Neisseria gonorrhoeae and Chlamydia trachomatis enter the

body from the outside via the cervical canal and travel to the uterus and pelvis via the lymphatic channels, uterine veins, or fallopian tubes. Mycobacterium tuberculosis enters through the lungs and is transported via the bloodstream.

71. **D** Signs and symptoms, such as lower abdominal pain, fever, chills, nausea, and vomiting may be confused with those of appendicitis or ectopic pregnancy. Ultrasound studies and cultures help in making the correct diagnosis.

72. **D** As with any infection in the lower abdominal region, peritonitis can be a potential complication if appropriate treatment is not prescribed and maintained. Because of the inflammatory process affecting the reproductive organs, patients with PID are at a higher risk for tubal ectopic pregnancies and subsequent infertility problems.

73. **C** The risk of acquiring PID is four to eight times greater in women who use an intrauterine device (IUD). During an episode of PID, many physicians recommend removal of the IUD once antibiotic therapy has been initiated. Abnormal menstrual cycles, stress, and continued use of antibiotics are not considered risk factors for PID.

74. **B** "I need to take all of the medication" indicates that the patient understands the discharge instructions involving continuing antibiotic therapy that the patient must finish taking all of the medication, even when the signs and symptoms, including vaginal discharge, have disappeared or she is feeling better. The patient does not need to be on bed rest or reduce her activity level during antibiotic therapy. The patient's sexual partner should also be treated to prevent the recurrence of infection.

75. **B** Depending on the infecting organism, the discharge instructions for this patient should include the education and treatment of all sexual contacts to prevent reinfection. Genetic counseling and education for stress reduction are not necessary in this situation. Follow-up urine and cervical cultures, not ultrasound studies, may be necessary.

76. **C** Characteristically, toxic shock syndrome has a rapid onset of nausea and vomiting followed by profuse diarrhea. Severe abdominal pain or rebound tenderness may occur. Fever in excess of 102°F (38.9°C) is an early sign and nearly always present. Volume loss with postural dizziness and hypotension develops quickly. Disorientation or altered consciousness without focal neurologic signs is sometimes prominent. Other symptoms may include photophobia, headache, diffuse muscle aches, joint stiffness, and sore throat. Toxic shock syndrome primarily affects previously healthy young women during their menstrual periods, although it may occur in non-menstruating women and in children. The nurse would not suspect ectopic pregnancy because the patient is menstruating. She also would not suspect vaginitis because the symptoms are too severe. Although the symptoms are similar to those of an ovarian cyst, the history of tampon use leads the nurse to suspect toxic shock syndrome over a cyst.

77. **B** The symptoms of toxic shock syndrome are accompanied by diffuse macular erythroderma that desquamates and progresses to marked peeling of the palms and soles about 10 days after onset.

78. **A** The toxin that causes toxic shock syndrome, Enterotoxin F, is secreted by Staphylococcus aureus, group I.

79. **B** The vagina is a favorable environment for the growth of S. aureus and its toxins, and it is believed that insertion of a tampon, contraceptive sponge, or diaphragm may traumatize the vaginal mucosa, thereby facilitating infection and absorption of the toxin. Extra-absorbent tampons seem to cause increased incidence because of increased absorbency and fewer tampon changes. The extra absorbency may cause occlusion of the menstrual flow and less frequent changes, permitting a contaminated environment for a longer time. Such contamination also may occur with contraceptive sponges and a diaphragm that is left in the vagina for 6 to 24 hours. The use of IUDs, douches, and oral antibiotics is not associated with toxic shock syndrome.

80. **A** An appropriate nursing diagnosis for this patient would be decreased cardiac output related to vasodilation and decreased myocardial contractility because the endotoxins released from bacteria produce vasodilation, which impairs myocardial contractility. The other diagnoses would be inappropriate because the patient already has an infection, not a potential for one, and because vaginal hemorrhage and seizures are not associated with toxic shock syndrome.

81. **A** The hypotension of toxic shock syndrome is frequently difficult to control, and immediate supportive care for shock should be initiated. Immediate volume replacement is imperative, or refractory hypotension with resulting vascular, cardiac, and renal abnormalities may result. Systolic pressure should be maintained at 90 mmHg. Treating fever and drawing blood for cultures are secondary nursing interventions to be performed after the patient has been stabilized. A spinal tap is not indicated for a patient with toxic shock syndrome.

82. **D** Adult respiratory distress syndrome, severe metabolic acidosis, and disseminated intravascular coagulation have developed in patients with toxic shock syndrome in response to vascular depletion, which causes decreased peripheral perfusion.

83. **A** About 40% of those with gonorrhea also are infected with chlamydia, which is commonly asymptomatic in women. Tetracycline (Tetracyn) is effective against chlamydia.

84. **C** Asking the patient what kind of sexual practices she engages in, such as oral or anal sex, may elicit information about infection in other areas of the body, which may be asymptomatic and treated differently. Although the other questions may be useful in eliciting information about the patient's sexual history, allowing the nurse to concentrate on specific areas for patient teaching, they are not useful in determining the course of treatment for this infection.

85. **B** Recurrence of sexually transmitted diseases does not place the patient at increased risk for renal disease. However, such a patient would be at increased risk for PID, which may result in infertility or ectopic pregnancy. High-risk sexual practices also place the patient at increased risk for contracting HIV.

86. **A** The patient's decision to use oral contraceptives would indicate the need for further patient teaching in this situation. Sexually active women with a history of sexually transmitted disease are recommended to use a barrier type of contraception, such as a condom, contraceptive sponge, or diaphragm, which may decrease the risk of recurrence. Oral contraceptives do not offer this kind of protection.

87. **D** The patient's should be alerted the Pyridium will turn the urine bright orange and a change in urine color should be expected. Antibiotics can reduce the effectiveness of oral contraceptives. Proper antibiotic teaching should include instructions to always complete the course as prescribed not just until symptoms subside. Often patients are instructed to drink enough fluids to keep their urine clear, however when on Pyridium the color change keeps the urine from being clear, thus patients are instructed to drink enough fluids so that they have the need to urinate frequently, approximately every 2 to 3 hours.

88. **C** The first message that must be conveyed is that the victim is in a safe, secure environment. Most sexual assaults occur in places known to the victim and, because the victim may know the attacker, even familiar surroundings may be perceived as threatening. The fact that sexual attacks commonly occur without warning contributes even more to the victim's fear and sense of loss of control. Telling the victim that all medical tests will be handled confidentially, that the examination will be done quickly, and that medications are available to prevent pregnancy may be conveyed after the patient's safety needs are met.

89. **D** Asking the victim whether she urinated or defecated, changed her clothes, or rinsed her mouth since the assault is an important part of the nursing history. Semen can be detected in urine and in a rectal swab specimen. In cases of oral assault, semen is likely to be found in oral secretions around the gum line. Such evidence as hair, blood, semen, and grass may be retained in clothing. The ultimate goal is to collect and maintain all evidence to ensure its admission into court.

90. **B** Having the victim fold each piece of clothing inward and place each article in a separate paper bag is the correct procedure. Folding rather than shaking the clothing will retain evidence and prevent contamination by staff members. Plastic bags should not be used because they may retain moisture and alter the evidence. If the victim consents, all clothing and other belongings should be retained for evidence, even if they had been removed during the assault. Minute pieces of hair, clothing, semen, blood, leaves, and dirt provide concrete evidence that should be identified by a qualified laboratory.

91. **C** The patient should return to her physician within 5 to 6 weeks because syphilis takes from 4 to 6 weeks to be detected serologically.

92. **D** The victim's basic needs of food, shelter, and clothing must be met to allow her to begin reestablishing control. Clear, concise, written instructions are necessary because the victim is unlikely to remember oral instructions. A list of referral telephone numbers is critical and should include at least one 24-hour resource.

93. **A** Potatoes do not provide a significant source of iron. Animal proteins and spinach are good sources.

94. **A** Creatinine is a direct measurement of kidney function and elevation can indicate renal insufficiency.

95. **B** Patients suffering from kidney stones alone, with no concurrent infection, do not have fever. Both flank pain and hematuria can be present with kidney stones or with kidney infections. Diaphoresis is common in patients suffering from acute kidney stones.

96. **D** Acute prostatitis is an infection of the prostate gland. Fever is common with infections. Lower back pain, dysuria and urinary frequency are all common findings with prostatitis. Incontinence is not a common finding but could indicate other urinary problems. Treatment for prostatitis would include antibiotic therapy.

97. **A** Irrigating the bladder increases the risk of infection by increasing the risk of introducing bacteria into the urinary tract. Using a closed drainage system is standard for indwelling catheters and should always be used absent any specific circumstance or order otherwise. Proper aseptic technique and gently cleaning the urinary meatus can also reduce the risk for infection.

98. **B** Kayexalate is a resin that binds to potassium in the GI tract and can decrease potassium levels until dialysis can be arranged. It cannot be guaranteed that furosemide would be effective in an end-stage renal patient. Hydrochlorothiazide is potassium sparing, and likely would not be effective in an end-stage renal patient. Amiodarone, although it manipulates the sodium potassium pump, it does not cause a loss in potassium, and is primarily used as an antiarrhythmic.

99. **A** Hyperkalemia is noted to cause tall, peaked T-waves on EKG.

100. **B** Tampon use, especially when left in longer than

recommended, is a known cause of toxic shock syndrome, caused by the Staphylococcus aureus bacteria. Vibrators, and other recreational accessories, could lead to a bacterial infection if not kept clean after use however the temporary usage results in a lowered chance of infection than a retained tampon.

NEUROLOGICAL EMERGENCIES

1. Which physiologic event precipitates most neurologic emergencies?

A. Head trauma
B. Cerebrovascular accident
C. Intracerebral hemorrhage
D. Increased intracranial pressure

2. The nurse understands that consciousness is determined by the:

A. Reticular activating system
B. Spinothalamic tract
C. Extrapyramidal tracts
D. Hypothalamus

3. Which method is the best way of determining a patient's level of consciousness in the emergency department (ED)?

A. Assessing pupillary reaction
B. Assessing vital signs
C. Assessing muscle strength in the extremities
D. Using the Glasgow Coma Scale

4. The nurse typically begins to assess level of consciousness by using:

A. Auditory stimulation
B. Tactile stimulation
C. Light pain
D. Deep pain

5. Which of the following is the most reliable index of a patient's neurologic condition?

A. Level of consciousness
B. Pupillary response
C. Vital signs
D. Motor function

6. Which symptom is least likely to be exhibited by a patient who sustains a cerebral concussion?

A. Dizziness
B. Loss of memory
C. Headache
D. Bizarre behavior

7. When planning discharge instructions for a patient with a cerebral concussion, the nurse should anticipate telling the patient that he can expect all neurologic symptoms to subside within:

A. 2 to 4 hours
B. 4 to 8 hours
C. 8 to 12 hours
D. 24 to 48 hours

8. Which condition would the nurse expect to note in a patient who has sustained a head injury and damage to the sixth cranial nerve?

A. Absent gag reflex
B. Fixed and dilated pupils
C. Nystagmus
D. Inward deviation of the eyes

9. A man is brought to the ED by ambulance after hitting his head when he dove into a 4' deep swimming pool. Which procedure would hold the highest priority after the patient's level of consciousness and vital signs have been checked?

A. Computed tomography (CT) scan of the head and cervical spine
B. X-ray of the cervical spine
C. Arterial blood gas measurements
D. Routine laboratory workup

10. The nurse assesses a comatose patient who is exhibiting decerebrate posturing. Which brain areas are likely to have been injured in this patient?

A. Cerebrum and cerebellum
B. Cerebrum and brain stem
C. Hypothalamus and brain stem
D. Cerebellum and hypothalamus

11. The nurse would anticipate a patient with a lesion at the lower midbrain level to demonstrate which breathing pattern?

A. Hyperventilation
B. Hypoventilation
C. Apneustic breathing
D. Cluster breathing

12. A 23-year-old man is brought to the ED after suddenly feeling ill while exercising with weights at a local health spa. While in the ED, he complains of a sudden, explosive headache. The nurse suspects:

A. Subarachnoid hemorrhage
B. Epidural hematoma
C. Basal skull fracture
D. Brain stem contusion

13. A man arrives at the ED via ambulance after sustaining a hemi-section of the spinal cord from a stab wound to the right side of the back. He experiences loss of movement on the right side and loss of pain and temperature sensations on the left. The nurse knows that this syndrome is called:

A. Brown-Sequard syndrome
B. Anterior cord syndrome
C. Partial cord syndrome
D. Central cord syndrome

14. Which statement accurately describes the mechanism of a generalized seizure?

A. The abnormal excessive firing of brain cells causes the clinical signs and symptoms of a seizure
B. The entire brain is involved in a seizure
C. The metabolism of the involved cells is greatly decreased during a seizure
D. The abnormal firing of neurons, once initiated, is perpetuated indefinitely until therapy is instituted

15. The nurse's highest priority when caring for a patient in a postictal state is to:

A. Obtain a complete family history
B. Begin an infusion of normal saline solution
C. Place the patient on his side
D. Call the physician

16. Which of the following is least likely to precipitate a seizure?

A. Head trauma
B. Heavy-metal ingestion
C. The patient's discontinuation of anticonvulsant therapy
D. Cerebral edema

17. Which nursing diagnostic category reflects the clinical problems associated with this patient's seizures?

A. Ineffective airway clearance
B. Altered tissue perfusion
C. Potential for injury
D. All of the above

18. When administering phenytoin intravenously, the nurse must:

A. Institute cardiac monitoring
B. Obtain a serum phenytoin level immediately after administration
C. Administer the drug in a dextrose solution
D. Administer the drug at a rate no faster than 500 mg/minute

19. Which life-threatening situation would the nurse expect to occur if phenytoin is administered by rapid IV bolus?

A. Ventricular tachycardia
B. Supraventricular tachycardia
C. Third-degree heart block
D. Electromechanical dissociation

20. Which information regarding phenytoin should the nurse include in discharge teaching?

A. Alcohol may cause phenytoin toxicity
B. Phenytoin must be taken even in the absence of seizures
C. Missed doses should not be made up
D. Aspirin, rather than acetaminophen, should be taken for headaches

21. Which statement about eclampsia is true?

A. Signs and symptoms typically occur during the third trimester but can occur up to 2 months postpartum
B. Signs and symptoms include hypertension, proteinuria, oliguria, and seizures
C. Eclampsia most commonly occurs in multigravida women
D. Eclampsia is idiopathic and not associated with any preexisting disease

22. A 21-year-old woman is admitted to the ED in a coma. She is accompanied by her husband, who states that she had a seizure. The patient is 1 week postpartum. Her vital signs are blood pressure 180/128 mmHg, pulse rate 120 beats/minute, and respiratory rate 12 breaths/minute. The physician diagnoses eclampsia. After the initial management of this patient, the nurse would expect the physician to order which medication?

A. Phenobarbital
B. Diazepam (Valium)
C. Magnesium sulfate
D. Phenytoin

23. Paramedics bring a middle-aged man who was found unconscious on the street to the ED. No identification or further information is available. Vital signs are blood pressure 160/90 mmHg, pulse rate 120 beats/minute, and respiratory rate 16 breaths/minute. Upon arrival, the patient begins experiencing sustained grand mal seizures and requires intubation. The nurse establishes an IV line. Which drug treatment is usually preferred to control status epilepticus?

A. 18 mg/kg of phenytoin
B. Diazepam 5 mg/minute IV every 5 to 10 minutes
C. 10 to 20 mg/kg of phenobarbital IV
D. 14 mg of lorazepam IV over 2 minutes

24. After a patient's seizure is controlled, the nurse would expect to administer all of the following except:

A. 50 mL of dextrose
B. 1 to 2 mg/kg of naloxone (Narcan) IV
C. 100 mg of thiamine IV
D. 2 mg of naloxone (Narcan) IV

25. Which drug is the treatment of choice to prevent seizures from traumatic head injury?

A. Diazepam (Valium)
B. Dexamethasone (Decadron)
C. Phenytoin (Dilantin)
D. Phenobarbital (Luminal)

26. A 60-year-old man with a history of seizures is brought to the ED because of recurrent seizure activity. While in the ED, he develops tonic-clonic movements of the right arm and leg. The nurse correctly determines that this patient is exhibiting a:

A. Grand mal seizure
B. Petit mal seizure
C. Jacksonian seizure
D. Psychomotor seizure

27. A 60-year-old man with a history of seizures is brought to the ED because of recurrent seizure activity. While in the ED, he develops tonic-clonic movements of the right arm and leg. Which postictal manifestation should the nurse anticipate and adjust for in the patient's plan of care?

A. Paralysis of the right side
B. Loss of consciousness
C. Incontinence
D. Seizure activity of the left side

28. A 25-year-old man, disoriented to time and place, is admitted to the ED. His co-worker states that the patient was hit on the head with a beam 2 hours ago and that the incident caused momentary unconsciousness. The patient was fine until 30 minutes ago, when he became tired and confused. Physical examination reveals a dilated nonreactive left pupil. Vital signs are blood pressure 160/80 mmHg, pulse rate 80 beats/minute, and respiratory rate 16 breaths/minute. Which diagnostic test would the nurse anticipate the physician to order initially?

A. Lumbar puncture
B. CT scan
C. Cervical spine X-ray
D. Cerebral angiography

29. Diagnostic studies reveal a temporal fracture with a pineal shift. The nurse would interpret this finding to indicate:

A. Subdural hematoma
B. Epidural hematoma
C. Subarachnoid hemorrhage
D. Intracerebral bleeding

30. A 25-year-old man, disoriented to time and place, is admitted to the ED. His co-worker states that the patient was hit on the head with a beam 2 hours ago and that the incident caused momentary unconsciousness. The patient was fine until 30 minutes ago, when he became tired and confused. Physical examination reveals a dilated nonreactive left pupil. Vital signs are blood pressure 160/80 mmHg, pulse rate 80 beats/minute, and respiratory rate 16 breaths/minute. Diagnostic studies reveal a temporal fracture with a pineal shift. The ED nurse would anticipate the medical treatment for this patient to include:

A. Direct intracranial pressure (ICP) monitoring in the intensive care unit (ICU)
B. Pharmacologic management
C. Lumbar puncture
D. Surgical evacuation of the clot

31. The primary objective in the plan of care for a patient with a traumatic head injury typically involves:

A. Decreasing the patient's ICP
B. Maintaining the patient's oxygenation
C. Maintaining the patient's body alignment
D. Hyperventilating the patient

32. Which independent nursing intervention best relieves increased ICP?

A. Elevating the head of the bed 30 degrees
B. Administering oxygen
C. Administering diuretics
D. Hyperventilating the patient

33. Which sign is typically the first indication of increased ICP?

A. Elevated systolic blood pressure
B. Elevated body temperature
C. Altered respiratory pattern
D. Altered level of consciousness

34. While caring for a patient with a head trauma, the nurse would assess for signs of uncal herniation. Which sign is an early indication of this condition?

A. Absent doll's eye reflex
B. Ipsilateral pupil dilation
C. Ataxic breathing
D. Impaired motor function

35. The nurse is aware that signs of increased ICP include:

A. Narrowing pulse pressure, rising systolic blood pressure, and bradycardia
B. Narrowing pulse pressure, rising systolic blood pressure, and tachycardia
C. Widening pulse pressure, rising diastolic blood pressure, and bradycardia
D. Widening pulse pressure, rising systolic blood pressure, and bradycardia

36. Although several nursing diagnostic categories would be applicable for a patient with increased ICP, which category is most appropriate for this patient?

A. Altered cerebral tissue perfusion
B. Increased cerebral perfusion pressure
C. Potential for brain injury
D. Increased intracranial adaptive capacity

37. The nurse knows that all of the following statements about epidural and subdural hematomas are false except:

A. Epidural bleeding occurs below the dura mater and above the arachnoid layer
B. Signs and symptoms of epidural bleeding develop more slowly than do those of subdural bleeding
C. Epidural hematomas usually are caused by arterial bleeding, and subdural hematomas usually are caused by injury to a vein
D. Temporal bone fractures are associated with subdural hematomas

38. When planning the care of a patient with increased ICP, the nurse includes appropriate interventions to prevent further worsening of the patient's condition. The nurse realizes that the patient's condition may worsen with the development of:

A. Hypoxemia, hypercapnia, and respiratory alkalosis
B. Hypoxemia, hypercapnia, and respiratory acidosis
C. Hypoxemia, hypocapnia, and respiratory alkalosis
D. Hypoxemia, hypocapnia, and respiratory acidosis

39. Which rationale best supports the use of mannitol in treating increased ICP?

A. It induces diuresis by raising the osmotic pressure of glomerular filtrate
B. It increases the rate of electrolyte excretion, particularly of sodium, chloride, and potassium
C. It increases plasma osmolality, thereby inducing diffusion of water from cerebrospinal fluid back into the plasma and intravascular space
D. It results in a shifting of intracellular fluid into the interstitial space, thus decreasing cellular edema

40. The nurse should include avoidance of which activity in the care plan of a patient with increased ICP?

A. Valsalva's maneuver
B. Coughing or sneezing
C. Isometric muscle contraction or hip flexion
D. All of the above

41. Which method of determining ICP is considered unsafe in a patient with a head injury?

A. Lumbar puncture
B. Epidural monitoring
C. Intraventricular catheterization
D. Subarachnoid screw insertion

42. A patient admitted to the ED after a motor vehicle accident is found to have a basal skull fracture with middle meningeal artery damage. The nurse would expect a patient who sustained damage to the middle meningeal artery to develop:

A. A subdural hematoma
B. A subarachnoid hemorrhage
C. An epidural hematoma
D. An aneurysm

43. A patient admitted to the ED after a motor vehicle accident is found to have a basal skull fracture with middle meningeal artery damage. The nurse assesses this patient for Battle's sign, which is best described as:

A. A postconcussion syndrome
B. An ecchymosis over the mastoid bone
C. Black and blue discoloration around the eyes
D. A superficial hematoma on the skull

44. A patient admitted to the ED after a motor vehicle accident is found to have a basal skull fracture with middle meningeal artery damage. This patient is also at risk for injury to the:

A. Oculomotor nerve
B. Olfactory nerve
C. Optic nerve
D. Ophthalmic nerve

45. The nurse would anticipate further assessment of a patient with a basal skull fracture to possibly reveal:

A. Otorrhea
B. Meningism
C. Facial paresis
D. Hemianopia

46. Which nursing measure will benefit a patient with a basal skull fracture?

A. Instructing the patient to blow his nose gently
B. Instructing the patient to avoid Valsalva's maneuver
C. Encouraging the patient to cough and breathe deeply
D. Carefully inserting a nasogastric tube

47. The nurse understands that raccoon's eyes usually indicate:

A. Meningitis
B. Intracerebral hemorrhage
C. Epidural hematoma
D. Anterior fossa fracture

48. A man is brought to the ED by emergency medical service after involvement in a motor vehicle accident. He is suspected of having a spinal cord injury. Spinal X-rays confirm a lesion at the C_5 to C_6 level. The nurse anticipates that the patient has:

A. Quadriplegia with intact triceps and biceps and intercostal breathing
B. Quadriplegia with gross arm movements and diaphragmatic breathing
C. Paraplegia with diaphragmatic breathing
D. Diaphragmatic and intercostal breathing with loss of intrinsic hand muscle power

49. Which nursing diagnosis would be the highest priority for a patient with a cervical spinal cord injury?

A. Impaired gas exchange related to pulmonary embolism
B. Dysfunctional grieving related to paralysis
C. Ineffective breathing pattern related to weakened respiratory muscles
D. Potential for multisystem dysfunction related to spinal shock

50. While in the ED, the patient develops spinal shock. This condition is defined as a state of:

A. Spastic paralysis caused by a lesion of the upper motor neuron
B. Inhibit ion of parasympathetic outflow
C. Sudden initiation of the facilitatory influences from higher brain centers
D. Transient reflex depression below the level of the lesion

51. Nursing assessment of the patient with a spinal cord injury reveals all of the following except:

A. Urinary incontinence
B. Bradycardia
C. Poikilothermy
D. Hypotension

52. One of the nurse's major concerns in caring for a patient with a spinal cord injury is to maintain optimal respiratory function. Which development would not lead to hypoventilation in this patient?

A. An injury below C_4 resulting in diaphragmatic breathing and decreased tidal volume
B. A cervical lesion at T_1 resulting in spinal shock
C. Paralysis of abdominal and intercostal muscles leading to ineffective cough and retention of secretions
D. Abdominal distension from gastric dilation, possibly restricting diaphragmatic excursion

53. When assessing the patient's motor function, the nurse determines spinothalamic tract function by:

A. Applying a tuning fork to a bony prominence and asking the patient to identify the vibration
B. Asking the patient to close both eyes and to touch his nose with his finger
C. Asking the patient to identify areas stimulated by pinprick
D. Testing the patient's position sense

54. Which assessment finding would indicate deterioration of this patient's respiratory status?

A. Arterial blood gas (ABG) measurements of pH 7.28, PCO_2 36 mmHg, HCO_3^- 18 mEq, and PO_2 86 mmHg
B. Inspiratory force of - 20 cm
C. Tidal volume of 500 mL
D. Bronchial breath sounds over the lung lobes

55. At which level does the phrenic nerve innervate the diaphragm?

A. C_2 to C_3
B. C_3 to C_5
C. T_1 to T_3
D. T_3 to T_4

56. In the patient with a spinal cord injury, early hypoventilation is best manifested by:

A. Poor respiratory exchange
B. Cyanosis
C. Shortness of breath while talking
D. ABG changes

57. A patient is admitted to the ED with possible spinal cord injury between T_4 and T_{12}. Which clinical finding would the nurse not expect to note?

A. Bladder and bowel incontinence
B. Paraplegia of the lower part of the body
C. Complete loss of motor function in the legs
D. Loss of feeling below the truncal dermatome level, corresponding with the site of cord damage

58. If a cervical spinal cord injury were suspected, the best way to open the patient's airway would be to:

A. Tilt the head forward, supporting the neck
B. Use a modified jaw-thrust maneuver
C. Log-roll the patient on his side and pull down the chin
D. Perform a tracheotomy

59. The nurse knows that loss of motor function in the right arm and leg may indicate a lesion in the:

A. Pyramidal tract of the left hemisphere
B. Spinocerebellar tract
C. Motor nerve fibers in the anterior horn of the spinal cord
D. Spinal cord at C_7

60. The most reliable technique for testing the motor strength of a patient's arm is to:

A. Observe for spontaneous movement
B. Test the patient's muscle reflexes
C. Ask the patient to squeeze the nurse's hands
D. Ask the patient to close his eyes and to raise his arms straight in front of him

61. A patient admitted to the ED with an injury to the left cerebral hemisphere may exhibit:

A. Left hemiparesis
B. Left homonymous hemianopia
C. Deviation of the eyes to the left
D. Left-sided hemiplegia.

62. The nurse understands that pinpoint pupils usually are indicative of a lesion in the:

A. Pons
B. Optic nerve
C. Medulla
D. Midbrain

63. An unconscious patient with pinpoint pupils is most likely to exhibit which breathing pattern?

A. Apneustic breathing
B. Biot's respirations
C. Ataxic breathing
D. Cheyne-Stokes respirations

64. Which patient assessment technique is the best way to check for meningeal irritation?

A. Flex the patient's leg at the hip and knee, then straighten the knee and watch for pain and resistance
B. Stroke the lateral aspect of the patient's sole and watch for dorsiflexion of the great toe
C. Check the patient's temperature; a reading above 102° F (38.9° C) indicates meningeal irritation
D. Check for papilledema

65. Which nursing action would be inappropriate for a patient who has just been diagnosed as having viral meningitis?

A. Institute seizure precautions
B. Institute isolation precautions
C. Monitor the patient's temperature frequently
D. Institute measures to control increased ICP

66. Which of the following findings is a common sign of meningococcal meningitis?

A. Petechiae
B. Hypothermia
C. Nystagmus
D. Hypertensive crisis

67. During a neurological assessment, the nurse understands all of the following clinical findings to be associated with meningeal irritation except:

A. Babinski reflex
B. Brudzinski's sign
C. Kernig's sign
D. Nuchal rigidity

68. The organism that most commonly causes meningitis in young adults is:

A. Haemophilus influenzae
B. Pneumococcus
C. Meningococcus
D. Streptococcus

69. The assessment findings with a patient who has neurogenic shock, would include:

A. Hypotension
B. Tachycardia
C. Cool, moist skin
D. Hyper-reflexia

70. All of the following interventions are appropriate for the patient in neurogenic shock except:

A. Elevate lower extremities and place antiembolic hose on patient
B. Insert gastric tube and indwelling urinary catheter
C. Administer steroids and atropine to elevate heart rate
D. Keep patient on backboard to prevent further neurological damage

NEUROLOGICAL EMERGENCIES: RATIONALE

1. **D** Increased intracranial pressure (ICP) commonly precedes most neurologic emergencies, such as head trauma, cerebrovascular accident, and intracranial hemorrhage. An ICP less than 10 mmHg is considered normal; any measurement above 15 mmHg is considered abnormal. Increased ICP can be caused by conditions that increase brain volume, such as hematomas, tumors, and cerebral edema; those that increase blood volume, such as hypercapnia; those that increase cerebrospinal fluid, such as hydrocephalus.

2. **A** The reticular activating system is responsible for maintaining consciousness by coordinating sensory input and responding, in proportion, to incoming stimuli. The spinothalamic tract is responsible for transmitting pain and temperature sensations to the brain. The extra-pyramidal tracts regulate and control voluntary motor activity. The hypothalamus is responsible for temperature regulation, behavior, autonomic responses, and control of the pituitary gland.

3. **D** The Glasgow Coma Scale (GCS) is the standard means of assessing a patient's level of consciousness in the emergency department (ED). The nurse uses the scale to assign a numeric value to the patient's ability to open his eyes, respond verbally, and demonstrate motor response to different stimuli. The totaled scores, ranging from 3 to 15, indicate the level of consciousness (alert, lethargic, obtunded, stuporous, semicomatose, or comatose); a total of 7 or less indicates a comatose state. Using the Glasgow Coma Scale allows the nurse to quickly determine any deterioration in the patient's neurologic status.

4. **A** The nurse typically begins to assess consciousness by using auditory stimulation and observing for a response. Because it is always best to start with the minimum amount of stimulation necessary to evoke a response, speaking to the patient is commonly the first step.

5. **A** Level of consciousness, the most important and reliable index of a patient's neurologic condition, is the earliest and most sensitive indicator of a change in neurologic status. Altered consciousness is the hallmark of cerebral injury.

6. **D** Bizarre behavior is characteristic of a patient with a cerebral contusion, not a cerebral concussion. A patient with a cerebral concussion may experience dizziness, loss of memory, and headaches. A cerebral concussion is a shock to the brain's soft tissues; a contusion involves bruising and laceration of brain tissue.

7. **D** All symptoms of a concussion should subside within 24 to 48 hours. Any problems lasting longer than that time indicate a more serious injury and require reevaluation by a physician.

8. **D** The nurse would expect to note inward deviation of the eyes because the sixth cranial (abducens) nerve controls this movement. The gag reflex is controlled by the ninth and tenth (glossopharyngeal and vagus, respectively) cranial nerves. Pupillary constriction and dilation is controlled by the third cranial (oculomotor) nerve. Nystagmus is caused by an interruption of cerebellar function.

9. **A** A view of C_7 is vitally important to determine whether the patient has a compression injury to the spinal cord and the level at which it has occurred. Although a cross-table lateral view could be obtained, the patient will need a CT scan of the head and neck in order to fully evaluate the cervical spine. Traditional practice was that patients were not moved until c-spine injury was ruled out, once ruled out they could be moved. However, the priority on this patient is the head injury and requires prompt evaluation via CT.

10. **B** Decerebrate posturing is indicative of a patient with damage to the brain stem and cerebrum, because both areas control motor function. The cerebellum coordinates muscle tone with movement and maintains equilibrium. The hypothalamus does not regulate motor function.

11. **A** Altered breathing patterns are directly related to specific levels of brain dysfunction. Central neurogenic hyperventilation, which is characterized by rapid, regular respirations (in excess of 24 breaths/minute) with an increase in depth of respiration, is typical of a patient with a lesion at the lower midbrain level. Apneustic breathing, which is characterized by prolonged inspiration with a 2 – 3 second pause at the end of inspiration, typically occurs in a patient with a lesion at the pons level. Cluster breathing, which is characterized by irregular breathing with periods of apnea at

irregular intervals, is associated with medullary damage. Hypoventilation typically occurs in a patient with metabolic or drug-induced coma, respiratory depression, or increased ICP.

12. **A** The patient is probably experiencing a subarachnoid hemorrhage caused by an arteriovenous malformation and brought on by strenuous activity. Epidural hematoma, basal skull fracture, and brain stem contusion typically occur because of traumatic injury.

13. **A** In Brown-Sequard syndrome, the damage is located on one side of the spinal cord. As a result, complete motor paralysis occurs on the same side (ipsilateral motor loss), with nearly complete loss of pain and temperature sensation on the opposite side below the level of the lesion (contralateral loss of pain and temperature sensation). In anterior cord syndrome, which may be caused by a forward dislocation or compression injury, the damage is mainly concentrated in the anterior aspect of the cord. Complete motor paralysis usually occurs below the level of the lesion, with complete loss of pain and temperature sensations. In central cord syndrome, the mechanism of injury usually is hyperextension of the cervical spine with compression, resulting in greater motor loss of upper extremities than of lower ones. No type of spinal cord damage is known as partial cord syndrome.

14. **A** The abnormal excessive firing of brain cells causes the clinical signs and symptoms of a seizure. Either a portion of or the entire brain may be involved. The metabolism of the involved cells is greatly increased during seizure activity. The abnormal firing of neurons may terminate as abruptly as it begins.

15. **C** Maintaining a patent airway is the primary nursing goal in this situation; placing the patient in a side-lying position with the head and body aligned ensures airway patency and helps prevent aspiration. An airway should be placed in the patient's mouth before a tonic phase begins. To prevent injury, objects should never be forced into the mouth during a seizure. The nurse should stay with the patient during the seizure and summon assistance if further equipment is needed. The nurse may need to establish an IV line to administer anticonvulsants. Once the patient is stabilized, the nurse may obtain a complete family history.

16. **B** Heavy metal ingestion is least likely to precipitate a seizure. Common precipitating events include the discontinuation of anticonvulsant therapy, which typically occurs as a result of the patient's forgetting to take the medication or not complying with the drug regimen; craniocerebral trauma; infections, particularly of the central nervous system; cerebral tumors; or metabolic brain disorders.

17. **D** All of these nursing diagnostic categories reflect the clinical problems associated with this patient's seizures, including ineffective airway clearance, altered tissue perfusion, and potential for injury. Appropriate nursing interventions would include inserting an artificial airway, providing supplemental oxygen, turning the patient to his side, initiating an IV line, administering prescribed drugs to stop the seizure activity, maintaining upright bed side rails, measuring the patient's temperature by the rectal route only, and protecting the patient's head during seizures.

18. **A** When administering phenytoin intravenously, the nurse should institute cardiac monitoring and observe the patient carefully. Therapeutic blood phenytoin levels of 10 to 20

mcg/mL can be achieved quickly by IV administration; however, rapid administration depresses the myocardium and can cause cardiac arrest. Because this patient had been taking this medication at home, the nurse would obtain a level before administration to provide a baseline level and prevent possible toxicity. Nystagmus with lateral gaze is the first sign of toxicity; ataxia, slurred speech, diplopia, lethargy, and coordination disturbances may result from acute overdose. IV Phenytoin must be administered slowly at a rate no faster than 50 mg/minute in a saline solution. If given in a dextrose solution, the drug will precipitate into crystals.

19. **C** Phenytoin is a myocardial depressant. Administering this drug by rapid IV bolus or in excessive doses may induce third-degree heart block and cardiac arrest.

20. **B** Phenytoin must be taken as ordered, even in the absence of seizures, because the drug is effective only when therapeutic blood levels are maintained. The patient should know the signs and symptoms of toxicity, such as slurred speech, confusion, diplopia, nausea, gingival hyperplasia, and fever. Because phenytoin is absorbed slowly from the GI tract, daily doses can be adjusted to the patient's convenience, and missed doses can be made up safely. The patient should be encouraged to wear a medical alert identification bracelet or necklace. The patient should be advised against using drugs that potentiate or inhibit phenytoin's action. Phenytoin's action may be potentiated by the concurrent use of aspirin, estrogen, disulfiram (Antabuse), chlordiazepoxide (Librium), or anticoagulants (especially dicumarol). Drugs that inhibit phenytoin's action include alcohol, antihistamines, barbiturates, hypnotics, and sedatives.

21. **B** Signs and symptoms of eclampsia include hypertension, proteinuria, oliguria, and seizures. These manifestations

typically occur during the third trimester but also can occur up to 2 weeks postpartum. Eclampsia, which is most common in primigravida patients, is associated with diabetes, hypertension, and renal disease.

22. **C** The nurse would expect the physician to order magnesium sulfate, the anticonvulsant of choice in treating eclampsia. Hydralazine (Apresoline) or nitroprusside sodium (Nipride) also may be ordered to control the patient's hypertension. Diazepam and other sedatives should be used judiciously in this condition.

23. **B** Of the drugs doses listed, the drug of choice here to manage status epilepticus would be diazepam, a rapid-acting anticonvulsant with fewer tendencies to produce hypotension. Phenytoin and phenobarbital would be indicated to prevent further seizures. Lorazepam can be used to treat seizures-and often is the drug of choice for adult active seizures, however the dose here is excessive. Although not listed, and not yet widely used, intranasal versed is now being recommended for status epilepticus.

24. **B** After the patient's seizure is controlled; secondary management should focus on finding the underlying cause of the seizure. If no one provides the ED team with this information, dextrose 50%, naloxone (Narcan), and thiamine should be administered. Dextrose is administered to reverse possible hypoglycemia. Naloxone (Narcan) is used to reverse potential drug opiate intoxication. Thiamine is commonly administered to alcoholic patients and those with a potential vitamin deficiency. All of these conditions can result in seizure activity. The dose of naloxone (Narcan) is up to 2mg IV push, the dose shown (1 to 2mg/kg) is excessive and would be incorrect.

25. **C** Phenytoin is the drug used to treat seizures resulting from head trauma because a therapeutic blood level is rapidly established. Phenytoin works by stabilizing the seizure threshold, thereby reducing seizure activity. Diazepam and phenobarbital should be avoided in the patient with head trauma because they cause sedation and will inhibit an accurate assessment of level of consciousness. Dexamethasone may be used to decrease cerebral edema; however, its action is decreased when used concurrently with phenytoin.

26. **C** Jacksonian seizures are characterized by tonic-clonic movement limited to one side of the body moving to the next. Grand mal seizures produce tonic-clonic movement of the entire body and loss of consciousness, followed by a postictal state of drowsiness. Petit mal seizures produce transient loss of consciousness with no postictal state. Psychomotor seizures, which are more common in children, are characterized by bizarre behavior with no loss of consciousness and by postictal drowsiness and amnesia about the seizure episode.

27. **A** A patient with Jacksonian seizures typically develops Todd's paralysis, transient postictal paralysis of the affected side. Unconsciousness and incontinence are associated with grand mal seizures.

28. **B** Once the patient's vital signs are stabilized, the nurse would expect an order for a CT scan of the head and cervical spine. A CT must be done to verify the extent of brain injury (as evidence by the patients confusion and momentary loss of consciousness).

29. **B** An epidural hematoma is commonly associated with a temporal fracture. The development of such a hematoma causes a contralateral pineal shift. These findings, along with a

nonreactive left pupil and a deteriorating level of consciousness, are indicative of an epidural hematoma.

30. **D** The nurse would anticipate the medical treatment for this patient to include surgical evacuation of the hematoma and ligation of the damaged vessel. Early diagnosis and immediate surgical treatment are directly related to a good prognosis.

31. **B** Although all these measures are important, the primary objective in caring for a patient with a traumatic head injury involves maintaining oxygen supply to the brain, as hypoxia and carbon dioxide retention cause cerebral vasodilation and increase ICP.

32. **A** All of these interventions decrease ICP. However, elevating the bead of the bed 30 degrees to allow for venous drainage by gravity, and is the only independent nursing intervention listed. The other interventions require an order.

33. **D** Altered level of consciousness is typically the first sign of increased ICP. It results from decreased blood supply to the cortex. Changes in vital signs and temperature are late indicators because the brain stem is not compressed until later stages of this condition.

34. **B** Ipsilateral pupil dilation is the earliest sign of uncal herniation. An expanding lesion of the lateral middle fossa, most commonly of the temporal lobe, causes shifting of the inner basal temporal lobe. This area contains the uncus, which is forced through the tentorium as pressure builds. The third cranial nerve and the posterior cerebral artery on the same side of the expanding temporal lobe lesion are frequently caught between the uncus and the tentorium. Ataxic or irregular respirations are seen in the later stages of herniation. An absent

doll's eye reflex indicates brain stem dysfunction and is a late sign of herniation. Impaired motor function is a common sign in various neurologic and neuromuscular diseases, such as cerebrovascular accident, multiple sclerosis, and myasthenia gravis.

35. **D** The classic signs of increased ICP involving the brain stem include widening pulse pressure, rising systolic blood pressure, and bradycardia. These three signs, known as Cushing's response, are a compensatory mechanism for maintaining blood pressure and cerebral blood flow when ICP increases. Vital signs, such as blood pressure and pulse rate are controlled in the vital centers of the brain stem. Hypertension stimulates the baroreceptors in the carotid and aortic bodies, stimulating the vagus nerve and producing bradycardia.

36. **A** Altered cerebral tissue perfusion is an appropriate nursing diagnostic category for this patient with increased ICP. Nursing interventions should focus on assisting with medical decompression of the cranial vault, ensuring adequate cerebral perfusion pressure, continuously monitoring the patient's neurologic status, preparing for surgical decompression, and instituting appropriate measures to prevent complications.

37. **C** Epidural hematomas usually are caused by arterial bleeding, and subdural hematomas usually are caused by injury to a vein. Epidural hematomas occur between the skull and the dura mater; subdural hematomas occur between the dura mater and arachnoid layer. Signs and symptoms develop more rapidly in epidural bleeding than in subdural bleeding because epidural bleeding is usually associated with arterial bleeding, whereas subdural bleeding results from venous bleeding. Approximately 85% of patients in whom epidural hematomas develop have sustained a skull fracture, with the most common site being the

temporal bone. The middle meningeal artery, located under the temporal bone, is usually the affected artery.

38. **B** Hypoxemia, hypercapnia, and respiratory acidosis are potent vasodilating factors in the body's attempt to increase oxygen supply to the brain. Cerebral vasodilation causes an increase in blood volume in the brain and a subsequent increase in ICP.

39. **C** Mannitol is used to treat increased ICP because it increases plasma osmolality, thereby inducing diffusion of water from cerebrospinal fluid (CSF) back into the plasma and intravascular space. Although mannitol induces diuresis by raising the osmotic pressure of the glomerular filtrate and increasing the rate of electrolyte excretion, neither of these actions decreases ICP. Shifting intracellular fluid to the interstitial space will not decrease edema.

40. **D** Valsalva's maneuver, an exertion against a closed epiglottis, increases intrathoracic pressure, impedes venous return from the brain, and increases ICP. Isometric muscle contractions, those that do not lengthen the muscle, cause a rise in systemic blood pressure, thereby elevating ICP. Coughing and sneezing elevate intra-abdominal and intrathoracic pressures. An increase in these pressures is transmitted to the spinal and intracranial subarachnoid spaces through the veins that communicate with the dural venous sinuses and intracranial subarachnoid space. The venous return from the cranial vault is impeded, resulting in an increase in ICP. Positions that obstruct venous return from the brain and increase ICP include extreme flexion of the hips, Trendelenburg's position, and angulation of the neck.

41. **A** Although a lumbar puncture is a means of measuring ICP, it is considered risky and therefore contraindicated in a patient with an expanding cerebral mass. A lumbar puncture will give accurate pressure readings only if CSF is flowing freely within the subarachnoid space. An expanding lesion, as well as adhesions and constrictions, will alter the flow of CSF and result in an inaccurate pressure reading. In addition, with increased ICP lumbar puncture may cause brain stem herniation by reducing spinal pressure. Epidural monitoring, intraventricular catheterization, and subarachnoid screw insertion are the three commonly used methods to measure ICP.

42. **C** The nurse would expect a patient who sustained damage to the middle meningeal artery to develop an epidural hematoma, which commonly results from arterial bleeding. A subdural hematoma commonly results from venous bleeding. A subarachnoid hemorrhage is commonly caused by a ruptured cerebral aneurysm, which involves the weakening of a vessel wall.

43. **B** Battle's sign, which is commonly associated with basal skull fractures involving the middle fossa, is best described as bleeding with resultant ecchymosis over the mastoid bone. Because this sign takes 24 hours to develop, it may be undetectable to the ED nurse. A basal skull fracture may involve the anterior, middle, or posterior fossa at the base of the skull.

44. **B** The patient with a basal skull fracture is also at risk for injury to the cranial nerves. Injury to the first cranial (olfactory) nerve is common and typically causes anosmia, or loss of the sense of smell. Other common cranial nerve injuries include those to the seventh (facial) nerve, which causes ipsilateral

facial paralysis, and the eighth (acoustic) nerve, which may lead to disturbances in hearing or equilibrium.

45. **A** Further assessment of the patient with a basal skull fracture may reveal cerebrospinal otorrhea or rhinorrhea. Cerebrospinal otorrhea occurs if the dura mater is torn and the tympanic membrane is ruptured; cerebrospinal rhinorrhea results if the tympanic membrane is intact; drainage samples from either site test positive for glucose. The best diagnostic test for CSF is the Halo test. If the drainage is bloody - human blood will contain glucose and this may give a false reading. A simple halo test is >95% accurate.

46. **B** The patient with a basal skull fracture will benefit from any nursing measure that aims to avert further tearing of the dura by preventing transient increases in ICP; therefore, the nurse should instruct the patient to avoid coughing and performing Valsalva's maneuver, The nurse should instruct the patient to avoid blowing his nose and to allow the fluid to drain freely. If rhinorrhea is significant, a small, loose dressing may be applied. Nothing should be put into the patient's nose or ears, including suction catheters or nasogastric tubes.

47. **D** Raccoon's eyes, bilateral ecchymoses from bleeding into the sinuses would usually indicate a basal skull fracture involving the anterior fossa. Anterior fossa fractures may also result in cerebrospinal rhinorrhea if the dura mater is torn.

48. **B** The nurse would expect a patient with a lesion at the C_5 to C_6 level to have quadriplegia with gross arm movements and diaphragmatic breathing. Such an injury would result in complete loss of motor power in the trunk and legs (quadriplegia), along with bladder and bowel retention. Although paralysis of intercostal respiration also occurs,

diaphragmatic respiration would continue without abdominal muscle action because the diaphragm is innervated via the phrenic nerve at the C_3 to C_5 level.

49. **C** The priority nursing diagnosis for a patient with a cervical spinal cord injury would be "Ineffective breathing pattern related to weakened respiratory muscles", because the nurse's immediate concern in such cases is always maintaining effective breathing.

50. **D** Spinal shock is a state of transient reflex depression below the level of the lesion. Although the pathophysiology of spinal shock is incompletely understood, the shock results, in part, from sudden withdrawal of facilitatory influences from higher brain centers. A loss of sympathetic outflow occurs in lesions higher than T_5. Flaccidity typically occurs during shock caused by a lesion of the upper motor neuron; spasticity returns after the shock subsides.

51. **A** Urine retention, rather than incontinence, is seen in spinal shock because of bladder atony. Spinal shock may result in such life-threatening symptoms as hypotension and bradycardia from sympathetic blockade. Poikilothermy results from the interruption of sympathetic pathways to the temperature-regulating centers in the hypothalamus. Spinal shock and neurogenic shock are frequently misunderstood. Spinal shock is just loss of deep tendon reflexes because the spinal cord is stunned. Spinal Shock produces flaccid paralysis and reflex emptying of the bladder (not atony) and may produce mild hypotension that typically does not require treatment. Neurogenic shock is caused by loss of sympathetic innervation and massive peripheral vasodilation occurs. BP drops but there is no sympathetic nervous system response so the parasympathetic nervous system takes over and the heart rate

drops (bradycardia). This is a form of distributive shock and can be life threatening. Poikilothermy can be present in any high-level spinal cord injury (T_6 and above) and is due to the reasons listed.

52. **B** A cervical lesion at T_1 accompanied by spinal shock would not lead to hypoventilation because spinal shock results in a transient reflex depression below this area; respiratory musculature should not be affected by this type of injury. A lesion at C_8/T_1 typically results in hand weakness and paraplegia. In the emergent and acute phases of SCI, secondary injuries can cause cord ischemia 2 levels up from the area of injury. This may impede ventilation because the intercostal muscles would be weak.

53. **C** To assess spinothalamic tract function, the nurse should ask the patient to close both eyes and then have him/her identify areas stimulated by a pinprick. The lateral spinothalamic tract conveys pain and temperature sensation, whereas the anterior spinothalamic tract conveys light touch, pressure, pain, and temperature sensation. Identifying vibrations and position assesses proprioceptive sensation. Point-to-point testing assesses coordination.

54. **D** Bronchial breath sounds over the patient's lung lobes indicate the development of pneumonia, probably the result of immobility, an ineffective cough, and a decreased vital capacity. The arterial blood gas (ABG) results indicate metabolic acidosis, which is not an indicator of the patient's respiratory status. An inspiratory force of -20 cm and a tidal volume of 500 mL are normal values.

55. **B** The phrenic nerve is innervated at C_3 - C_5 (spinal nerves), which corresponds to C_4 (bone). Complete lesions at this level would result in respiratory paralysis.

56. **D** In spinal cord injury, early hypoventilation is manifested by ABG level changes. Poor values indicate inadequate oxygenation and ventilation. Cyanosis, a late sign of hypoventilation, may not be an accurate indicator because it may never develop in an anemic patient and is difficult to assess in a black patient.

57. **A** The nurse would not expect the patient with a possible spinal cord injury between T_4 and T_{12} to have bladder and bowel incontinence. An injury to this area typically results in paraplegia of the lower part of the body, including complete loss of motor function in the legs. However, the patient can perform all activities of daily living, achieve mobility with a wheelchair, and transfer easily. The T_{11} to L_2 level is a particularly important area of the cord; sympathetic motor fibers exiting the spinal cord at this level innervate the trigone muscle of the bladder. Thus, injury at this level produces loss of voluntary bowel and bladder control, resulting in retention.

58. **B** If a cervical spinal cord injury is suspected the patient's airway should be opened by a modified jaw-thrust maneuver. This is the safest approach to opening the airway of a patient with a suspected neck injury. The modified jaw-thrust maneuver is accomplished by grasping one of the angles of the patient's lower jaw in each hand and lifting both hands, thus displacing the mandible forward. If the lips close, the lower lip can be retracted with the thumb. The head of the bed should not be tilted because paralysis may ensue. Pulling down the chin alone will not open the airway. A tracheotomy would not be indicated at this time.

59. **A** Loss of motor function in the right arm and leg may indicate a lesion in the pyramidal tract of the left hemisphere. The lateral corticospinal (pyramidal) tract is the most important upper motor neuron tract. Damage to this area results in contralateral motor loss. Middle cerebral artery syndrome is by far the most common of all cerebral occlusions. If the main stem of the middle cerebral artery is occluded, a massive infarction of most of the hemisphere results.

60. **D** The most reliable technique for testing upper extremity motor strength is for the nurse to ask the patient to close his eyes and raise his arms straight in front of him, palms up. The nurse should watch how well this position is maintained. By asking the patient to squeeze her hands, the nurse can assess equality of strength in hand grasps, but this is less accurate than that of arm extension. Observing for spontaneous movement does not assess strength. Testing reflexes assesses the intactness of the reflex arcs.

61. **C** A patient admitted with an injury to the left cerebral hemisphere would exhibit contralateral findings, such as right-sided hemiparesis and hemiplegia, and right homonymous hemianopia (loss of vision in the right half of both visual fields). In an injury to the left cerebral hemisphere accompanied by right-sided visual loss, the eyes deviate to the left to permit better visualization.

62. **A** Pinpoint pupils usually are indicative of a lesion in the pons. Small, bilateral, nonreactive pupils may result from the loss of sympathetic innervation. Parasympathetic innervation remains, causing pupillary constriction. A lesion in the midbrain may result in midposition, nonreactive pupils. Bilateral fixed and dilated pupils are seen in severe cerebral anoxia.

63. **A** Apneustic breathing and pinpoint pupils occur in the patient with an injury, or lesion, of the pons. In apneustic breathing, the patient experiences a prolonged inspiration with a pause at the end of the inspiratory and expiratory cycle.

64. **A** One of the best techniques for assessing meningeal irritation is to elicit Kernig's sign by flexing the patient's leg at the hip and knee, then straightening the knee and watching for pain and resistance. In a patient with meningitis, pain and spasm of the hamstrings occur when any attempt is made to extend the knee. Eliciting Brudzinski's sign is another effective technique to assess meningeal irritation. A positive sign is indicated by the flexing of both legs at the hips and knees in response to passive flexion of the neck and head onto the chest. A stiff neck (nuchal rigidity) and photophobia are other symptoms of meningeal irritation.

65. **B** Instituting isolation precautions is unnecessary and therefore inappropriate for a patient who has just been diagnosed as having viral meningitis. Appropriate interventions would include monitoring the patient's temperature frequently, because fever increases ICP, and instituting seizure precautions, because seizure activity is common in patients with central nervous system infection. A major responsibility in caring for a patient with viral meningitis involves monitoring and managing increased ICP.

66. **A** A common sign of meningococcal meningitis is petechiae. Petechiae, rash, purpuric lesions, or ecchymoses develop in 50% of patients with this condition. Patients with bacterial meningitis may also have fever, headache, lethargy, confusion, irritability, and neck stiffness.

67. **A** Signs of meningeal irritation include: Brudzinski's sign, Kernig's sign and nuchal rigidity. A Babinski's reflex is not associated with meningeal irritation. It is a reflex that indicates pyramidal tract damage, an alteration in the motor tracts of the brain.

Brudzinski's sign: Adduction and flexion of the legs as the patient's neck is flexed

Kernig's sign: When the patient's hip is flexed and the knee is at a right angle, the extension of the patient's leg elicits pain in the hamstring and neck.

Nuchal rigidity: Resistance to flexion of the neck

68. **C** Meningococcus most commonly causes meningitis in your adults. Meningococcal meningitis, which spreads via the nasopharynx by intimate contact or droplets, is the most contagious form of the disease and causes the highest mortality. Haemophilus influenzae is the most common cause of meningitis in children and adults over 45.

69. **A** A patient with neurogenic shock would display the findings of: Hypotension, profound bradycardia, warm, dry skin resulting from the loss of sympathetic response and areflexia.

70. **D** The patient must be removed from the backboard as soon as possible to prevent skin breakdown. To enhance venous return to the heart, elevate the lower extremities and place antiembolic hose. Insertion of gastric and urinary catheters, as well as administration of steroids and atropine, are in the plan of care for the patient with neurogenic shock

OBSTETRIC EMERGENCIES

1. The nurse knows that a slow rate of continuous postpartum vaginal bleeding usually indicates:

A. Cervical laceration
B. Clots in the uterus
C. Retained placental fragments
D. Too-vigorous uterine massage

2. Two hours later, the bleeding decreases but continues to be heavier than normal. The fundus is soft and located above and to the right of the umbilicus. The most appropriate initial nursing intervention would be to:

A. Notify the physician and prepare the patient for a dilation and curettage
B. Record the findings on the patient's chart
C. Encourage voiding and assist the patient in using a bedpan
D. Assist the patient in getting out of bed and encourage her to ambulate

3. A patient has delivered a baby, 1 hour afterwards. A blood pressure of 90/60 mmHg, pulse rate 92 beats/minute, and respiratory rate 16 breaths/minute is noted. She complains of light-headedness and appears restless. The fundus is firm with a moderate amount of lochia rubra. The appropriate nursing action would be to stay with the patient, alert other staff, and:

A. Place the patient in modified Trendelenburg's position and initiate fluid resuscitation
B. Increase IV fluids to 150 mL/hour
C. Obtain a specimen for a second CBC with differential
D. Massage the fundus to remove clots

4. A 26-year-old woman is admitted to the ED with complaints of severe right lower quadrant abdominal pain and moderate, bright-red vaginal bleeding that began as spotting this morning. The patient has not menstruated for 2 months. She has had five or six episodes of nausea without vomiting in the morning. She states she has swollen breasts and occasionally feels fatigued. She thinks she is pregnant but has not yet had a pregnancy test. Her medical history reveals an episode of pelvic inflammatory disease (PID) 3 years ago, which was treated with a course of antibiotic therapy. Vital signs, which are taken every 15 minutes, remain stable: blood pressure is 110/70 mmHg, pulse rate 100 beats/minute, respiratory rate 24 breaths/minute, and temperature 100.6°F (38.1°C). She is pale, but alert and responsive. The physician orders a CBC, type and cross match for 2 units of blood, a radioimmunoassay, and a pelvic ultrasound. The nurse begins an infusion of 1,000 mL of Lactated Ringer's solution, as ordered. Within 2 hours, the laboratory and ultrasound data confirm an ectopic pregnancy. Over 90% of all ectopic pregnancies are located at which site:

A. Fallopian tube
B. Cervix
C. Abdominal cavity
D. Retroperitoneal area

5. Which finding indicates the potential for development of an ectopic pregnancy?

A. Amenorrhea for 8 weeks
B. Nausea without vomiting
C. History of PID
D. Positive radioimmunoassay of human chorionic gonadotropin

6. Which clinical sign of ectopic pregnancy would the nurse expect to note in a patient:

A. Back pain
B. Shoulder and neck pain
C. Leg cramping
D. Intestinal cramping

7. Which nursing action is essential to performing a pelvic ultrasound?

A. Monitoring the patient's vital signs every 15 minutes
B. Increasing the patient's fluid intake before the test
C. Obtaining informed consent
D. Placing the patient on her right side

8. Of the following, which assessment finding indicates that the patient is at risk for postpartum hemorrhage?

A. Blood pressure
B. Home birth
C. High parity
D. Neonatal birth weight

9. Which finding suggests postpartum hemorrhage related to a vaginal laceration?

A. Extramural delivery of an infant weighing 6 lb, 5 oz. (2.9 kg)
B. Vital signs, restlessness, and pallor
C. Blood loss of greater than 500 mL
D. Bright-red bleeding and a firm fundus

10. A 33-year-old woman, P6/G6, is admitted to the ED on a stretcher. She arrived by ambulance approximately 1 hour after an extramural delivery of a healthy, 6lb, 5oz (2.9-kg) girl at home. While assisting with transferring the patient from the ambulance stretcher to the ED stretcher, the ED nurse notes that the sheets under the patient are saturated with bright-red blood. The patient is pale and restless. Her blood pressure is 90/60 mmHg, pulse rate 108 beats/minute, respiratory rate 28 breaths/minute, and temperature 99.6 F (37.5 C). The fundus is firm at the umbilical level. The patient's perineal pad is completely saturated with lochia rubra. Blood loss is estimated at greater than 500 mL. After examining the patient, the physician diagnoses postpartum hemorrhage caused by a vaginal laceration. The priority nursing action at this time would be to assess the patient's:

A. Vital signs
B. Need for oxytocin therapy
C. Response to fundal massage
D. Response to verbal stimuli

11. Which finding would the nurse expect to note when assessing a patient who is bleeding from abruptio placentae?

A. Premature labor
B. Severe abdominal pain
C. Nontender uterus
D. Boggy uterus

12. Any third-trimester vaginal bleeding calls for close fetal monitoring. Which fetal heart rate pattern would alert the nurse to the deterioration in a client's condition?

A. Late decelerations below the normal baseline level
B. Accelerations, to 160 beats/minute, lasting 15 seconds
C. Stable heart rate of 120 beats/minute
D. All of the above

13. If impending shock were suspected in a pregnant patient with vaginal bleeding, the initial nursing action would be to stay with the patient and alert the other staff. The next action would be to:

A. Start an infusion of dextrose 5% in water
B. Monitor the fetal heart rate
C. Position the patient on her right side
D. Massage the fundus

14. During the nursing assessment of an antepartal patient, which blood pressure change would signal the onset of mild preeclampsia?

A. An increase in systolic pressure of 30 mmHg or greater
B. A blood pressure reading of 140/90 mmHg or greater
C. Any increase in diastolic pressure above 90 mmHg
D. A minimum of three consecutive blood pressure measurements above the patient's baseline

15. A woman in the 38th week of pregnancy arrives at the emergency department (ED) complaining of painless vaginal bleeding that occurred, without warning, upon arising this morning. Her abdomen is soft, and her uterus is nontender. The fetal heart rate is assessed at the umbilical level at 120 bears/minute. Based on the patient history and physical findings, the nurse would suspect that the patient has:

A. Abruptio placentae
B. Disseminated intravascular coagulation
C. Spontaneous abortion
D. Placenta previa

16. A woman in the 38th week of pregnancy arrives at the emergency department (ED) complaining of painless vaginal bleeding that occurred, without warning, upon arising this morning. Her abdomen is soft, and her uterus is nontender. The fetal heart rate is assessed at the umbilical level at 120 bears/minute. An appropriate nursing diagnosis for this patient would be:

A. Fluid volume deficit related to uterine rupture
B. Fluid volume deficit related to uterine hemorrhage
C. Altered peripheral tissue perfusion related to abnormal coagulation
D. Spiritual distress related to neonatal death

17. A woman in the 38th week of pregnancy arrives at the emergency department (ED) complaining of painless vaginal bleeding that occurred, without warning, upon arising this morning. Her abdomen is soft, and her uterus is nontender. The fetal heart rate is assessed at the umbilical level at 120 bears/minute. The nurse's highest priority in caring for this patient involves:

A. Preparing for a potential cesarean section
B. Maintaining the patient on strict bed rest and observing for further bleeding
C. Assessing for signs of shock caused by blood loss
D. Avoiding pelvic examinations or the insertion of any foreign objects into the vagina

18. A woman is brought to the ED while in labor. Her membranes had ruptured earlier. Uterine contractions are now occurring every 2 to 3 minutes, lasting approximately 60 to 90 seconds. With the next contraction, the patient experiences the urge to bear down. Pelvic examination indicates the cervix is fully dilated and 100% effaced, the fetal station is + 2, and the presenting part is the head. Which equipment should be available for the delivery?

A. Sterile gloves and scissors, two sterile Kelly clamps, warm blankets, a bulb syringe, and a bag-valve-mask device
B. Sterile gloves and a basin, a sterile Kelly clamp, and a DeLee suction apparatus
C. Sterile gloves and scissors, a sterile Kelly clamp, and 1% lidocaine solution
D. Sterile gloves and scissors and two sterile Kelly clamps

19. Which sign indicates imminent delivery?

A. Bulging of the perineum
B. Crowning of the fetal head
C. Receding of the fetal head between contractions
D. Involuntary bowel movements

20. The nurse instructs the patient to pant or breathe through contractions during the delivery. The primary rationale for this intervention is to:

A. Help the patient to cope with the pain of contractions
B. Avoid fetal hypoxia or distress
C. Avoid a too-rapid or uncontrolled delivery
D. Assist the physician in a more efficient and safe delivery

21. The patient gives birth to a girl. The physician performs an initial neonatal assessment and assigns an Apgar score of 8. Which statement about the Apgar scoring system is true?

A. Scores are assigned immediately after delivery and 10 minutes later
B. Scores are based on assessment of the neonate's heart rate, respiratory effort, muscle tone, reflex irritability, and skin color
C. A score of 1 to 3 is considered excellent
D. All of the above

22. The nurse would expect the first sign of placental separation to be:

A. Lengthening of the umbilical cord
B. A gush of blood from the vagina
C. Rising of the fundus as it contracts and separates from the placenta
D. Shakes and chills

23. A woman in the 36th week of pregnancy arrives at the ED complaining of a persistent headache and a feeling of indigestion. Her blood pressure is 150/100 mmHg. Her ankles show 2+ pitting edema. Urinalysis reveals 3+ proteinuria. She is placed in a quiet, private ED evaluating room, and the physician is notified. While waiting for the physician, the nurse assesses the patient for the possible development of eclampsia. Which finding would the nurse expect to note in a patient with this condition?

A. Blood pressure of 150/100 mmHg
B. Generalized edema
C. Seizures
D. 3+ proteinuria

24. Which intervention would be the nurse's highest priority when caring for an eclamptic patient?

A. Turn the patient on her right side to prevent aspiration
B. Insert an IV line for medication administration
C. Monitor the patient's vital signs continuously
D. Maintain a patent airway and administer supplemental oxygen

25. While waiting for the physician, the nurse assesses a patient for the possible development of eclampsia. The priority nursing diagnosis for this patient at this time would be:

A. Altered renal tissue perfusion related to hypertension
B. Fluid volume excess related to hypertension and edema
C. Fluid volume deficit related to uterine hemorrhage
D. Potential for injury related to seizures

26. The primary rationale for placing a patient, with possible preeclampsia, in a quiet, private room is to:

A. Prevent onset of early labor
B. Reduce external stimuli
C. Protect the patient from becoming emotionally upset by seeing other patients
D. Protect her from infection

27. The physician orders magnesium sulfate at 1 g/hour via a continuous infusion. During the infusion, the nurse should monitor for, and immediately report:

A. A blood pressure of 120/80 mmHg
B. A urine output of 50 mL/hour
C. A respiratory rate less than 12 breaths/minute
D. Increased serum calcium levels

28. Approximately 1 hour prior to arrival at the ED, a 29-year-old has given birth to a normal, healthy girl. Since arriving in the ED, the patient has completely saturated five perineal pads. Her blood pressure is 100/70 mmHg, pulse rate 82 beats/minute and regular; and respiratory rate, 18 breaths/minute. She has no sign of syncope or light-headedness and has not lost consciousness. Blood specimens are sent to the laboratory for a complete blood count (CBC) with differential, electrolyte levels, and type and cross match. Two units of packed red blood cells are available, if necessary. The nurse palpates the fundus and determines that it is soft. Which nursing intervention would be most appropriate at this time?

A. Recheck the patient's vital signs
B. Massage the fundus gently until firm
C. Request an order for oxytocin (Pitocin)
D. Assess the amount of bleeding

29. A patient, post deliver in the ED of a healthy baby boy has had excessive bleeding, with stable vital signs and asymptomatic. No transfusion was necessary, however, blood is available should it be needed. After palpating the fundus, and discovering it is soft, the patient is to be admitted to the medical-surgical unit for further observation. The nurse explains to the patient the reason for the admission. Which of the following best indicates that the patient has understood the explanation:

A. The patient seems to have understood the nurse's explanation
B. The patient verbalizes an understanding of the reason for the admission
C. The patient is resting quietly while awaiting admission
D. The patient's blood pressure stabilizes at 110/70 mmHg

30. Postpartum hemorrhage can occur after either vaginal or C-section deliveries and can be seen anytime from immediately after delivery to several weeks postpartum. What is the most common cause of early postpartum hemorrhage?

A. Retained placental tissue
B. Lacerations of the cervix or vagina
C. Uterine atony
D. Uterine rupture

OBSTETRIC EMERGENCIES: RATIONALE

1. **A** A slow rate of continuous postpartum vaginal bleeding usually indicates a cervical laceration. Lacerations of the vagina, perineum, and labia also can occur. Continued bleeding is typically observed despite efficient postpartum uterine contractions. This requires immediate vaginal inspection because continuous bleeding can lead to hemorrhagic shock. In this situation, the potential for lacerations is increased because the delivery was spontaneous and unattended at home. Retained placental fragments usually result in vaginal bleeding at a fast rate, as may over massaging the uterus. Clots in the uterus may slow or stop bleeding until they are passed.

2. **C** The most appropriate initial action in this situation would be to encourage voiding and assist the patient in using a bedpan. Positioning of the uterus to the right of the umbilicus is a sign of bladder distension, which increases uterine pressure and, in some cases, vaginal bleeding. If the patient cannot urinate on the bedpan, catheterization may be necessary to empty the bladder and control bleeding. Afterward, the nurse should record the amount of urine obtained, the status of the uterus, the presence of bleeding, and the patient's comfort level on the patient's chart.

3. **A** The appropriate nursing action in this situation would be to place the patient in modified Trendelenburg's position because the patient is showing signs of a fluid volume deficit. In this position, the patient's legs would be higher than her head, which would increase circulation back to the heart. Increasing IV fluids, as ordered, and obtaining a new specimen for a CBC and differential are appropriate subsequent interventions. The nurse should keep in mind, however, that this CBC might not be

indicative of the immediate blood loss because it may take several hours for the hemoglobin and hematocrit to drop. Massaging the fundus at this time would be unnecessary because it is already firm. Additionally, the priority is volume resuscitation. The rate of 150 mL/hour is likely not sufficient. The patient should not remain in Trendelenburg for any long period as the baroreceptors in the carotid bodies and in the aortic arch will sense that the pressure is normal and could inhibit the body's compensatory response.

4. **A** Although ectopic pregnancies can also develop at the cervix, ovary, retroperitoneal area, and abdominal cavity, approximately 90% develop in the fallopian tubes. A tubal ectopic pregnancy may result from any condition that causes narrowing or constriction within the fallopian tube. Under such circumstances, the lumen of the fallopian tube is large enough to permit spermatozoa to ascend but not large enough to permit the fertilized ovum to pass downward.

5. **C** A patient with a history of pelvic inflammatory disease (PID), such as the one in this situation, is at increased risk for ectopic pregnancy. Kinking of the fallopian tube, segmental narrowing of the tube, and partial agglutination of the opposing surfaces of the tube can be caused by endometriosis, developmental defects, or inflammatory disorders, such as PID. A positive radioimmunoassay of human chorionic gonadotropin and nausea (with or without vomiting) are signs of pregnancy.

6. **B** The nurse would expect to note shoulder and neck pain that may radiate into sharp lower abdominal pain. Such pain is commonly precipitated by activities that increase abdominal pressure, such as defecation.

7. **B** Increasing the patient's fluid intake before the test is essential for a pelvic ultrasound because filling the bladder lifts the uterus and allows for better visualization of the uterus and other structures. Monitoring vital signs is unnecessary. An informed consent is not required. Usually, the patient is placed in a supine position for this procedure.

8. **C** High parity is considered a predictive assessment factor associated with potential postpartum bleeding; other factors include rapid labor, an overdistended uterus, and a high neonatal birth weight. Any relaxation of the uterine muscle fibers, as occurs in a high-parity patient, gives rise to a continuous oozing of blood, one of the forms of postpartum hemorrhage. Assessing the patient before delivery helps determine the patient's risk of postpartum hemorrhage. In the obstetric designation P6G6, the first number indicates the number of pregnancies; the second indicates the number of full-term deliveries. Blood pressure and home birth are not associated with postpartum hemorrhage.

9. **D** Vaginal lacerations are particularly likely to cause serious bleeding. Bright-red arterial blood and a firm fundus suggest postpartum hemorrhage related to a vaginal laceration; however, a vaginal inspection is necessary to confirm the diagnosis. A firm fundus indicates that the uterine muscle is contracted and an unlikely source of bleeding.

10. **A** The priority nursing action in this situation would be to assess the patient's vital signs for onset of shock. When hemorrhaging occurs, the body activates certain compensatory mechanisms, such as tachycardia and vasoconstriction, to delay the onset of shock. The patient's condition and size determine the amount of blood loss that can be tolerated. However, when hemorrhaging is profuse, compensatory mechanisms can fail

and shock ensues. As shock deepens, restlessness, diaphoresis, cool and clammy skin, tachypnea, unconsciousness, and death may follow. Assessing for response to verbal stimuli would be appropriate if the patient were unconscious or losing consciousness. Oxytocin administration and fundal massage would be inappropriate in this situation because they do not stop bleeding from a vaginal laceration.

11. **B** The bleeding in abruptio placentae is typically accompanied by severe abdominal pain related to changes in the uterus as the placenta separates from the myometrium. This is described as uteroplacental apoplexy, or Couvelaire uterus; a boardlike abdomen accompanies the pain. An extremely tense and painful abdomen indicates placental bleeding into the myometrium; an enlarging uterus may indicate blood accumulating behind the placenta.

12. **A** Any significant changes in the baseline fetal heart rate, which is normally 120 to 160 beats/minute, are significant, particularly late decelerations of any degree. Periodic late decelerations are indicative of fetal hypoxia or anoxia. Accelerations to 160 beats/minute, lasting 15 seconds, and a stable fetal heart rate of 120 beats/minute are considered normal. Periodic baseline accelerations are indicative of an adequate fetal-placental circulation. Any situation that disturbs maternal hemodynamics or the uteroplacental blood flow will eventually affect fetal well-being. Continuous or frequent monitoring with a Doppler ultrasound stethoscope or bell stethoscope is necessary.

13. **B** In this situation, the priority action would be to monitor the fetal heart rate for significant changes from the normal baseline rate and for late decelerations that may indicate dysfunction in uteroplacental blood flow. Positioning the

patient on her left side while monitoring the fetal heart rate minimizes compression of the ascending vena cava by the gravid uterus. Such compression can impede blood return to the right atrium, resulting in a drop in cardiac output and hypotension. An alternative would be to place the patient in a supine position with the right hip elevated. Supplemental oxygen should be provided. An IV infusion of isotonic fluid, such as normal saline or Lactated Ringer's solution, should be started to administer fluids and to allow for medication administration. Massaging or stimulating the fundus is always contraindicated to avoid putting pressure on the presenting part, particularly if it is the placenta.

14. **A** Mild preeclampsia is indicated by an increase in systolic pressure of 30 mmHg or more and an increase in diastolic pressure of 15 mmHg or more on two occasions, at least 6 hours apart. The patient should be maintained on bed rest in the left lateral position during these 6 hours. A pre-pregnancy or first-trimester blood pressure reading is necessary as a baseline level to assess any blood pressure changes in the second or third trimester. Blood pressure normally decreases in the second trimester because of blood volume expansion.

15. **D** Based on the patient's history and physical findings, the nurse would suspect that this patient has placenta previa. Painless vaginal bleeding is the hallmark of placenta previa in women who carry until midterm or later. The degree of placental placement over the internal cervical os determines the bleeding's severity and the onset of the initial episode. Bleeding associated with spontaneous abortion occurs earlier in a pregnancy, usually before the 20th week. Abruptio placentae is usually associated with pain. Disseminated intravascular coagulation most commonly occurs postpartum.

16. **B** An appropriate nursing diagnosis for this patient would be Fluid volume deficit related to uterine hemorrhage because the patient has suffered blood loss caused by premature separation of the placenta from the uterine wall. The other diagnoses are inappropriate because neither uterine rupture nor abnormal coagulation has occurred. Although the fetus is certainly compromised, the situation does not indicate that neonatal death has occurred.

17. **C** The highest priority would be to assess for signs of shock caused by blood loss. This is best accomplished by monitoring the patient's vital signs and obtaining a blood specimen for a complete blood count (CBC) and type and cross match. Two units of blood should be available in case the patient's hemoglobin and hematocrit values decrease significantly. IV fluids, such as Lactated Ringer's or normal saline solution, should be started to replace lost fluids and to prepare an access site for blood transfusion if this becomes necessary. When stabilized, the patient should be restricted to complete bed rest. Perineal pads should be counted to assess further blood loss. A cesarean section may be unnecessary if bleeding is not severe and fetal well-being is maintained. If no emergency exists, the physician should assess maturity of the fetus before delivery is performed. Pelvic examinations are contraindicated in the emergency department because manipulating the cervix without knowing the cause of the problem may result in placental tearing. Any pelvic examination of a patient with suspected placenta previa should be performed in the labor and delivery suite under a "double set-up"; that is, the patient is prepared and draped for a cesarean section and all personnel are ready to operate should hemorrhage occur.

18. **A** The nurse's priorities in an imminent or emergency delivery include establishing effective respirations in the

neonate, maintaining asepsis, and preventing hypothermia. Sterile gloves, scissors, and two sterile Kelly clamps are preferable to maintain asepsis and to clamp and cut the umbilical cord. Warm, dry blankets are used to dry the neonate's face, nose, and mouth and to wrap the neonate's head and body for warmth. If the fetal head is delivered slowly while the thorax is being squeezed in the birth canal, seepage of fluid into the neonate's nose and mouth can occur. A bulb syringe is used to suction the mouth, then the nose. Suctioning the nose first may elicit a reflex inhalation of amniotic fluids into the respiratory tract before the mouth has been cleared. If no respirations are noted, a bag-valve-mask device is used for resuscitation.

19. **B** Crowning, the process by which the vaginal opening completely encircles the neonate's head, is a sign of imminent delivery, especially in a multiparous patient. In a nulliparous patient, delivery may occur up to 30 minutes after crowning occurs. If the amniotic sac is still intact at this point, the nurse will tear it to prevent the neonate from aspirating amniotic fluid with his first respiration. Bulging of the perineum may occur during contractions as the fetus moves down the birth canal; this may not be an indication of imminent delivery. If the fetal head recedes between contractions, the fetus still needs to move further down the vagina before delivery. Although feces may be excreted during contractions, this does not signify immediate delivery.

20. **C** The patient usually is instructed to continue to pant or breathe through contractions and to bear down only when asked to do so, to avoid a too-rapid or uncontrolled delivery, which consequently prevents fetal hypoxia or distress and assists the physician in a more efficient and safe delivery. The nurse typically uses one hand to apply gentle pressure on the

advancing head to control the delivery and prevent a precipitous birth; she uses the other hand to support the patient's perineum and receive the neonate's head as it emerges. Depending on the patient, one or more contractions may be necessary to distend maternal tissues and allow passage of the head through the introitus. The nurse should be sure to maintain a supportive and calm attitude at this time. Usually, the head is delivered between contractions. Breathing through contractions may help the patient to maintain control over the situation and help her to cope with the pain of contractions.

21. **B** The Apgar scoring system, a means of measuring neonatal transition to extrauterine life, is based on assessment of the neonate's heart rate, respiratory effort, muscle tone, reflex irritability, and skin color. Typically, two assessments are performed – one immediately after delivery and another in 5 minutes. At each assessment, the individual categories are rated 0 (poor) to 2 (excellent), then added to reveal the total Apgar score. A score of 0 to 3 indicates that the neonate is in poor condition; 4 to 6, fair condition; and 7 to 10, excellent condition. The heart rate, the most important parameter of a neonate's condition, is typically 150 to 180 beats/minute during the first few minutes after delivery, then quickly subsides to 130 to 140 beats/minute. A rate below 100 beats/minute indicates neonatal asphyxia, for which resuscitative measures may be necessary. Respiratory effort should be assessed with the heart rate; crying is a good indicator of a normal condition. Muscle tone, the degree of flexion and muscle resistance, may be assessed with normal handling after delivery. A normal neonate should not appear flaccid or floppy. Reflex irritability may be assessed by eliciting a cough or gag reflex with the first suctioning effort or by eliciting a startle reflex by tickling the neonate's feet. Most neonates do not appear pink immediately after delivery. Commonly, the extremities are blue and the

torso, pink (acrocyanosis). Providing warmth to the neonate typically reverses this condition.

22. **B** The first sign of placental separation is typically a gush of blood from the vagina. This is followed by lengthening of the umbilical cord and rising of the fundus as the uterus contracts and separates from the placenta. Pushing on the fundus or pulling on the umbilical cord is contraindicated before delivery of the placenta. A patient may feel an uncomfortable contraction as the placenta passes through the cervix. After the placenta is delivered, it must be examined for completeness and the presence of all cotyledons. Shaking and chills are benign phenomena that may occur during the transitional stage of labor or post partum; they are not associated with placental separation.

23. **C** The nurse would expect to note seizures in an eclamptic patient. Choices A, B, and D are all signs of pre-eclampsia. The patient is noted to have progressed from pre-eclampsia to eclampsia at the onset of seizure. Such seizures occur because of the hyper reflexivity associated with preeclampsia. The patient in this situation is exhibiting signs of severe preeclampsia (headache, hypertension, edema, hyperreflexia, proteinuria, and sudden weight gain); however, the severity of symptoms is not always indicative of the potential for seizures. Although seizures are not necessarily life-threatening to the patient, they may result in fetal hypoxia. Efforts toward delivering the fetus should be made after a seizure occurs.

24. **D** The priority action in managing an eclamptic patient is to establish a patent airway and provide supplemental oxygen. The patient should also be positioned on her left side to reduce compression of the inferior vena cava by the enlarged uterus, thereby increasing the blood supply to the fetus. After a patent

airway has been established, the nurse should insert an IV line for medication administration and monitor the patient's vital signs, especially the blood pressure, continuously.

25. **D** Because this patient is at greatest risk for seizures from the hyper reflexivity associated with preeclampsia, the priority nursing diagnosis would be Potential for injury related to seizures. The other diagnoses are inappropriate because altered renal perfusion and fluid volume excess have not been indicated and uterine hemorrhage is not associated with preeclampsia.

26. **B** The primary rationale for placing the patient in a quiet, private room is to reduce external stimuli, because the reduction of environmental stimuli plays an important role in limiting central nervous system (CNS) stimulation and preventing seizures.

27. **C** The nurse should monitor for and immediately report a respiratory rate of less than 12 breaths/minute, because respiratory depression may indicate that the patient is receiving too much of the medication. Magnesium sulfate, a CNS depressant, reduces synaptic activity at the neuromuscular junction and helps prevent convulsions. Assessment parameters include respirations, deep tendon reflexes, and urine output. An absent or sluggish patellar reflex also suggests overdose. Serum magnesium levels should be checked every 4 to 6 hours to maintain therapeutic levels of 4 to 7 mg/dL; levels above 20 mg/dL can result in cardiac arrest. Usual dosage is 4 to 6 g IV, given over 10 minutes, followed by a continuous infusion of 1 to 2 g/hour; or 4 g IM every 4 hours. Calcium gluconate should be available at the bedside to reverse the effects of magnesium sulfate, if necessary. A blood pressure of 120/80 mmHg and a urine output of 50 mL/hour are normal. Use of magnesium sulfate may result in hypocalcemia.

28. **B** The most appropriate nursing intervention at this time would be to massage the fundus until it is firm. Bleeding soon after delivery usually is caused by uterine atony. Massaging the fundus stimulates the myometrium to contract, promoting hemostasis, and clot expulsion. The nurse should always use two hands to massage the fundus: one hand to anchor the lower uterine segment just above the symphysis pubis, and the other hand to gently massage the fundus. Anchoring the lower segment of the uterus provides support because the uterus may be relaxed after delivery. Using gentle massage helps prevent partial or complete uterine prolapse. If massage is ineffective, oxytocin may be ordered; over massage may cause muscle fatigue and relaxation. Some physicians routinely use IM or IV oxytocin after delivery to aid in uterine contraction. Nipple stimulation from breastfeeding also helps to promote uterine tone and hemostasis. Rechecking vital signs and the amount of bleeding are considered additional secondary interventions.

29. **B** The best indication that the patient has understood the nurse's explanation is a verbalization of her understanding of the reason for admission. Explaining to the patient the reason for treatment and care and ensuring that the patient understands the reason are part of the nurse's responsibilities. Because the nurse is the health professional who typically spends the most time with the patient and can best evaluate the patient's comprehension, the nurse is liable for the patient's understanding. The nurse must document that the patient can verbalize an understanding of what is taught or, if it is a specific skill, demonstrate what has been taught. Noting that the patient seems to understand the explanation is based on the nurse's perception, not the patient's acknowledgment that she understands. Objective data, such as a blood pressure measurement or observing that the patient is resting quietly, do not reflect that learning has occurred.

30. **C** Uterine atony, loss of tone of the uterine musculature, accounts for the vast majority (nearly 90%) of all postpartum bleeding complications. Retained placental tissue, uterine rupture, and lacerations of the cervix and/or vagina are all common complications but occur with much less frequency.

ORGAN DONATION

1. In terms of organ donation, the word tissue commonly refers to:

A. All organs
B. Organs, eyes, and bone
C. Skin only
D. Eyes, bone, skin, and heart valves

2. The emergency department nurse knows that the responsibilities of an organ procurement coordinator include:

A. Managing the organ donor
B. Communicating with the donor's family
C. Coordinating organ retrieval
D. All of the above

3. Which statement about brain death is true?

A. It is defined as the irreversible cessation of entire brain function, including brain stem function
B. A patient in a deep coma is considered brain-dead
C. A patient in a persistent vegetative state is considered brain-dead
D. Brain death is not a necessary criterion for organ retrieval

4. Brain death should be declared:

A. Before retrieving organs and discontinuing ventilator support
B. After retrieving organs but before discontinuing ventilator support
C. After retrieving organs and discontinuing ventilator support
D. None of the above

5. Legally, the time of death is when:

A. The second brain-death note is placed on the donor's chart
B. The ventilator is turned off in the operating room
C. The first brain-death note is placed on the donor's chart
D. The donor's heart is removed during organ retrieval

6. The nurse is aware that most organ donors die from:

A. Severe head injuries
B. Cardiopulmonary arrest
C. Myocardial infarction
D. Respiratory arrest

7. Consent for organ donation must be given by:

A. The potential donor before his death
B. The legal next of kin
C. Any member of the potential donor's family
D. The physician

8. The nurse understands that kidney donations usually are accepted from persons:

A. Aged 2 to 60
B. Aged 15 to 50
C. Under age 50
D. Of any age

9. For solid organ retrieval to be effective, the donor must have:

A. An intact heartbeat
B. Adequate blood pressure
C. Mechanical ventilator support
D. All of the above

10. A urine output greater than the IV fluid intake in a potential organ donor is indicative of which condition?

A. Fluid overload
B. Diabetes insipidus
C. Polyuric phase of renal failure
D. Adequate renal function

11. Which condition does not initially contribute to hypotension in an organ donor?

A. Brain stem herniation
B. Collapse of peripheral vascular resistance
C. Therapeutic dehydration
D. Disseminated intravascular coagulation

12. Which situation would not fall under the jurisdiction of the medical examiner?

A. Death by homicide
B. Death by suicide
C. Death by accidental traumatic injury
D. Death by a witnessed cardiac arrest in a person known to have cardiovascular disease

13. Which rationale best describes the reason for administering 1 g of methylprednisolone sodium succinate (Solu-Medrol) IV to a potential organ donor?

A. To decrease the body's inflammatory response
B. To stabilize the kidney membrane during organ retrieval
C. To help prevent infection
D. To prevent tissue rejection

14. The nurse knows that evaluation of a potential organ recipient is based on all of the following criteria except:

A. Urgency of need
B. ABO blood-group compatibility
C. Sex
D. Tissue typing

15. The nurse is aware that most people over age 65 are ineligible for heart transplantation because:

A. They are not within the age limit for organ recipients
B. They typically have little or no health insurance
C. They typically have poor health
D. Their life expectancy will not increase substantially to warrant transplantation

16. Who may be considered for tissue donation?

A. Any patient who dies in a hospital
B. An individual referred within 6 to 12 hours after a cardiac-
   related death
C. Deceased patients of any age
D. All of the above

17. Which age group is the established parameter for lung
donation?

A. Newborn to age 40
B. Ages 2 to 50
C. Ages 4 to 60
D. Ages 10 to 50

18. Which age group is the established parameter for bone
donation?

A. Ages 2 to 50
B. Ages 15 to 65
C. Ages 20 to 50
D. All ages

19. Which age group is the established parameter for eye
donation?

A. Newborn to age 65
B. Ages 6 to 55
C. Ages 10 to 90
D. All ages

20. When caring for a potential organ donor, the nurse should keep in mind that norepinephrine (Levophed) and epinephrine should not be used as vasopressors because they:

A. Are extremely potent vasoconstrictors and may cause kidney and liver damage
B. Cannot be metabolized by a dying patient
C. Are ineffective in a brain-dead patient
D. Cause donor reactions

21. The nurse knows that the cost of organ retrieval is paid by the:

A. Donor's family
B. Donating hospital
C. Transplant center
D. Federal government

22. Which conditions are not considered contraindications for organ donation?

A. Urinary tract infection and intracranial cancer
B. Sepsis and IV drug abuse
C. Metastatic cancer
D. Human immunodeficiency virus infection and heroin addiction

23. The goals of donor maintenance include ensuring:

A. Adequate ventilation
B. Hemodynamic stability
C. Asepsis
D. All of the above

24. When discussing organ donation with a potential donor's family, the nurse should focus on:

A. Details about the intended recipient
B. Details relating to the surgical procedure
C. The monetary value of the organs to be transplanted
D. The positive aspects of transplantation

25. Which organ is commonly associated with the term living related donor?

A. Liver
B. Heart
C. Kidney
D. Pancreas

26. Which nursing intervention is most appropriate for kidney donor maintenance?

A. Maintaining a systolic blood pressure of 100 to 110 mmHg
B. Maintaining a urine output greater than 100 mL/hour
C. Maintaining adequate ventilation
D. All of the above

27. When should the organ procurement agency be notified about a potential donor?

A. After consent is obtained
B. When the operating room is ready
C. As soon as a potential donor is identified
D. When the physician orders

28. The nurse would expect all of the following patients to be considered potential organ donors except:

A. A 35-year-old man with acquired immunodeficiency syndrome and a self-inflicted gunshot wound to the head
B. A 2-year-old near-drowning victim with hypoxic encephalopathy
C. A 56-year-old man with a massive intraventricular hemorrhage
D. A 14-year-old boy with massive head injuries and chest trauma

29. The nurse is aware that a thorough medical history can prove invaluable because:

A. It can help predict future organ functioning in the recipient
B. It can give important information to the recipient about the donor
C. It can help determine the existence of a disorder that may preclude organ donation
D. It is necessary for accurate record keeping

30. The nurse knows that a potential organ donor under age 5 may require extended observation because:

A. A young child has increased resistance to brain damage and may recover
B. Federal law mandates it
C. This type of observation is comforting to the parents
D. Test results of a young child typically are difficult to interpret

ORGAN DONATION: RATIONALE

1. **D** In terms of organ donation, tissue typically refers to eyes, bone, skin, and heart valves. Tissue transplantation does not require a heart-beating donor, whereas organ transplantation does.

2. **D** An organ procurement coordinator is responsible for managing the organ donor, coordinating organ retrieval, and communicating with the deceased donor's family. Other responsibilities include public and professional education and the development of organ donation programs in hospitals.

3. **A** Brain death is the irreversible cessation of entire brain function, including brain stem function. Clinical criteria for establishing brain death include the absence of all cortical brain stem function, including cerebral responses to light, noise, motion, and pain; reflexes or muscle activity; spontaneous respirations; and cranial nerve reflexes and responses. Neither a comatose patient nor a patient in a persistent vegetative state is considered brain-dead because brain stem function still exists. A patient in a persistent vegetative state typically has severe, irreversible damage to the higher brain centers; however, the brain stem remains intact.

4. **A** Brain death should be declared before retrieving organs and discontinuing ventilator support. Two attending physicians are necessary to declare a patient brain-dead. In many cases, however, brain death is a necessary criterion for organ retrieval.

5. **A** Legally, the time of death is when the second brain-death note is placed on the patient's chart. No notation or pronouncement of death should be made in the operative note.

The potential donor must be declared brain-dead before entering the operating room.

6. **A** Most organ donors die from severe head injuries. Some, patients who die from cardiopulmonary reasons are excluded from organ donation, but in many cases may donate tissue.

7. **B** In the absence of consent by the patient, the consent for organ donation must then be given by the legal next of kin, including (in order of priority) the patient's spouse, an adult brother or sister, the patient's legal guardian at the time of death, and a representative appointed by a court of competent jurisdiction who has ascertained that no person of higher priority exists who objects to organ donation. The Anatomical Gift Act states that a driver's license or living will can be used as consent.

8. **A** Kidney donations usually are accepted from persons aged 2 to 60. Because the kidneys of children under age 2 are immature, they usually are unacceptable for donation; this policy, however, may vary, depending on the procurement center. The kidneys of those over age 60 are at increased risk for kidney disease and therefore are unacceptable for donation.

9. **D** For solid organ (heart, kidney, lung, or liver) retrieval to be effective, the organ donor must have an intact heartbeat, adequate blood pressure, and effective mechanical ventilator support. These criteria are necessary to maintain the proper organ function and adequate tissue oxygenation and perfusion required for effective organ procurement.

10. **B** A urine output greater than the IV fluid intake in a potential organ donor indicates diabetes insipidus. This endocrine disorder, commonly seen in those who have

sustained a severe head injury, typically results from the impaired ability of the hypothalamus to produce antidiuretic hormone (ADH) or the posterior pituitary gland to secrete ADH because of increased intracranial pressure. Decreased or absent ADH levels prevent the kidneys from reabsorbing water back into systemic circulation. This causes an increase in urine output, which is typically greater than the patient's fluid intake.

11. **D** Disseminated intravascular coagulation (DIC) does not contribute to the development of hypotension in an organ donor; this disorder commonly results from prolonged hypotension but does not cause it. Hypotension, the most common complication during postmortem organ donor management, may result from brain stem herniation, collapse of peripheral vascular resistance, and therapeutic dehydration. In an organ donor, brain stem herniation may impair the medulla's vasomotor center, resulting in decreased blood vessel tone and eventual collapse of peripheral vascular resistance. Hypotension typically results from therapeutic dehydration caused by such intravascular depletion. Prolonged hypotension in an organ donor may cause cardiac death, acute tubular necrosis in transplanted kidneys, or DIC.

12. **D** A witnessed cardiac arrest in a person known to have cardiovascular disease would not normally fall under the jurisdiction of the medical examiner. The medical examiner would be responsible for investigating any death resulting from an unknown cause, a suspected homicide, a suicide, or an accidental traumatic injury. The medical examiner typically gives consent for organ retrieval except when removal of a particular organ may inhibit the investigation.

13. **B** Methylprednisolone sodium succinate is commonly administered IV to a potential organ donor because it stabilizes

the kidney membrane during the retrieval process. This medication should be given immediately before retrieving the organ in the operating room.

14. **C** Sex is not one of the criteria used when evaluating a potential organ recipient, because it has no bearing on the selection process. The most important criterion governing recipient selection is urgency of need, followed by ABO blood-group compatibility and tissue typing. Blood-group compatibility is the most important physiologic criterion involved in the selection process. Age usually is the second factor considered. Body size also is a necessary criterion for matching heart and liver recipients. Body size and tissue typing are necessary criteria for kidney transplants.

15. **C** With few exceptions, those over age 65 are ineligible for heart transplantation because they typically have poor health. Because of the tremendous shortage of organ donors, transplant candidates must be chosen carefully, with special consideration given to the potential recipient's overall health status. The ability to comply with changes in diet, drug regimens, and life-style also must be evaluated when considering a potential candidate.

16. **D** A patient of any age who dies in a hospital or a person who is referred within 6 to 12 hours after a cardiac death may be considered for tissue donation. If the tissue is not used for transplantation, it may be used for research.

17. **D** The age parameters for lung donation are ages 10 to 50. This range provides for lung maturity as well as optimal lung health.

18. **B** The age parameters for bone donation are ages 15 to 65. Before age 15, bone growth typically is incomplete. After age 65, bone strength tends to deteriorate, particularly in women, from osteoporosis.

19. **D** No age limit exists for eye donation. Eye tissue not used for corneal transplantation may be used for research.

20. **A** Norepinephrine and epinephrine should not be used as vasopressors in a potential organ donor because they are extremely potent vasoconstrictors and may cause kidney and liver damage. In case of severe hypotension, however, they may be used. The extreme vasopressor action of these medications produces marked vasoconstriction, resulting in acute tubular necrosis of the kidneys, and severely decreases blood flow to the liver, causing irreversible organ engorgement.

21. **C** The cost of organ retrieval is paid by the receiving transplant center. The donor's family, the donating hospital, and the federal government do not pay for organ donation retrieval.

22. **A** Urinary tract infection and intracranial cancer are not considered contraindications for organ donation. If a potential organ donor has evidence of a urinary tract infection, the ureters can be cultured during the retrieval process; the recipient can then be treated with appropriate antibiotics. A patient with intracranial cancer can donate organs as long as the cancer is confined to the cranium. Although pneumonia is a contraindication for lung donation, it does not affect other types of donation. Such conditions as sepsis, IV drug abuse, human immunodeficiency virus (HIV) infection, and metastatic cancer are contraindications for all types of organ donation.

23. **D** The goals of donor maintenance include ensuring adequate ventilation, hemodynamic stability, and asepsis. Adequate ventilation and hemodynamic stability are necessary for proper tissue perfusion and oxygenation. Asepsis is necessary because the organ recipient is immunosuppressed and likely to become further suppressed once antirejection drugs have been started; the introduction of microorganisms to his already-compromised system may be detrimental.

24. **D** When discussing organ donation with a potential donor's family, the nurse should limit the discussion to the positive aspects of transplantation as well as to answering their questions about brain death. Details about the potential organ recipient are strictly confidential. The family should not be concerned with surgical techniques or the monetary value of organs. They should understand that organ donation involves no cost or monetary compensation. Primary nursing concerns include offering the family clear, concise, and nontechnical explanations as well as supportive measures, such as a quiet, private room; pastoral support; and time alone with the donor.

25. **C** Living related donor is the term used to describe a person who donates one kidney to a blood relative, typically a son, daughter, mother, father, sister, or brother.

26. **D** Nursing interventions related to kidney donor maintenance include maintaining a systolic blood pressure of 100 to 110 mmHg, a urine output greater than 100 mL/hour, and adequate ventilation. All these interventions are necessary to ensure proper kidney perfusion and function and tissue oxygenation.

27. **C** The organ procurement agency should be notified as soon as a potential donor is identified. The procurement coordinator

is specially trained to assess the person and to approach the family tactfully.

28. **A** A 35-year-old man with acquired immunodeficiency syndrome (AIDS) and a self-inflicted gunshot wound to the head would not be an acceptable candidate for organ donation because AIDS, which is caused by HIV, is a contraindication for all types of organ donation. All of the other patients in this situation are likely candidates for organ donation.

29. **C** A thorough medical history of a potential organ donor can prove invaluable because it can help determine the existence of a disorder that may preclude organ donation. A good medical history can give evidence of chronic renal impairment, previous myocardial injury, or alcohol abuse, which could exclude the patient as a kidney, heart, or liver donor.

30. **A** A child's brain is typically more resilient to brain damage than an older child's or adult's and may recover even after brain function appears lost. Electroencephalograms and cerebral arteriography may be necessary.

ORTHOPEDIC EMERGENCIES

1. Which early complication should the nurse assess for in a patient with a femoral shaft fracture:

A. Delayed union
B. Nonunion
C. Fat embolism
D. Infection

2. The nurse knows that the most serious complication of a femoral shaft fracture to assess for in a child would be:

A. Post-traumatic avascular necrosis
B. Volkmann's ischemia of nerves and muscles
C. Nonunion
D. Progressive coxa vara

3. Which primary treatment would the nurse expect a child between ages 2 and 9 with an uncomplicated femoral shaft fracture to receive?

A. Bryant's skin traction
B. Fixed skeletal traction
C. A double-hip spica cast
D. Intramedullary nailing

4. Which pelvic fracture is considered stable (minor)?

A. Straddle fracture
B. Malgaigne's hemipelvis fracture-dislocation
C. Combined hemipelvis fracture
D. Fracture of the ipsilateral rami

5. The nurse would prepare all of the following patients with a pelvic fracture for surgery except for the patient with:

A. A bilateral pelvic fracture
B. An open pelvic fracture
C. A major vessel injury
D. Hypovolemic shock

6. The nurse would expect which patient to be at highest risk for a pelvic fracture:

A. A 16-year-old boy who sustained a football-related injury
B. An 80-year-old woman who fell while walking in a nursing home
C. A 30-year-old man who was involved in a motorcycle accident
D. A 30-year-old man who fell from a window, landing on his feet

7. Which complication is considered most severe in a patient with a fractured pelvis?

A. Pneumothorax
B. Ruptured bladder
C. Intestinal perforation
D. Bleeding from iliac vessels

8. Which technique would be inappropriate for stabilizing a severely displaced pelvic fracture in the early resuscitative period?

A. External fixation
B. Internal fixation
C. Medical antishock trousers (MAST, or a pneumatic antishock garment) application
D. Skeletal traction

9. The nurse notes blood at the urethral meatus while assessing a male patient with a pelvic fracture. This indicates that:

A. Indwelling urinary catheterization is necessary
B. Indwelling urinary catheterization is contraindicated
C. The bladder has been traumatized
D. The patient has a retroperitoneal hematoma

10. The principle clinical effects of MAST for a patient with multiple injuries, including a pelvic fracture, include all of the following except:

A. Hemostasis (tamponade)
B. Autotransfusion
C. Decreased venous return
D. Increased peripheral vascular resistance

11. Which finding would the nurse expect to see in a patient with an impacted femoral neck fracture:

A. Groin pain on the affected side and limited range of motion in the affected leg
B. Shortening and external rotation of the affected leg
C. Severe leg pain and inability to bear weight
D. Severe thigh swelling

12. Which type of injury would most likely be placed in traction?

A. Tibia/Fibula fracture
B. Mid-shaft femur fracture
C. Obvious deformity to the ankle
D. Dislocated patella

13. A patient arrives at the ED on a stretcher via an ambulance after involvement in a head-on automobile accident. The mechanism of injury was a force to the flexed knee with the hip in flexion. The patient reports that his knee struck the dashboard. During assessment, the nurse notes the affected leg is shortened, internally rotated, and adducted. The patient complains of severe hip pain on the affected side. Based on the assessment findings, the nurse suspects that this patient has:

A. A posterior hip dislocation
B. An anterior hip dislocation
C. A central acetabular fracture-dislocation
D. A pelvic fracture

14. The nurse knows that the prognosis for a patient with a posterior hip dislocation will have a successful recovery if the injury is reduced within the first:

A. 6 hours
B. 12 hours
C. 18 hours
D. 24 hours

15. A patient arrives at the ED on a stretcher via an ambulance after involvement in a head-on automobile accident. The mechanism of injury was a force to the flexed knee with the hip in flexion. The patient reports that his knee struck the dashboard. During assessment, the nurse notes the affected leg is shortened, internally rotated, and adducted. The patient complains of severe hip pain on the affected side. Which nursing diagnosis is most appropriate for this patient?

A. Potential fluid volume deficit related to hemorrhage from pelvic fracture
B. Potential for injury related to sciatic nerve damage
C. Altered patterns of urinary elimination related to urethral trauma
D. Alteration in tissue perfusion of affected leg related to compartment syndrome

16. A patient arrives at the ED on a stretcher via an ambulance after involvement in a head-on automobile accident. The mechanism of injury was a force to the flexed knee with the hip in flexion. The patient reports that his knee struck the dashboard. During assessment, the nurse notes the affected leg is shortened, internally rotated, and adducted. The patient complains of severe hip pain on the affected side. Which of the following is an expected outcome for the above nursing diagnosis:

A. The patient will have normal hemoglobin and hematocrit levels
B. The patient will have no sign of blood at the urethral meatus
C. The patient will maintain a urine output of at least 30 mL/hr
D. The patient will be able to move the affected leg with intact sensation

17. A 24-year-old man who is wearing a football uniform enters the ED. He is holding his right arm by his side and appears to be uncomfortable. He reports that he was injured during a game and developed sudden, severe right shoulder pain. The patient resists any passive movement and has a loss of shoulder symmetry. Based on the above assessment, the nurse suspects that the patient has:

A. An anterior shoulder dislocation
B. A posterior shoulder dislocation
C. A fractured clavicle
D. An acute tear of the rotator cuff

18. The nurse determines that no injury has occurred to the ulnar nerve based on which assessment finding:

A. Ability to oppose the thumb
B. Intact sensation to the smallest finger
C. Intact sensation to the palmar aspect of the thumb
D. Intact sensation to the tip of the index finger

19. When relaying discharge instructions, the nurse should advise the patient to apply which treatment over the next 48 hours:

A. Ice
B. Moist heat
C. Heating pad
D. Ethyl chloride spray

20. Which statement indicates that the patient understands the nurse's discharge instructions for a shoulder dislocation?

A. "I should apply the treatment for 2 hours at a time"
B. "I should return to the hospital if my arm feels numb"
C. "I should expect the pain to get real bad"
D. "I should move my arm around as much as I can tolerate"

21. A 25-year-old man is transported to the ED after striking a lamppost while driving a motorcycle. His vital signs are stable, and he is alert and oriented. His right leg is splinted. The nurse examines the patient's leg and notes gross deformity. About 2" (5 cm) of the tibia is exposed, and dirt and shreds of denim are found in the open wound. The foot is warm, the dorsalis pedis and posterior tibial pulses are strong. Sensations are intact. X-rays reveal a comminuted fracture of the midshaft tibia and fibula. The nurse would expect the physician to order all of the following treatments for this patient except:

A. Antibiotic administration
B. Preparation for surgery
C. Cast application
D. Continuous leg splinting while the patient is in the ED

22. A 25-year-old man is transported to the ED after striking a lamppost while driving a motorcycle. His vital signs are stable, and he is alert and oriented. His right leg is splinted. The nurse examines the patient's leg and notes gross deformity. About 2" (5 cm) of the tibia is exposed, and dirt and shreds of denim are found in the open wound. The foot is warm, the dorsalis pedis and posterior tibial pulses are strong. Sensations are intact. X-rays reveal a comminuted fracture of the midshaft tibia and fibula. Which nursing diagnosis is most appropriate for the patient in this situation?

A. Fluid volume deficit related to vascular injury of the right lower leg
B. Altered tissue perfusion related to nerve damage of the right lower leg
C. Potential for infection related to wound contamination
D. Altered cerebral tissue perfusion related to cranial trauma

23. While caring for a patient who suffered a femur fracture three days earlier, you notice a rash to the chest. Several minutes later you notice tachypnea restlessness and confusion. The most likely cause to be alert for is:

A. Sepsis
B. Hypovolemia
C. Fat embolism
D. Pneumonia

24. A middle-aged man presents to the emergency room with complaints of elbow pain after a participating in a company basketball tournament. The nurse should expect care of this patient to include:

A. Evacuation of collected fluids from the joint
B. Instruction of proper antibiotic prescription use
C. Preparation for corticosteroid injection
D. Application of a compression dressing

25. What type of skull fracture is one in which the skull breaks into many small pieces?

A. Comminuted
B. Depressed
C. Compound
D. Basilar

26. To achieve the best outcomes and maintain the most tissue viability, an amputated limb should be cooled to what temperature before reattachment?

A. 0.0 C
B. 4°C
C. 14°C
D. 20°C

27. Which of the following would not be among the recommended treatment for a patient with an acute shoulder dislocation?

A. Manual reduction
B. Immobilization
C. Heating pad for pain relief
D. Cold compress to reduce swelling

28. When would be appropriate to advise the use of a heating pad for relief of pain with a strained muscle?

A. Immediately after the injury
B. In the first 48 hours after the injury
C. After the first 48 hours since the injury has passed
D. Never

29. Which one of the following fractures in an 8-month-old child is most likely associated with physical abuse?

A. Spiral leg fracture
B. Compressed vertebral fracture
C. Monteggia's fracture
D. Galeazzi fracture

30. The definition of a greenstick fracture is:

A. A type of pathologic fracture.
B. A fracture only on one side of the shaft of a bone.
C. A fractured bone that is exposed outside the skin.
D. Characterized by a spiral break on a bone

1. **C** The nurse should assess for development of fat embolism, caused by the mobilization of fat from the bone marrow into the vascular bed, and for shock - early complications in a patient with a femoral shaft fracture. Because the femur is the largest bone in the body and the shaft is extremely strong, the patient would have to sustain a violent, direct injury to fracture the femoral shaft. Internal hemorrhage and ensuing shock should be expected and must be treated expeditiously. The patient typically has a markedly swollen and deformed thigh with this type of fracture. Considerable soft tissue damage and blood loss of up to 1,000 mL is common. Because a femoral shaft fracture is completely unstable, the leg should be immobilized with Thomas' splint during the emergency treatment phase. Splinting helps to relieve pain and prevent additional injury to the soft tissue. The patient is likely to have associated injuries in the same leg; X-rays of the joints above and below the injury must be taken. Persistent knee stiffness is a troublesome late complication. The quadriceps muscle or patella may adhere to the distal femur and require surgical release. Nonunion, delayed union, and infection are considered late complications. Nonunion without infection is rare. Delayed union is an indication for bone grafting.

2. **B** In a child, the most serious complication of a femoral shaft fracture is Volkmann's ischemia of nerves and muscles, which typically results from femoral arterial spasm secondary to an intimal tear. Signs and symptoms include pain, pallor, puffiness, pulseless, paresthesia, and paralysis. Analgesics typically mask these signs and should be avoided. The nurse should assess for severe, constant pain, especially in the calf. This pain may be worsened by excessive traction. If Volkmann's ischemia is suspected, encircling bandages should

be removed, thereby restoring circulation. Nonunion and progressive coxa vara may occur in a child with a femoral neck fracture. These complications typically result from nonuse or inadequate use of internal skeletal traction. Post-traumatic avascular necrosis, a complication that develops in about 30% of children with this type of injury, may result from disruption of the blood supply to the femoral head at the time of injury.

3. **C** The nurse would expect a child between ages 2 and 9 to be treated with a double-hip spica cast after stabilization for 24 hours in Buck's traction. Bryant's skin traction, an overhead traction applied to both legs, is typically used for children under age 2. This type of traction is not used in older children because of the high risk of femoral arterial spasm and ensuing Volkmann's ischemia of nerves and muscles. Fixed (balanced-suspension) skeletal traction is typically used for children over age 9 or for whom a hip spica cast is impractical. Intramedullary nailing would be considered only after the child is skeletally mature, typically, by age 18, although X-rays should confirm skeletal maturity.

4. **D** A fracture of the ipsilateral rami is considered a stable (minor) pelvic fracture. Stable fractures, which are uncommon in patients with multiple trauma, commonly result from low-energy or well-localized injury to the pelvis. They typically fall into one of two categories: fractures involving individual bones without a break in the continuity of the pelvic ring (such as an avulsion fracture or a fracture of the pubic bone, ischium, iliac wing, sacrum, or coccyx) or fractures with a single break in the pelvic ring (such as a fracture of two ipsilateral rami or a fracture near or subluxation of the sacroiliac joint). Unstable (major) pelvic fractures, most common in patients with multiple trauma, result in a double break of the pelvic ring. Such fractures include straddle fractures, which involve a break of

the bilateral superior and inferior rami and are commonly associated with a high incidence of complications; Malgaigne's hemipelvis fracture dislocation, which involves double vertical breaks in the pelvic ring, and combined hemipelvis fractures.

5. **A** The nurse would not expect to prepare a patient with a bilateral pelvic fracture for surgery. This type of fracture is usually reduced by skeletal traction of the legs. Direct surgical management of pelvic fractures would be indicated for a patient with an open fracture or major vessel injury or for a patient in hypovolemic shock. An open fracture requires debridement, removal of contaminated material, and application of an external fixation device. Internal fixation may be performed later, after cardiopulmonary stability has been achieved. Major vessel injury, although uncommon in a patient with blunt pelvic trauma, is commonly associated with hypovolemic shock and thus requires surgical control. Severe shock after blunt trauma also requires endotracheal intubation, chest tube insertion, institution of two large-bore IV lines, application of medical antishock trousers (MAST, or a pneumatic antishock garment), and blood volume replacement once bleeding sites are identified and blood loss is estimated.

6. **C** The nurse would expect a 30-year-old man who was involved in a motorcycle accident to be at highest risk for a fractured pelvis. Any patient involved in a motorcycle or an automobile accident, either as a passenger or a pedestrian, should be considered at high risk for this type of fracture. Others at risk include those involved in crush injuries to the abdomen. A football-related injury usually involves the shoulders or knees. An injury sustained by an older person while walking usually involves the hip. Landing on the feet after falling from a window usually results in spinal trauma.

7. **D** The most severe complication in a patient with a fractured pelvis would be bleeding from the iliac vessels. Other, less severe complications include damage to the gastrointestinal or genitourinary systems, such as intestinal perforation or ruptured bladder. Pneumothorax usually is not associated with pelvic fractures unless chest trauma has also been incurred.

8. **B** Internal fixation would be inappropriate for stabilizing a severely displaced pelvic fracture in the early resuscitative period. Because a severely displaced pelvic or acetabular fracture typically involves massive hemorrhage (the patient may incur a blood loss of as much as 5,000 mL), appropriate methods of stabilization include external skeletal fixation (application of a Hoffman device), MAST application, or skeletal traction. External skeletal fixation, perhaps the optimal method of treating pelvic ring fractures, helps to decrease post traumatic bleeding when the device is applied during the early resuscitative period. This type of fixation also relieves fracture pain and provides adequate immobilization. MAST immobilizes the fracture and prevents further damage to retroperitoneal tissues from sharp bony fragments. External compression of the pelvic ring forces bone fragments against one other and slows bleeding from cancellous bone. MAST may partially reduce the fracture and decrease intrapelvic volume, thereby resulting in tamponade of the retroperitoneal space. Pelvic ring fractures also may be treated with skeletal traction, a pelvic sling, or a hip spica cast. Because these devices involve prolonged bed rest, late pulmonary, urologic, and soft tissue complications are possible. Open reduction and internal fixation should be carried out within the first week, after the patient is hemodynamically stable. This method is not used during the early resuscitative period because of the procedure's complexity and the likelihood of significant blood loss.

9. **B** Blood at the tip of the urethral meatus in a male patient indicates urethral injury; therefore, indwelling urinary catheterization is contraindicated until the continuity of the urethra bas been confirmed. Blood at the urethral meatus or vagina in a female patient may indicate an occult open fracture of the pelvis. Although, pelvic fractures have been associated with injuries to the rectum, bladder, and male urethra. Bladder trauma typically results in hematuria, not frank bleeding from the urethral meatus. Although retroperitoneal bleeding is difficult to assess, signs and symptoms may include ecchymoses, tenderness over the flank area, and signs of fluid loss.

10. **C** Decreased venous return is not one of the clinical effects of MAST application for a patient with multiple injuries. Clinical effects include hemostasis (tamponade), autotransfusion, and increased peripheral vascular resistance. Though MAST use is controversial the combined effects of its use can produce decreased blood loss, increased venous return, and improved mean arterial pressure. Hemostasis occurs because the external pressure reduces the vessel wall pressure, allowing a clot to form. The volume of autotransfusion using MAST has been estimated at 250 to 1,000 ml.

11. **A** The nurse would expect to note groin pain on the affected side and limited range of motion in the affected leg of a patient with an impacted femoral neck fracture. The patient with this type of fracture typically complains of pain in the groin or medial knee and walks with a painless limp; he may feel slight discomfort with active or passive range of motion. Limited range of motion typically results from muscle spasms associated with this type of injury. No shortening or external rotation of the leg should be noted on physical examination. Shortening and external rotation of the affected leg is

commonly associated with displaced femoral neck fractures and intertrochanteric fractures. In a displaced femoral neck fracture, the patient typically has severe pain and cannot bear weight on the affected leg because of the instability of the fracture. Because blood infiltrates the joint rather than the soft tissue, swelling usually is not noted. In an intertrochanteric fracture, the thigh will appear swollen from extracapsular bleeding into the soft tissues.

12. **B** Skeletal traction is most commonly used to treat fractures of the femur, most commonly in the pre-hospital, pre-surgical setting to reduce pain and assure unimpaired circulation beyond the fracture. A dislocated patella can often be reduced manually in the ED by the physician with minimal medication. Prompt reduction, either manually followed by splinting, or surgical with pinning, is the preferred treatment for major fractures, as opposed to prolonged traction, which requires prolonged immobilization of the patient.

13. **A** Based on the findings, the nurse would suspect that the patient has a posterior hip dislocation. This type of injury may occur when force is applied against the flexed knee with the hip in flexion, such as occurs when the knee strikes the dashboard during an automobile accident. The higher the degree of hip flexion, the greater the chance of a simple dislocation. Assessment typically reveals a shortened, internally rotated, and adducted leg. Associated knee and femur injuries are common. Major complications include sciatic nerve injury and avascular necrosis of the femoral head. In an anterior hip dislocation, which occurs with forced abduction (as in a fall, an automobile accident, or a blow to the back while squatting), leg shortening is rare. Assessment typically reveals abduction, external rotation, and either flexion or extension of the affected leg, depending on the type of anterior dislocation. Early reduction is

essential. In a central acetabular fracture-dislocation, which occurs from a blow to the lateral side of the trochanter and pelvis with the force exerted on the femoral head, the patient typically has a slightly shortened affected leg, muscle spasms, and limited range of motion. This type of injury is commonly associated with other serious injuries, such as pelvic and abdominal trauma. Pelvic X-rays are recommended, because pelvic fractures are the second leading cause of traumatic death. The mechanism of injury for pelvic, sacral, and coccygeal fractures is direct trauma through the femur. The nurse should suspect a pelvic fracture if the patient has pain, crepitus, or tenderness over the symphysis pubis, anterior spine, iliac crest, sacrum, or coccyx. The patient must be observed for signs of shock and hemorrhage.

14. **A** The prognosis for a patient with a dislocated hip without a fractured acetabulum will be favorable if the injury is reduced within the first 6 hours. A poor prognosis can be expected if the hip remains out of the acetabulum for more than 24 hours. If the patient suffers from sciatic nerve injury, only partial resolution may occur after reduction; typically, sensation to the bottom of the feet returns, but footdrop does not resolve.

15. **B** The most appropriate nursing diagnosis in this situation is Potential for injury related to sciatic nerve damage. The nurse must assess sciatic nerve function and distal pulses in the patient with a hip dislocation because of the high risk of sciatic palsy associated with this type of injury. The other diagnoses are inappropriate because pelvic fractures and urethral trauma are more commonly seen with central acetabular fracture; in this situation, trauma to the knee forced the femoral head out of the acetabulum posteriorly. Also, the patient is at low risk for compartment syndrome with this type of injury.

16. **D** The expected outcome for a patient with potential for injury related to sciatic nerve damage is that the patient will be able to move the affected leg with intact sensation. This outcome indicates that nursing interventions to prevent sciatic nerve damage have been successful. Absence of footdrop would be another indication that injury has not occurred.

17. **A** Based on the assessment findings, suspect that the patient has an anterior shoulder dislocation. Approximately 50% of all major joint dislocations occur at the shoulder, 95% of which are anterior dislocations. An anterior dislocation occurs with abduction, extension, and external rotation of the shoulder. The patient typically resists passive and active abduction of the arm. Loss of shoulder symmetry is typically noted, and the humeral bead can be palpated anteriorly. Assessing the patient's neurovascular status before reduction is important with this type of injury. Posterior shoulder dislocations are difficult to diagnose. They typically occur with violent internal rotation, as occurs during a seizure. The patient may complain of shoulder pain and an inability to lift the arm. Examination typically reveals limited abduction and external rotation. The deformity is less noticeable than with an anterior dislocation. A neurovascular assessment is essential before reduction in this type of injury. Clavicular fractures commonly result from falling onto a shoulder or an outstretched hand or from a direct blow to the clavicle. Diagnosis usually is based on the patient's history, the location of pain, and the degree of deformity noted during inspection and palpation. Acute tears of the rotator cuff commonly result from falling on a shoulder, throwing an object, or lifting a heavy object. Abduction of the shoulder may be impossible, and tenderness may be noted over the area where the rotator cuff is inserted into the tuberosities. Passive range of motion should be unrestricted with this type of injury. X-ray findings are normal in most cases.

18. **B** Intact sensation to the smallest finger is a good indication that no injury has occurred to the ulnar nerve. Intact sensation to the palmar aspect of the thumb reflects an intact radial nerve. Intact sensation to the tip of the index finger and ability to oppose the thumb reflect a functioning median nerve.

19. **A** Cold therapy, such as ice, is indicated for the first 48 hours to reduce swelling and relieve pain. Heat applied to the injured area increases swelling. Although very rarely used, cold sprays, such as ethyl chloride, are not recommended for home use. In the rare case they are indicated and ordered, they should be applied only by a health care professional because of the risk of a cold thermal injury.

20. **B** The patient's acknowledgment that he should return to the hospital if his arm feels numb indicates that he has understood the discharge instructions for a shoulder dislocation. Any patient with this type of injury should be advised to seek medical attention if numbness, tingling, or extreme pain occurs because prompt treatment can prevent neurovascular damage. Ice packs should be applied for 20 to 30 minutes at a time, to prevent frostbite. The arm should be kept immobile in a sling to reduce such complications as pain, neurovascular injury, and recurrence of the dislocation.

21. **C** The nurse would not expect the physician to order cast application for this patient. The patient will require surgery to reduce and fixate the fracture. Antibiotics are necessary because of the gross contamination to the leg. Continuous leg splinting is necessary until the patient is in the operating room, to prevent neurovascular injury.

22. **C** The most appropriate nursing diagnosis in this situation would be potential for infection related to wound contamination

because of the open wound and debris noted during assessment. The other diagnoses are inappropriate because there is no evidence of neurovascular injury or cranial trauma at this time.

23. **C** Patients sustaining fractures involving the pelvis or long bones are at risk for the development of fat emboli within the first 24 to 48 hours after injury. Signs include a petechial rash to the chest and altered level of consciousness due to hypoxia caused from the embolism. Though femur fractures pose a risk for major bleeding which could lead to hypovolemia, this would be an acute rather than late concern. Bed bound patients are at risk for pneumonia and should be encouraged to perform deep breathing exercises (incentive spirometry) while immobilized. Sepsis is a concern with open fractures. A, B, and D while possible, are less likely in this scenario.

24. **D** Injuries occurring from repetitive motion likely indicate inflammation of the tendons. The most appropriate intervention for a tendonitis injury would be rest and support with a mild compression dressing to reduce motion and promote healing. Corticosteroids would be considered for more chronic injuries. Evacuation of fluid from the joint would be consistent with treatment for bursitis. Antibiotics are not indicated for repetitive motion tendonitis injuries.

25. A In a comminuted skull fracture, the skull breaks in to multiple small pieces. A depressed fracture occurs where the broken piece of skull is pushed inward and may be putting pressure on the brain. These types of fractures can sometimes cause damage to the underlying brain tissue. A compound fracture occurs in conjunction with a laceration on the surface of the scalp and extends to tear the meninges of the brain. A basilar fracture occurs at the base of the brain and can cause a lot of damage to the brainstem, depending on the severity of the fracture.

26. **B** 35°F to 39°F (2°C to 4° C) is the correct range. The body part should be irrigated with Lactated Ringer's solution, cool sterile water, or normal saline solution to remove debris; prolonged irrigation should be avoided. X-rays of the injured extremity and the amputated part should be done. Afterward, the amputated part should be wrapped in sterile gauze, put into a sterile container, and then placed on top of ice in a large container. Another acceptable method would involve wrapping the amputated part in a sterile sponge that has been moistened in a physiologic solution, placing it in a plastic bag or cup, and inserting it into an ice bath at 35°F to 39°F (2°C to 4° C). Placing the part directly on ice does not provide the homogeneous cooling that occurs with insertion in an ice bath. The specimen container must also be labeled with the patient's name.

27. **C** Treatment for an acute shoulder dislocation includes reduction of the affected area, immobilization using, brace or sling, and cold compresses to reduce swelling. Application of heat is not advised and would not be an appropriate intervention.

28. **C** With most simple muscle strains or sprains, ice should be

applied to the area for the first 48 hours. After the first 48 hours has passed, heat can then be applied for 15 to 20 minutes, as needed throughout the day.

29. **A** An 8 month old child is likely not old enough to walk yet and is not likely to fracture a bone on his own. In this age group, a spiral leg fracture is suggestive of physical abuse. Spiral fractures occur in older children and adults with a twisting injury while bearing weight. A Galeazzi fracture occurs commonly in adults, resulting either from a fall or a blow to the lateral wrist and distal radius. A Monteggia's fracture occurs on the proximal ulna and includes dislocation of the head of the radius.

30. **B** A greenstick fracture is a break, which occurs only on one side of the shaft of a bone. This is common in children because their bones are flexible. When stressed to the breaking point, the bone bends and cracks but not completely through. The term comes from the association with a living, or green, stick of wood. When it is bent, it cracks on one side, but it doesn't break all the way through.

PSYCHIATRIC AND PSYCHOLOGICAL EMERGENCIES

1. The physician/NP/PA diagnoses the patient as having a manic bipolar disorder. The nurse is aware that signs and symptoms supporting this diagnosis include:

A. Looseness of association, agitation, suspiciousness, and irregular menses
B. Flight of ideas, hyperactivity, social isolation, and increased appetite
C. Rhyming, grandiosity, insomnia, and decreased appetite
D. Pressured speech, anxiety, delusions of persecution, and refusal to eat or drink

2. While waiting for the patient to be admitted to the medical-surgical unit, the nurse would expect the physician to order:

A. Chlorpromazine hydrochloride (Thorazine) 100 mg PO
B. Lithium carbonate (Eskalith) 300 mg PO
C. Imipramine hydrochloride (Tofranil) 50 mg IM
D. Chlordiazepoxide hydrochloride (Librium) 25 mg PO

3. While sitting in the waiting area, the patient strikes herself in the head, saying, "Somebody has to help me. I can't take this any longer." Which action is most appropriate at this time?

A. Alert the security team that the patient may become agitated, and ask them watch her closely
B. Approach the patient with two other staff nurses, and ask. "What seems to be the problem?"
C. Walk over to the patient and say, "I understand you think there is a radio in your brain. How did that happen?"
D. Sit next to the patient and say, "I'm a nurse. I saw you hitting your head. Can you tell me what you are experiencing right now?"

4. A patient becomes increasingly agitated and begins pacing the floor, hitting her head harder and yelling, "Stop it. I'm a good girl. Stop saying those things about me." The nurse suspects that the patient is experiencing:

A. Auditory hallucinations
B. Delusions of persecution
C. Obsessive ideation
D. Looseness of association

5. A 40-year-old woman walks into the ED and says to the admissions secretary, "Are there any doctors here who can take the radio out of my brain?" The secretary tells the patient to have a seat and calls for the nurse. The nurse should plan to focus further assessment on the patient's:

A. Vital signs
B. Orientation to time, place, and person
C. Receptivity to treatment
D. Content of thought

6. Which nursing action would be most appropriate if a patient were to become uncontrollable and require restraint?

A. Address the patient in a warm, reassuring manner
B. Administer medication while the patient is being restrained by two security guards
C. Restrain the patient with the help of at least three other trained personnel
D. Administer medication to avoid restraint

7. The nurse knows that safe nursing care for a restrained patient includes:

A. Allowing the patient to rest undisturbed until calm
B. Talking to the patient about what precipitated the restraint
C. Continuous observation and monitoring of vital signs
D. Performing range-of-motion exercises every ½ hour until the patient is released from the restraints

8. His mother, who states that she can no longer manage him at home, brings a 30-year-old man to the ED. According to the mother, the patient, who has been in and out of psychiatric hospitals since age 19, acts infantile; he refuses to dress or wash without her help and has frequent episodes of urinary and fecal incontinence. In the examining room, the patient grimaces and poses in front of a glass cabinet. He does not respond when his name is called. The nurse determines that the best way to approach this patient would be to:

A. Walk over to him, place a hand on his shoulder, and repeat his name
B. Ask him what he is doing
C. Tell him to stop making faces and to explain what is wrong
D. Repeat his name louder, then move closer and wait for a sign that he is aware of her presence

9. When the patient is questioned about why his mother brought him to the hospital, he replies, "I had to go on a trip. The sky is empty now. The man's name is Big Bob." The nurse knows that this response demonstrates:

A. Looseness of association
B. Flight of ideas
C. Neologism
D. Echolalia

10. During the admission interview, the patient has an episode of urinary incontinence. The best way to handle this situation would be to:

A. Ignore the incontinence to avoid embarrassing the patient
B. Firmly remind the patient that men do not urinate in their pants
C. Have the patient remove his wet pants and put on a gown and a diaper to prevent further urine leakage
D. Say, "You are wet. Let me help you change into this dry gown"

11. The patient says to the nurse, "Is it better to eat or to drink? To sleep or to wake? To sing or to dance? Which is better?" The nurse knows that these questions indicate:

A. Ambivalence
B. Confusion
C. Autism
D. Regression

12. The mother informs the nurse that she feels guilty about bringing her son back to the hospital. She says, "He doesn't like to be here; he always begs me to take him home once he's here. Why can't I take care of him at home?" Which statement offers the best support for the mother?

A. "Don't feel guilty. You've certainly done your best for him. Let us help him now"
B. "I understand how much you care about your son and can see that you're able to recognize when you need help in managing him"
C. "Patients like your son never really recover; they typically require repeated hospitalizations"
D. "It must have been an awful strain taking care of your son all these years. Perhaps you should consider a group home"

13. The nurse is aware that schizophrenia is one of a group of psychotic reactions characterized by:

A. Marked psychomotor disturbance, which may involve stupor, negativism, excitement, rigidity, or posturing
B. Incoherence, grossly disorganized actions, prominent delusions, and hallucinations
C. Alternating episodes of psychosis and apparent normalcy
D. Basic disturbances in relationships with others and an inability to communicate and think clearly

14. Nursing assessment of a patient diagnosed with paranoid schizophrenia requires careful inquiry and observation of the patient's:

A. Reality perception and ability to communicate on multiple levels
B. Ability to communicate and interact with others during periods of total self-absorption
C. Ability to think, perceive, symbolize, communicate, and make decisions
D. Ability to interact in established relationships

15. A 32-year-old man, accompanied by two police officers, is brought to the emergency department (ED) in handcuffs. He had been standing on the rooftop of a six-story office building, shouting obscenities and yelling, "You are all doomed to die for what you've done to me." The priority nursing action at this time would be to evaluate the patient's:

A. Orientation to time, place, and person
B. Vital signs
C. Threat to the safety of self and others
D. History of psychiatric illness

16. A 32-year-old man, accompanied by two police officers, is brought to the emergency department (ED) in handcuffs. He had been standing on the rooftop of a six-story office building, shouting obscenities and yelling, "You are all doomed to die for what you've done to me." The patient is agitated and complains about the handcuffs and the presence of the police officers. The most helpful approach for the nurse to take in this situation is one that is:

A. Calm and firm, but nonthreatening
B. Relaxed, casual, and friendly
C. Authoritarian and directive
D. Permissive and comforting

17. A 32-year-old man, accompanied by two police officers, is brought to the emergency department (ED) in handcuffs. He had been standing on the rooftop of a six-story office building, shouting obscenities and yelling, "You are all doomed to die for what you've done to me." After the patient is evaluated by the nurse and the psychiatric resident, the officers remove the handcuffs. Which statement would be most appropriate at this time?

A. "If you promise to be good, we won't have to restrain you anymore"
B. "We will remove the handcuffs now; you will not be restrained as long as you can control yourself"
C. "I know that the handcuffs are uncomfortable, so we will take them off now"
D. "Because you have calmed down, we will remove the handcuffs"

18. A 32-year-old man, accompanied by two police officers, is brought to the emergency department (ED) in handcuffs. He had been standing on the rooftop of a six-story office building, shouting obscenities and yelling, "You are all doomed to die for what you've done to me." The patient appears anxious and guarded during the interview. The nurse knows that such anxiety may be reduced by:

A. A detailed explanation of the entire admission procedure
B. Approaching the patient confidently and offering simple, direct explanations
C. Limited interaction and focus on physical assessment rather than conversation
D. A warm attitude and the use of touch to demonstrate caring

19. A 32-year-old man, accompanied by two police officers, is brought to the emergency department (ED) in handcuffs. He had been standing on the rooftop of a six-story office building, shouting obscenities and yelling, "You are all doomed to die for what you've done to me." Admitting this patient for psychiatric observation would most likely be made on the basis of:

A. The patient's history of previous psychiatric hospitalizations
B. The patient's anxiety level
C. The need to evaluate the patient's homicidal and suicidal ideation more thoroughly
D. The fact that the patient was brought in by the police

20. A 30-year-old woman is brought to the ED by her husband, who reports that she has not eaten or slept in 7 days and that she has become progressively elated over the past 3 weeks. The patient is wearing only shorts, a T-shirt, and sneakers, despite that fact that it is 20°F (6°C) outside. The nurse notes that the patient is shivering and confronts her about her clothing. The patient says, "Well, it must be summer somewhere, and that's where I want to be." Which response would be most appropriate?

A. "It is obvious that your judgment is impaired. You are dressed inappropriately"
B. "Where would you like to be, instead of here?"
C. "Please put this robe on. You don't want to catch pneumonia, do you?"
D. "You are shivering and appear chilled. Put this robe on"

21. While waiting to be examined, a patient begins singing loudly and walking around "entertaining" the other patients. The best approach at this time is to:

A. Assign three available nursing assistants to keep the patient from annoying others
B. Recognize that this behavior is characteristic of bipolar disorder
C. Lead the patient to a quiet area
D. Obtain an order for medication to control her behavior

22. During the admission interview, the nurse asks the patient about her sleeping and eating patterns. The patient replies, "I live on love. I thank the stars above. Sleep is cheap. Food ruins the mood." The nurse knows that this response is indicative of:

A. Grandiose delusion
B. Auditory hallucination
C. Word salad
D. Clang association

23. When assessing the patient's thought content, the nurse should focus primarily on:

A. Delusions
B. Complex fantasies and self-absorption
C. The degree of negative verbalization toward significant others
D. Objective data elicited from the patient's psychiatric history

24. During the interview, the nurse should ask such questions as "Do you dream vividly? Do you see light flashes or figures that others cannot see? Do you hear voices when no one is present? If so, whose voices? Are the voices clear? Abusive? Accusatory? Can you stop the voices?" These questions are important because:

A. The patient's major defense mechanisms are an indication of his level of psychosis
B. Assessing for hallucinations is integral to determining the patient's perception
C. Elicited emotional responses provide an assessment of the appropriateness of the patient's affect (mood)
D. The psychotic patient can never distinguish between what is real and unreal

25. When caring for a psychotic patient, the ED nurse must be:

A. Nonthreatening, to enable the patient to express emotions appropriately
B. Goal-directed, to ensure the gathering of data necessary for the treatment plan
C. Nonjudgmental, to provide an atmosphere of trust and open communication
D. Flexible, to enable the nurse to adjust the care as the situation demands

26. A 36-year-old man is brought to the ED anxious, trembling, and crying. He states he began feeling depressed and disinterested in life 1 year ago, after learning that his partner wanted a separation because of his relationship with another man. The patient claims that he was not angry with his partner and blames himself for his infidelity. During the relationship, he developed few personal interests, having little time between his career and domestic responsibilities. After separation arrangements began, he became aware of intense feelings of sadness, fatigue, grief, hopelessness, and worthlessness and had recurrent thoughts of death. Family history reveals that the patient's mother had suffered from chronic illness and depression. A diagnosis of distorted grief reaction, major depression, is made. The nurse understands that a maladaptive or pathologic response to loss is likely to occur when a person:

A. Does not successfully complete the normal grieving process associated with loss
B. Does not resolve the social situations that precipitated feelings of powerlessness and low self-esteem
C. Cannot use coping mechanisms and ego strengths successfully
D. Does not balance intrapersonal and interpersonal needs successfully

27. The nurse is aware that a patient with a delayed or distorted grief reaction must experience the feelings and thoughts he initially avoided if he is ever to complete the grieving process and accept his loss. In this situation, the most appropriate way to help the patient through the grieving process would be to:

A. Encourage the patient to undergo psychotherapy with her former partner to work through his loss
B. Gently encourage the patient to discuss his loss, then support him during the grieving process
C. Encourage the patient to increase his social contacts and accept his ego strengths
D. Explain to the patient that grieving is time-limited and that the emotional pain eventually will resolve

28. The patient tells the nurse that he is afraid to face his feelings and express emotion; he fears that his condition will worsen if he remembers the past and its accompanying pain. When teaching this patient about the grieving process, the nurse should:

A. Reassure the patient that he will not cry forever, lose permanent control, or go crazy if he grieves
B. Reassure the patient that the expression of active feelings is a natural part of the grieving process
C. Discourage the patient from blaming himself for the divorce
D. Encourage the patient to express repressed feelings toward himself and his former partner through role-playing

29. Which test can help diagnose depression?

A. Serotonin level test
B. Serotonin suppression test
C. Dexamethasone suppression test
D. Monoamine oxidase inhibitor suppression test

30. The nurse knows that sadness is the major affect associated with grief and depression. Other characteristic affects include:

A. Euphoria with varying degrees of dysphoria
B. Self-absorption, crying, and psychomotor agitation or retardation
C. Irritability, agitation, hostility, anger, apathy, lethargy, shame, self-doubt, and anhedonia (total lack of pleasure)
D. Low energy level; withdrawal; and demanding, regressive, and infantile behavior with periodic crying

31. The physician prescribes phenelzine sulfate (Nardil) 15 mg PO stat and advises the patient to set up an appointment with the outpatient mental health department in 2 weeks. Which information should the nurse include in the discharge instructions for this patient:

A. Follow-up instructions, including the need to undergo a thorough physical examination and psychotherapy
B. Signs and symptoms of potential adverse effects, including blurred vision, constipation, tachycardia, and delayed micturition
C. Signs and symptoms of potential adverse effects, including hypothalamic crisis and hyperglycemia
D. Dietary precautions

32. A patient in an acute psychotic or organic state who demonstrates assaultive, violent, or homicidal behavior typically does so because he:

A. Possesses an explosive personality
B. Imagines being threatened by outside forces
C. Acts out of rage, frustration, or anger because he cannot think before acting
D. Succumbs to violent impulses and reenacts old conflicts to get what he wants

33. Which patient is most likely to exhibit violence?

A. A patient with organic brain syndrome
B. A criminal
C. A substance abuser
D. A psychotic patient

34. The nurse knows that the best means of predicting the threat of violent behavior is via:

A. The patient's psychomotor activity
B. The patient's affect and accompanying changes in speech and motor activity
C. The degree of violence to which the patient has been subjected
D. Observation and intuition

35. Upon which criteria would the nurse determine that a patient is potentially assaultive?

A. Disorientation, visual and auditory hallucinations, and memory impairment
B. Diagnosis of psychosis and a history of violent behavior, particularly violence that resulted in a recent criminal incarceration
C. Diagnosis of manic depression with psychotic features and possession of a weapon, such as a gun or knife
D. Increased motor agitation, threatening statements or gestures, intensification of affect, and use of alcohol or addictive drugs

36. The immediate goal when caring for an assaultive or homicidal patient is to:

A. Administer a fast-acting sedative, as ordered
B. Help the patient to regain or prevent further loss of control
C. Restrain the patient according to hospital policy and help him to regain control
D. Provide the patient with opportunities for appropriate release of frustrations

37. Which is the most effective means of managing an overtly violent patient:

A. Speaking to the patient calmly but firmly
B. Using a team approach
C. Calling in the psychiatric resident or a supportive family member to speak to the patient
D. Restraining the patient, then administering a psychotropic medication

38. Most state mental health laws are specific about the length of time a patient legally may be restrained, commonly stipulating that restraints:

A. Cannot be used for longer than 24 hours
B. Cannot be used if the patient has cardiac or respiratory disease or insufficiency
C. Can be used only after a psychiatrist evaluates the patient
D. May be applied if the patient poses a danger to himself or others, provided the risk of danger is reevaluated every few hours

39. While the nurse applies sterile dressings to the wounds of a 42-year-old male, who has attempted suicide, the patient says, "It makes sense. I don't have anybody. I want to put myself out of this misery. Next time, I'll succeed." Which nursing action would be essential during the initial interview of this patient?

A. Help the patient to reevaluate her life and to make immediate, realistic changes
B. Inform the patient that a professional mental health practitioner will be assigned to care for and watch over her
C. Assess the need for psychotropic medications
D. Listen carefully to what the patient says about the nature of the suicidal intent

40. When assessing a suicidal patient's behavior, the nurse should pay particular attention to the suicide method because:

A. Certain suicide methods are gestures, a means of engaging in attention-seeking behavior, and not meant to be taken seriously
B. Most nonlethal methods reflect the patient's intrapsychic hope that someone will rescue her from self-destruction
C. Although all suicide threats and attempts must be taken seriously, more vigorous and vigilant nursing attention is indicated when the patient plans or attempts a highly lethal means
D. Most nonlethal methods reflect the patient's wish to discover whether anyone cares enough to prevent his self-destruction

41. All of the following statements about suicide are true except:

A. Most people who talk about committing suicide do not go through with their plan
B. Suicide occurs equally among all levels of society
C. Most suicides occur within 3 months after the beginning of improvement, when the person has the energy to put morbid thoughts and feelings into action
D. Although a suicidal person is extremely unhappy, he is not necessarily mentally ill

42. Because a severely depressed patient is at high risk for suicide, the nurse must carefully investigate all factors that may contribute to depression, including the patient's medication regimen. Which commonly prescribed drugs can cause depression?

A. Chlordiazepoxide hydrochloride, diazepam (Valium), doxepin hydrochloride (Sinequan), imipramine hydrochloride
B. Clonidine hydrochloride (Catapres), methyldopa (Aldomet), propranolol (Inderal), reserpine (Serpasil)
C. Clonidine hydrochloride, diazepam, methylphenidate hydrochloride (Ritalin), protriptyline hydrochloride (Vivactil)
D. Amitriptyline hydrochloride (Elavil), chlorpromazine hydrochloride, phenelzine sulfate, tranylcypromine sulfate (Parnate)

43. The physician and the nurse concur that a patient should be hospitalized because she cannot control her destructive impulses without medical assistance. Which is the most appropriate intervention to include in the plan of care to ensure the patient's physical safety:

A. Provide the patient with a quiet room to decrease stimuli
B. Institute suicide precautions
C. Keep the patient in a locked room
D. Administer psychotropic medications, as ordered, to help the patient gain better control and reduce her self-destructive impulses

44. Which characteristic is shared by most suicidal patients?

A. Psychosis
B. Guilt
C. Ambivalence
D. Anger

45. Which groups are at highest risk for self-destructive behavior?

A. Alcoholics, previous suicide attempters, terminally ill patients, members of minority groups, and psychotic patients
B. Adolescents, psychotic patients, substance abusers, and newlyweds
C. Psychotic patients, previous attempters, clergy members, adolescents, and terminally ill patients
D. Psychotic patients, depressed individuals, and preadolescents

46. A 12-year-old girl is admitted to the ED with dysuria, scant vaginal bleeding, and a 2-cm linear laceration on the posterior aspect of her left thigh. She has not had menarche. The mother reports that her daughter has a Poor relationship with her peers and that she has recently become more withdrawn. The parents are divorced; the patient and her mother recently moved in with a maternal uncle to help ease financial difficulties. The nurse suspects that the patient is a victim of child abuse. The nurse knows that child abuse is most prevalent among children of which age group:

A. Infants
B. Toddlers
C. School-age children (ages 5 to 12)
D. Adolescents

47. The nurse would expect a hospitalized child-abuse victim to exhibit all of the following behaviors except:

A. Always wanting to know what will happen next
B. Seeming constantly alert to potential danger
C. Looking to adults for reassurance
D. Seeming less afraid of other children

48. All of the following factors increase a child's risk for abuse except:

A. Mental retardation
B. Physical handicap
C. Prematurity
D. First-born status

49. The nurse should suspect child abuse or neglect if a 2-year-old child presents with:

A. Symmetrical bruises on both knees
B. A finger laceration and clinging behavior
C. Bruises in various stages of healing on both arms
D. A partial-thickness burn to the fingers of one hand

50. Which cause of death is most commonly associated with child abuse?

A. Abdominal trauma
B. Asphyxiation
C. Head trauma
D. Malnutrition

51. The nurse would suspect which child of suffering from neglect?

A. An uneducated older child
B. A young child whose parents provide little or no supervision
C. An infant who is diagnosed with failure to thrive
D. All of the above

52. Which statement about sexual abuse is true?

A. Incest that begins and ends before adolescence is more difficult to manage than incest that occurs during adolescence
B. A child typically recovers more easily from sexual abuse when the abuser is a family member
C. Boys have more difficulty adjusting to sexual abuse than girls do
D. Boys receive more family support than girls when incest is discovered

53. Which assessment findings best support a diagnosis of child abuse?

A. Occasional accidents from lack of adult supervision
B. Sexually transmitted disease in a young child
C. Pregnancy in late adolescence
D. Excessive anger by a daughter toward her father

54. Which of the following should be the nurse's primary concern when caring for an abused child:

A. Helping the child to establish peer relationships
B. Ensuring the continuation of parental contact
C. Demonstrating acceptance of and affection for the child
D. Recommending appropriate behavior modification for the child

55. Which factor should be the nurse's primary consideration when planning the care of a child admitted to the hospital because of child abuse?

A. The nurse's personal feelings about the parents and their expectations for the child
B. The child's developmental level
C. The child's peer relationships
D. Community support and foster parent needs

56. Which nursing action is most appropriate in cases of suspected child abuse?

A. Assume that the physician caring for the child will suspect abuse and report it to the appropriate agency
B. Confront the parents directly and report findings to the appropriate agency
C. Assume responsibility for reporting suspected abuse to the appropriate agency
D. Assign responsibility for reporting suspected abuse to a social worker

57. The nurse is aware that parents who abuse their children typically:

A. View violence as an acceptable method of behavior modification
B. Are socially involved with their neighbors
C. Have had good relationships with their parents
D. Are self-sufficient

58. Which statement about abuse or neglect is true?

A. A neglectful parent is likely to restrict a child's social activities
B. An abusive parent is unlikely to restrict a child's social activities
C. Only a small percentage of neglected children are also abused
D. All of the above

59. All of the following treatment objectives for an abused child and his family are appropriate except:

A. Helping the parents to understand their needs
B. Teaching the child to express his needs in a direct manner
C. Encouraging the parents and child to increase their isolation and focus upon them
D. Redistributing power within the family so that no one assumes total control

60. Which observation should the ED nurse report when referring an 8-year-old girl who has been sexually abused to the community health nurse?

A. The child received 50,000 units/kg of procaine penicillin IM
B. Results of the Venereal Disease Research Laboratory test revealed that no further studies are indicated
C. A urine specimen for human chorionic gonadotropin levels was obtained for pregnancy testing
D. Pelvic examination revealed an intact hymen

61. Which of the following personality disorders is seen in most patients with somatization disorder?

A. Histrionic
B. Antisocial
C. Narcissistic
D. Schizoid

62. A young woman is brought to the emergency department by her friend. The friend states she has not been eating, sleeps most of the day, has not showered and cries inconsolably since the death of a close friend. The patient reports she was just seen last week by her primary care physician and given a new prescription for sertraline (Zoloft). What is your first nursing priority?

A. Inform her that these medications can take several weeks to become effective and to continue taking them as prescribed.
B. Facilitate obtaining a new prescription or higher dose,
C. Refer her to the psychiatric unit.
D. Assess for suicidal ideation.

63. A teenage girl is brought to the emergency department after a fainting episode in school. During your assessment you begin to suspect either anorexia or bulimia. What physical or laboratory results would lean you more toward a diagnosis of bulimia?

A. Emaciated appearance
B. Dental Caries
C. Electrolyte imbalance
D. Dry skin

64. A female college student is brought to the emergency department by her family after having been witnessed taking a full bottle of Tylenol. She reports she took the medication because she was upset and "just wanted to sleep." What drug would you anticipate giving this patient?

A. Naloxone
B. Diazepam
C. N-acetylcysteine
D. Flumazenil

65. A 42-year-old man arrives in the emergency department and states, "Jesus told me to come here." The client is likely suffering from which component of psychosis?

A. Auditory hallucination
B. Visual hallucination
C. Flight of ideas
D. Grandiosity

PSYCHIATRIC AND PSYCHOLOGICAL EMERGENCIES: RATIONALE

1. **C** Rhyming, grandiosity, insomnia, and decreased appetite are all signs and symptoms of a manic disorder. While agitation, flight of ideas, hyperactivity, pressured speech, and anxiety may occur during a manic episode, irregular menses, social isolation, increased appetite, and refusal to eat or drink are not characteristic of this disorder. In severe cases (i.e. Stage III - Delirious Mania) psychotic symptoms such as suspiciousness, looseness of association, and delusions of persecution may also occur.

2. **A** The nurse would expect the physician to order chlorpromazine hydrochloride, an agent commonly prescribed to control hyperactivity. Lithium carbonate, which is used to prevent or control mania, takes 7 to 10 days to achieve therapeutic blood levels. Imipramine hydrochloride, an antidepressant, would not be prescribed in this situation.

3. **D** The appropriate action would be to sit next to the patient and say, "I'm a nurse. I saw you hitting your head. Can you tell me what you are experiencing right now?" This enables the nurse to acknowledge the patient's distress and to reassure the patient that someone understands and wishes to help. Measures that place the patient on the defensive, such as alerting the security team, approaching the patient with two other staff nurses, or confronting the patient head-on, should be avoided.

4. **A** The nurse would suspect auditory hallucinations because the patient appears to be responding to what she is hearing.

5. **D** The nurse should plan to focus on the patient's content of thought. Such assessment should reveal the nature of the

hallucinations and enable the nurse to protect the patient and others from potential violent outbursts.

6. **C** If the patient were to become uncontrollable and require restraint, the appropriate action would be to restrain the patient with the help of at least three other trained personnel. Restraints are used to protect the safety of the patient and staff. At least four persons trained in restraining patients can do this safely and efficiently. Medication should have been given earlier in an attempt to prevent any escalation of the patient's agitated behavior to the point where restraints were required.

7. **C** A restrained patient requires continuous observation and close monitoring of vital signs. Talking about the event at this point will further agitate the patient rather than calm her. Range-of-motion exercises are not as important as checking for circulation, respirations, and hydration; also, performing range-of-motion exercise would require the release of restraints, which may be unsafe.

8. **D** The nurse should repeat the patient's name louder, then move closer and wait for a sign that the patient is aware of her presence. The nurse should avoid startling the patient by not touching him or asking questions before she identifies herself and establishes a relationship.

9. **A** This type of response indicates looseness of association, a thought process characterized by obscure links in thought content. In flight of ideas, the links, although weak, are more evident. In this situation, the patient is not demonstrating neologisms (fabricated words) or echolalia (repetitious speech).

10. **D** The best response in this situation would be to say, "You are wet. Let me help you change into this dry gown." The nurse

should be aware that the patient's self-esteem may be fragile during such regressive episodes and that sensitively helping the patient changing his clothes is the best approach. Having the patient put on a diaper may embarrass him. Ignoring the incontinence may be interpreted as not caring.

11. **A** These questions demonstrate ambivalence, which is characterized by statements of opposing or dual behaviors.

12. **B** The most supportive statement would be "I understand how much you care about your son and can see that you're able to recognize when you need help in managing him." This acknowledges the mother's concern and decision to bring her son to the hospital. The nurse should not deny the mother's feelings, imply that there is no hope, or promote feelings of guilt.

13. **D** Schizophrenia is one of a group of psychotic reactions characterized by basic disturbances in relationships with others and an inability to communicate and think clearly. Withdrawal, fluctuating moods, disordered thinking, and regressive tendencies often evidence the patient's thoughts, feelings, and behavior.

14. **C** Nursing assessment of a patient with psychosis requires careful inquiry and observation of the patient's ability to think, perceive, symbolize, communicate, and make decisions. Such assessment should focus on alterations in thought content and processes, perception, affect (mood), and psychomotor behavior; changes in personality, coping styles, and sense of self; lack of self-motivation; psychosocial stressors; and degeneration of adaptive functioning.

15. **C** Ensuring the safety of the patient and others is always the top priority. Evaluating the patient's orientation to time, place, and person, vital signs, and psychiatric history are part of the total assessment.

16. **A** The most helpful approach would be one that is calm and firm, but nonthreatening. Taking this approach should help to lessen the patient's fear and anxiety. The patient may view the other approaches as suspicious or threatening.

17. **B** The most appropriate statement would be "We will remove the handcuffs now; you will not be restrained as long as you can control yourself." This statement clearly informs the patient about what will be done and sets appropriate limitations. The nurse should avoid asking the patient to make promises that he may be unable to keep.

18. **B** Anxiety interferes with a patient's ability to concentrate and comprehend complex information. Therefore, the nurse should approach the patient confidently and offer simple, direct explanations. Performing a physical assessment and touching the patient may be interpreted as intrusive and threatening and, therefore, should be avoided at this time.

19. **C** Because the patient had been threatening others, he must undergo a thorough evaluation for homicidal and suicidal ideation. The patient's history of previous psychiatric hospitalizations and the fact that he was brought in by the police would be insufficient grounds to warrant admission for further psychiatric evaluation.

20. **D** The most appropriate response would be "You are shivering and appear chilled. Put this robe on." Such a response allows the nurse to comment on her observation and to suggest

an appropriate behavior in a matter-of-fact, nonjudgmental way. Telling the patient that her judgment is impaired degrades the patient; asking where she would like to be provides no meaningful information. Direct statements are useful in this type of emergency. Allowing the patient to rebuttal a comment may not permit the best treatment for a person's care.

21. **C** The best approach in this situation would be to lead the patient to a quiet area, thereby decreasing environmental stimuli and reducing hyperactivity. The patient should receive constant supervision; however, assigning three nursing assistants may be over stimulating for the patient. The nurse should avoid obtaining an order for medication until the patient has been thoroughly evaluated.

22. **D** This response is indicative of clang association, a form of clanging rhyme that is common in manic disorders. Auditory hallucinations and word salad (meaningless combination of words) are seen in schizophrenia. The patient does not show evidence of grandiose delusions.

23. **A** Delusions typically constitute the major disturbance in thought content of a patient with psychosis and therefore should be the nurse's primary focus. Although some patients report delusions spontaneously, specific questioning commonly is required. During the interview, the nurse should look for clues suggestive of delusions, such as evasiveness, suspicion, and oversensitivity.

24. **B** The nurse should include such questions in the patient interview to assess for hallucinations, the most common perceptual disturbance manifested in psychosis. Such hallucinations may be auditory or visual. During auditory hallucinations, the patient may hear the voices of family

members or strangers making derogatory or insulting remarks. The patient also may hear voices telling him to do something (command hallucinations) that may be dangerous to self or others.

25. **D** The emergency department (ED) nurse must be flexible when caring for any patient who behaves in a suspicious, withdrawn, or regressed way or who has a thinking disorder. Because such a patient typically communicates in an unpredictable fashion and is in control of himself at various times, the nurse must adjust the care as the situation demands.

26. **A** A maladaptive or pathologic response to loss implies that something has prevented the patient from completing the normal grieving process associated with loss. Pathologic grief reactions may take on one of two forms: a distorted reaction or a delayed reaction. A distorted reaction is characterized by failure to successfully engage in the physical and psychological distress normally associated with loss. In this situation, the patient is suffering from depression, a type of distorted grief reaction characterized by the abnormal extension or overelaboration of sadness and grief.

27. **B** The most appropriate way to help this patient would be to gently encourage him to discuss his loss, and then support him during the grieving process. Those who fail to grieve sometimes do so because they have no available and supportive social matrix. The nurse can direct this patient to various support groups within the hospital and community.

28. **A** When teaching the patient about the grieving process, the nurse should reassure the patient that he will not cry forever, lose permanent control, or go crazy if he grieves. He should explain that such untoward consequences typically occur only

when a patient fails to grieve. If the patient complains that the past is the past and should remain buried, the nurse should reply that the past is very much in the present because it has not really been buried. Grieving is necessary to put the past in proper perspective.

29. **C** The dexamethasone suppression test gained considerable attention as a diagnostic marker for endogenous depression, as well as for its implications for treatment and prognostic factors. Most studies have found that 40% to 50% of patients suffering from endogenous depression or from major depressive disorders with melancholia demonstrate early recovery from cortisol suppression after the administration of dexamethasone. There are other tests that are done, along side a dexamethasone suppression test that helps to rule out other diagnoses that may be an underlying factor to a patient's depression.

30. **C** Besides sadness, other characteristic affects associated with grief and depression include irritability, agitation, hostility, anger, apathy, lethargy, shame, self-doubt, and anhedonia (total lack of pleasure). Assessment of a depressed patient typically involves a thorough mental examination that includes a careful evaluation of affect. The nurse should assess for ambivalence and hopelessness, which may indicate dire feelings of emptiness, worthlessness, and a lack of self-respect and confidence. Self-blame and low self-esteem are also present. The patient may be emotionally labile, crying easily one moment and laughing the next.

31. **D** When giving discharge instructions to a patient with a prescription for phenelzine sulfate (Nardil), the nurse must include information about necessary dietary precautions. Because of the dangers of hypertensive reactions resulting from the tyramine content of this monoamine oxidase inhibitor, the

patient should be advised to avoid ingesting aged cheese, sour cream, beer, wine (especially Chianti), yogurt, yeast, pickled herring, aged meat, meat tenderizer, and chicken liver. Chocolate and caffeine also have been implicated in blood pressure elevation and therefore should be avoided. The nurse also should advise the patient to note and report early signs of an impending hypertensive reaction, including headache, palpitations, neck stiffness, sweating, nausea, and photophobia.

32. **B** In an acute psychotic or organic state, assaultive, violent, or homicidal behavior typically occurs because the patient imagines being threatened by outside forces. He cannot correctly perceive the reality of his environment and acts in response to real or imagined threats.

33. **D** A psychotic patient is most likely to exhibit violence. Such a patient typically suffers from acute attacks of paranoia (psychotic episodes) that may result from a functional mental disorder or an organic brain syndrome. The patient's thought pattern is projective (the patient projects his thoughts to those around him) and leads to the development of delusions, which are typically persecutory in nature. The patient's reality perception is impaired; if uncorrected, this could lead to persistent delusions that cause the patient to perceive his environment as hostile and destructive. Violence may ensue as the patient attempts to protect himself in such an environment.

34. **D** The nurse's best means of predicting the threat of violent behavior is via observation and intuition. By observing the patient's behavior and mannerisms, the nurse can gauge whether the patient is acting strangely or in a potentially destructive way. For example, the nurse might note a patient suddenly beginning to pace, mumble angrily, and make threatening gestures-all warning signs of potential violence. Although

direct observation of dangerousness is a good indication of potential violence, the nurse also needs to rely on intuition to evaluate the potential for violence. Such intuition commonly is based on the nurse's gut instincts and feelings in a particular situation as well as on previous experience in similar situations. Thus, a nurse who witnessed the same warning signs in a previous situation is likely to sense the possibility of danger more readily than an inexperienced nurse would.

35. **D** The criteria for determining whether a patient is potentially assaultive include increased motor agitation, threatening statements or gestures toward real or imagined objects, intensification of affect, and use of alcohol or addictive drugs, as well as a history of assaultive behavior or diagnosis of acute organic brain syndrome.

36. **B** The immediate goal when caring for an assaultive or homicidal patient is to help the patient regain or prevent further loss of control. The other interventions may be appropriate but are not the immediate goal.

37. **B** The most effective means of managing an overtly violent patient is a team approach. The team, whose presence serves as a constant reminder of discipline and external control, aims to help the patient to understand his feelings. This is accomplished by helping him to control or set limits on impulsive aggressive behavior, examine the immediate situation that prompted the impulse reaction, and learn alternative methods of reacting in similar situations or other ways to discharge aggressive energies on an ongoing basis.

38. **D** Most state mental health laws stipulate that restraints may be applied if the patient poses a danger to himself or others, provided the risk of danger is reevaluated every few hours and

the restraints are continued only until more humane methods (such as sedative administration) become effective. In some instance, however, more humane methods are impossible. For example, when treating a violent patient who is intoxicated or who has overdosed on drugs, administering a sedative is impossible until the alcohol or drug is metabolized; restraints with continued observation might be necessary. In many states, the only legal form of restraint is a camisole (strait-jacket) or restraining sheet. Four-point restraint (both wrists and ankles tied separately) is illegal in many states. However, when no other method works, four-point restraint may be used, provided that one limb is untied at a specified interval and the restraints are rotated, much in the manner of rotating tourniquets. Health professionals may never use handcuffs, which are commonly used by the police to restrain violent patients brought to the ED.

39. **D** During the initial interview, the nurse should listen carefully to what the patient says about the nature of the suicidal intent. After evaluating the information, the nurse should assess the patient's feelings of adequacy in coping with immediate and chronic stressors, her degree of hope, and her overall view of life and the immediate situation.

40. **C** When assessing suicide behavior, the nurse should place heavy emphasis on the lethality of the suicide method chosen or used by a patient who has threatened or attempted suicide. Although all suicide threats and attempts should be taken seriously, more vigorous and vigilant nursing attention is indicated when the patient plans or tries a highly lethal means, such as shooting, hanging, or jumping from a high place. Less lethal means include carbon monoxide poisoning and drug overdose, which allow time for discovery once the suicidal action has been taken. Such assessment also should focus on whether the patient has made a specific plan and whether the

means to carry out the plan is readily available. Typically, the patient at highest risk for suicide is one who plans a violent death (such as a gunshot to the head), has a specific plan of action (for example, shooting himself as soon as his wife leaves the house to go shopping), and has the means readily available (such as a loaded handgun in a desk drawer).

41. **A** One of the misconceptions about suicide is that most people who talk about committing suicide do not actually follow up on their plan. In reality, 8 out of 10 persons who commit suicide give definite warnings of their suicidal intentions. Almost no one commits suicide without letting others know how he is feeling. Another misconception is that those who attempt suicide are fully intent on dying. The fact is that most people who attempt suicide are undecided about living and dying and gamble with death, relying on others to save them.

42. **B** When investigating the source of a patient's depression, the nurse must not overlook the possibility that the patient's medication regimen may be responsible. Commonly prescribed drugs that may cause depression include clonidine hydrochloride, methyldopa, propranolol, and reserpine. Other common depression-causing drugs include asparaginase (Elspar), baclofen (Lioresal), carisoprodol (Soma), chloramphenicol (Chloromycetin), dantrolene sodium (Dantrium), diazepam, diethylstilbestrol (DES), gentamicin sulfate (Garamycin), guanethidine sulfate (Ismelin), hydralazine hydrochloride (Apresoline), indomethacin (Indocin), pentazocine hydrochloride (Talwin), phenytoin (Dilantin), tamoxifen citrate (Nolvadex), and trimethobenzamide hydrochloride (Tigan), as well as anorectants, barbiturates, estrogen-containing products, and sulfonamides.

43. **B** The most appropriate intervention to include in the plan of care to ensure the patient's safety is to institute suicide precautions. Such precautions include searching the patient's personal effects for toxic agents, such as drugs or alcohol; removing any sharp instruments from the room, including razor blades, knives, letter openers, and glass bottles; removing all cords and sheets from the room and all straps, belts, neckties, stockings, and pantyhose from the patient's clothing; and instituting one-on-one observation.

44. **C** A common characteristic shared by most suicidal patients is ambivalence. Within each of these patients is a struggle between self-preserving and self-destructing forces. This is most apparent when patients threaten or attempt suicide, and then try to get help. When discussing the possible outcomes of suicide, many patients focus on life-related outcomes, such as relief from an unhappy situation, rather than on death.

45. **A** The groups at highest risk for self-destructive behavior include alcoholics, previous suicide attempters, terminally ill patients, members of minority groups, psychotic patients, police officers, physicians, adolescents, and elderly people. Of those who attempt suicide, three times as many men as women die; although more women attempt to kill themselves, they typically choose less effective means than men do.

46. **A** Child abuse is most prevalent among infants because they are typically defenseless, nonverbal, and at times difficult to manage.

47. **C** The nurse would not expect a hospitalized child-abuse victim to look to adults for reassurance. In most cases, the abused child shows a wariness and distrust of adults because adults are the most common abusers. The nurse would expect

the abused child to attempt to gain some control over the environment by wanting to know what will happen next and remaining alert to potential danger. Other children are typically nonthreatening to the abused child, who may easily settle into the hospital environment.

48. **D** A child's first-born status does not increase his risk for abuse. Maltreatment is commonly noted in children who are mentally retarded or physically handicapped. A contributing factor in both of these cases appears to be the increased difficulty in caring for these children. The increased incidence of abuse among premature children is attributed to ensuing medical problems, financial stress, and interruption of the bonding process.

49. **C** One of the hallmarks of chronic physical abuse is the appearance of bruises in various stages of healing on a child's arms or legs. When assessing for possible abuse, the nurse should keep in mind that ecchymotic areas normally appear reddish purple (initially), then green (within 5 to 7 days), and then yellowish brown (within 1 to 3 weeks) before they finally disappear (in about 4 weeks). The nurse would not suspect abuse in the other situations because symmetrical bruises on both knees commonly result from a 2-year-old's tendency to fall on his knees; lacerations are an atypical finding in an abused child, especially one who demonstrates clingy behavior suggestive of the need for parental support; intentionally burned areas typically are symmetrical and full-thickness and usually involve the feet and buttocks, not the fingers of one hand.

50. **C** Head trauma, especially involving a subdural hematoma, is the most common cause of death in child abuse. Abdominal trauma with bruising or rupture of the abdominal viscera is the second leading cause of death in abused children. Asphyxiation,

although reported as the cause of death in some situations, seldom occurs. Malnutrition, a commonly reported finding in abuse, rarely is a cause of death, except in children who are isolated from society.

51. **D** Lack of education or supervision and failure to thrive are recognized forms of child neglect. Other categories include abandonment, nutritional, medical, or dental neglect, and inappropriate or insufficient clothing.

52. **C** Boys have more difficulty adjusting to sexual abuse than girls do because this type of abuse is more common among girls, for whom support networks have been established. Incest that begins and ends before adolescence is less difficult to manage than incest that occurs during adolescence, possibly because younger children are not as cognizant of society's norms. A child typically recovers more easily from sexual abuse when the abuser is outside the family, because the child does not have to face the abuser on an ongoing basis. Also, the child's family typically assumes a protective role when the abuser is a nonfamily member.

53. **B** Sexually transmitted disease in a young child indicates child abuse. Child abuse can take many forms: physical, sexual, and emotional. Physical and behavioral indicators may include bruises, welts, burns, fractures, dislocations, lacerations, abrasions, dysuria, vaginal or penile discharge, wariness of physical contact with adults, feeding disorders, self-stimulation, withdrawal, or unusual sexual knowledge or behavior. Frequent accidents because of lack of adult supervision may indicate neglect. Pregnancy in early adolescence is indicative of sexual abuse; commonly, the child fails to disclose the paternal source. Excessive anger from a daughter directed toward the mother

may be another indicator of sexual abuse; this results from the perceived failure of the mother to protect the daughter.

54. **C** The nurse's primary concern when caring for an abused child should focus on demonstrating acceptance of and affection for the child through consistent caregiving. The nurse should keep in mind, however, that the abused child might not readily return acceptance and affection because his previous efforts had been met with frustration, neglect, or abuse. As a result, the abused child will not easily establish a trusting relationship with an adult. The nurse must demonstrate affection while attempting to modify negative methods of interaction and discipline and to provide the child with appropriate ways to display anger and frustration. An abused child typically has little difficulty establishing peer relationships. Depending on the nature and severity of the abuse, parental rights and contact may be terminated.

55. **A** The most important factor to consider when planning the care of a child who has been admitted to the hospital because of child abuse is the nurse's personal feelings about the parents and their expectations for their child. The nurse, the primary health care professional responsible for the abused child's care, must be careful to examine her feelings toward the parents and refrain from expressing any negative feelings. Once the nurse has come to terms with her feelings, she can proceed with planning interventions. Appropriate interventions should focus on helping the parents to establish realistic expectations for the child and promoting adequate parental problem-solving skills with appropriate discipline. In many cases, parents have unrealistic expectations for the child and thus need information about appropriate growth and development. Self-help groups may benefit abusive families by helping the parents to gain personal insight and learn appropriate methods of releasing

frustration. Crisis centers or hotlines may decrease the incidence of child abuse, but only on a short-term basis. An abused child typically adjusts well to new environments and makes friends without difficulty. Poor peer relationships, when they occur, tend to be more common among sexually abused children. If foster care is necessary, the foster parents should be encouraged to visit the hospitalized child and participate in care. They should be encouraged to show affection for and acceptance of the child to help the child develop a sense of trust.

56. **C** In many states, nurses are legally responsible for reporting all cases of suspected child abuse to the appropriate agency. The nurse is typically the primary health care professional caring for an abused child in the hospital setting. Because of the intimate nature of the nurse-patient relationship, the nurse may have more insight into the child's relationship with his parents. Consequently, the nurse is in a better position to recognize the signs of possible abuse and typically assumes an active role in reporting and preventing child abuse. Direct confrontation with the parents is not recommended, because this may escalate the anger and fear of the parents, who may remove the child from the hospital before the proper authorities arrive.

57. **A** Parents who abuse or neglect their children typically view violence as an acceptable method of behavior modification. Various factors can precipitate or fuel violence in such parents, including mental or physical handicaps, low self-esteem, and poor coping mechanisms. Abusive parents tend to be socially isolated and have minimal support systems. Most are not in a position to be self-sufficient; this, coupled with their social isolation, fosters a non-supportive environment that can lead to

abuse. Studies indicate that parents who abuse their children commonly were abused themselves.

58. **C** Only a small percentage of neglected children are also abused. A child suffering from neglect typically is ignored; therefore, abuse is less likely to occur. An abusive parent tends to restrict the child's social interactions to minimize the risk of discovery, whereas a neglectful parent typically allows the child to interact freely.

59. **C** The parents and child should be encouraged to expand their relationships, thereby improving support mechanisms. The child must be taught to express his needs directly, thus eliminating confusion and fostering realistic expectations. Helping the parents to understand themselves, redistribute power within the family, and share responsibilities helps to strengthen the family unit.

60. **D** When referring this patient to the community health nurse, the ED nurse should report that a pelvic examination revealed an intact hymen. Although the condition of the hymen neither proves nor disproves penetration, this information has legal significance and must be reported. A child's hymen may rupture as a result of various non-coital activities or accidents, or it may have enough elasticity for penetration without laceration. Nevertheless, a pelvic examination must be performed whenever penetration is suspected. Hair sampling and swabs for spermatozoa and gonorrhea also must be obtained. A serologic Venereal Disease Research Laboratory test for syphilis is required and should be repeated 1 to 2 months after the initial examination. The administration of 100,000 units/kg of procaine penicillin IM for a child and 4.8 million units for an adolescent are recommended. After

menarche, urine should be obtained for human chorionic gonadotropin testing to determine possible pregnancy.

61. **A** Somatization disorder refers to a constellation of physical symptoms that cannot be explained by a known medical condition. Pain, gastrointestinal, sexual, and neurologic symptoms predominate. An integral part of the diagnosis is that the patient is not faking the symptoms--the patient is truly is experiencing them, and will argue against any evidence that indicates somatization.

62. **D** While all of the above actions may be appropriate, the very first priority when dealing with a patient with acute depressive disorder would be to assess for suicidal ideation. Once it has been determined the patient is not suicidal, additional interventions and teaching can be considered. A is true, but it would not be the first priority in this case. B would likely not be considered for at least 4 to 6 weeks as the medication takes several weeks to become effective. C May be appropriate depending on the circumstances but suicidal risk must be assessed first.

63. **B** Patients with bulimia often go through periods of binge eating followed by induced purging, fasting, or laxative abuse to compensate for the large amount taken in by the binge period. Patients with either mild or severe bulimia can maintain a normal body weight and generally do not have the emaciated appearance common to anorexic patients. Bulimia often causes dental caries and loss of enamel due to frequent exposure to gastric acids during vomiting. Electrolyte imbalances and dry skin can be seen in both anorexia and bulimia. B is the correct answer.

64. **C** N-acetylcysteine is the only drug that can neutralize the hepatotoxic metabolites that form due to the excessive ingestion of Tylenol. Naloxone is used to treat an opiate overdose, such as heroin or morphine. Flumazenil is used to treat an overdose from benzodiazepines. Diazepam would also be incorrect.

65. **A** The most common symptom of psychosis is auditory hallucination, usually from an authoritative figure.

RESPIRATORY EMERGENCIES

1. In a patient with atelectasis, the nurse would expect to hear bronchial breath sounds over the:

A. Carina
B. Middle of the right lung lobe
C. Right main-stem bronchus
D. Left main-stem bronchus

2. While percussing a patient's lung fields, the nurse notes consolidated areas. These areas typically produce which sound?

A. Tympany
B. Flatness or dullness
C. Hollowness
D. Hyperresonance

3. The nurse knows that bronchovesicular breath sounds are normally auscultated over the:

A. Large bronchi
B. Lung periphery
C. Entire lung surface area
D. Trachea

4. When auscultating a patient, the nurse notes decreased vesicular breath sounds. This is an indication of:

A. Pulmonary fibrosis
B. Pleural effusion
C. Chronic obstructive pulmonary disease
D. All of the above

5. Which technique is commonly used to determine the degree of respiratory excursion?

A. Cardiothoracic ratio on chest X-ray
B. Percussion
C. Palpation
D. Auscultation

6. Which of the following is the most common cause of upper airway obstruction in an unconscious adult?

A. Food
B. Dentures
C. Bronchospasm
D. Relaxed tongue

7. Which assessment finding is a symptom of complete upper airway obstruction?

A. Hoarseness
B. Inability to speak
C. Forceful cough
D. Wheezing

8. Which nursing action is most appropriate in the initial management of a conscious adult with complete upper airway obstruction by a foreign body?

A. Administering four quick back blows with the heel of the hand between the victim's scapulae
B. Administering abdominal thrusts until the object is relieved, or until the patient loses consciousness.
C. Allowing the victim to expel the foreign body through vigorous coughing
D. Administering artificial respiration

9. Which action would be the nurse's highest priority when a nurse witnesses a patient suddenly go into respiratory arrest?

A. Auscultate for breath sounds
B. Feel for a radial pulse
C. Insert an oropharyngeal airway
D. Open the patient's airway

10. Which statement about endotracheal intubation for a patient in respiratory arrest is true?

A. It is necessary to ensure adequate ventilation
B. It should be performed as the initial step in airway management
C. It should be attempted only after other oxygenation methods have failed
D. It should be performed within 2 minutes of the onset of respiratory arrest

11. Which statement about esophageal obturator airway management is true?

A. It may damage the trachea
B. It requires visualization of the airway for insertion
C. It should be removed before endotracheal intubation is performed
D. Its removal is commonly followed by immediate regurgitation

12. The nurse assesses a patient at risk for respiratory failure. All of the following are early signs of respiratory failure except:

A. Restlessness
B. Tachycardia
C. Cyanosis
D. Tachypnea

13. When assessing a patient with acute respiratory failure resulting from impaired ventilation, the nurse would initially expect to note:

A. Hypoxia
B. Hypoxia and hypercapnia
C. Hypercapnia
D. Hypocapnia

14. Acute respiratory failure in a patient with essentially normal lung tissue usually is indicated by:

A. Shortness of breath, a PaO_2 of 80 mmHg, and a $PaCO_2$ of 40 mmHg
B. Diaphoresis, chest pain, and shortness of breath
C. A $PaCO_2$ greater than 50 mmHg and a PaO_2 less than 50 mmHg
D. A $PaCO_2$ less than 40 mmHg and a PaO_2 greater than 50 mmHg

15. A side-effect of Naloxone (Narcan) when administered rapid IV push is:

A. Respiratory Failure
B. Pinpoint pupils
C. Cardiac arrest
D. Projectile vomiting

16. Which statement about the aspiration of gastric contents is true?

A. An unconscious patient is at low risk for aspiration because regurgitation is impossible in this state
B. Aspiration of gastric contents is more common in adults than children
C. Adult respiratory distress syndrome can occur as a result of aspiration because of the high pH of gastric contents
D. Aspiration of gastric contents commonly results from attempts to ventilate an obstructed airway

17. Which factor should be the nurse's most important consideration in efforts to prevent aspiration?

A. Level of consciousness
B. Body position
C. Degree of gastric distention
D. Cardiac sphincter integrity

18. A 34-year-old woman is found unconscious in the emergency department (ED) waiting room. She is diaphoretic and apneic, with a slightly irregular pulse rate of 88 beats/minute. She is ventilated effectively with oxygen. Which drug treatment would the nurse expect the physician to order next?

A. Lidocaine (Xylocaine)
B. Naloxone
C. Epinephrine
D. Dextrose

19. Which statement about airway management is true?

A. Nasotracheal intubation is a logical choice in a patient with maxillofacial injury
B. Cricothyroidotomy is the formation of an opening for an artificial airway above the vocal cords
C. Tracheotomy is a less hazardous procedure than cricothyroidotomy
D. The carina is the landmark by which proper depth of endotracheal intubation should be measured

20. Which is the most common cause of impaired gas exchange after blunt chest trauma?

A. Apnea or hypopnea
B. Flail chest
C. Pulmonary contusion
D. Phrenic nerve paralysis

21. Fracture of the scapula or first or second rib indicates a serious force of injury and a high probability of underlying tissue damage. The nurse knows that, in the emergent phase of care, pulmonary contusion is best indicated by:

A. Auscultation
B. Arterial blood gas analysis
C. Radiographic studies
D. Dyspnea assessment

22. Which assessment finding is indicative of hypoxia?

A. Deterioration in level of consciousness
B. Change in urine output
C. Peripheral vasoconstriction
D. Delayed capillary refill time

23. The nurse knows that an increase in negative pressure inside the pleural space will result in:

A. Lung collapse
B. Tension pneumothorax
C. Normal inspiration
D. Normal expiration

24. The nurse would suspect dyspnea in a patient with a stab wound in the left upper abdominal quadrant to result from:

A. Pain and anxiety
B. Peritoneal irritation
C. Gastric rupture
D. Associated chest injury

25. Development of sudden subcutaneous emphysema and a crunching or crackling sound associated with auscultation of the apical heart rate is indicative of:

A. Empyema
B. Mediastinal air leak
C. Pericarditis
D. Fat embolism

26. The nurse's discharge instructions for a patient with a rib contusion and a minor rib fracture include information on the need to report fever, dyspnea on exertion, sputum production, or chest pain should any of these symptoms occur. These symptoms are indicative of:

A. Pneumonia or costochondritis
B. Empyema
C. Pulmonary hypertension
D. Pneumothorax

27. Which size chest tube should be prepared for a suspected hemothorax in an adult?

A. #20 French
B. #28 French
C. #36 French
D. #44 French

28. Autotransfusion usually is indicated for a patient with which condition?

A. Left-sided hemothorax with hypotension
B. Hypotension secondary to spinal cord injury
C. Avulsion amputation of the left thigh and leg
D. Hepatic hemorrhage secondary to a gunshot wound

29. A woman with a history of coronary artery disease is standing outside a supermarket when she suddenly complains of chest pain and collapses in full cardiac arrest. Bystanders initiate basic life support measures until emergency medical technicians (EMTs) arrive. The paramedics properly intubate and ventilate the patient; an automatic chest compressor also is used. One of the paramedics radios the ED nurse, and informs that the patient is not responding. Which factor is probably not contributing to the patient's unresponsiveness?

A. Pericardial tamponade
B. Hypocapnia
C. Tension pneumothorax
D. Volume deficit

30. A 25-year-old man drives to the ED after falling off a roof and landing on his right side on a concrete abutment. His chief complaints are dyspnea and significant chest pain. All of the following nursing actions would ensure proper ventilation and perfusion in this patient except:

A. Splinting the affected side with a pillow
B. Encouraging slow, deep breathing
C. Positioning the patient on his right side
D. Positioning the patient on his left side

31. Which injury constitutes flail chest?

A. Single fractures of the fourth, fifth, sixth, and seventh left lateral ribs
B. Single fractures of the seventh and eighth left and right anterior ribs
C. Fractured xiphoid process
D. Fractured sternum

32. The nurse knows that flail chest is easiest to assess:

A. When the thoracic fracture occurs posteriorly
B. When the thoracic fracture occurs anteriorly
C. In a conscious patient with well-developed musculature
D. Immediately after the injury

33. In a patient with a massive flail chest, all of the following factors are indications for ventilatory support except:

A. Advanced age and obesity
B. Progressive breathing fatigue
C. Hypercapnia, hypoxia, and dyspnea
D. Imminent abdominal surgery

34. In a patient with multiple rib fractures, which nursing intervention would be appropriate to encourage optimal ventilation?

A. Binding the chest wall
B. Frequently administering low-dose narcotics, as ordered
C. Performing postural drainage and incentive spirometry
D. Encouraging forceful coughing after chest percussion

35. A 50-year-old man is admitted to the ED with a diagnosis of suspected pulmonary embolus. He is dyspneic and anxious. The physician plans to start heparin therapy. Which laboratory test results are consistent with a diagnosis of pulmonary embolism?

A. A PaO_2 of 70 mmHg and an elevated lactic dehydrogenase (LDH) level
B. A normal LDH level and a PaO_2 of 70 mmHg
C. A white blood cell (WBC) count of 10,000/mm^3 and a PaO_2 of 85 mmHg
D. A WBC count of 20,000/mm^3 and a PaO_2 of 85 mmHg

36. Which nursing diagnosis would be the highest priority for a patient with a diagnosis of pulmonary embolism?

A. Anxiety related to hypoxia and pain
B. Pain related to pulmonary ischemia
C. Potential for injury related to hemorrhage from anticoagulant therapy
D. Impaired gas exchange related to altered pulmonary tissue perfusion

37. When the nurse dorsiflexes the patient's foot, the patient complains of calf pain. The nurse correctly interprets this response as an indication of a positive:

A. Trousseau's sign
B. Homans' sign
C. Kehr's sign
D. Babinski's reflex

38. Which electrocardiographic finding would the nurse expect to find in a patient with pulmonary embolism?

A. Sinus tachycardia
B. Increased R waves in lead V_1
C. First-degree atrioventricular block
D. Left axis deviation

39. The nurse practitioner orders heparin therapy for a patient diagnosed with pulmonary embolism. Which statement about the use of heparin therapy for pulmonary embolism is true?

A. Heparin helps to dissolve existing clots
B. Heparin reduces the risk of secondary thrombi formation
C. The heparin dosage is based on the patient's prothrombin time
D. Bolus administration is preferred for the high-risk patient

40. The nurse would anticipate initial emergency treatment for a patient with mild to moderate respiratory distress secondary to chronic obstructive pulmonary disease (COPD) to include:

A. Administration of 30% oxygen via facemask and bronchodilator therapy
B. Administration of 50% oxygen via humidity mask and bronchodilator therapy
C. Administration of 100% oxygen via facemask and 2 mg of morphine sulfate IV push to decrease anxiety
D. Endotracheal intubation and positive-pressure ventilation

41. Which nursing intervention would be appropriate for a patient with respiratory distress secondary to COPD?

A. Place the patient in a supine position in preparation for endotracheal intubation
B. Place the patient in high-Fowler's position or leaning upright over an over a bed table
C. Administer morphine sulfate, as ordered, to decrease anxiety
D. Perform postural drainage and chest percussion

42. A 69-year-old man is admitted to the ED with difficulty breathing. He has a 50-pack-year history of smoking. Upon examination, the nurse notes the patient's reliance on accessory muscles for breathing and his barrel chest. Which history finding is the most significant factor contributing to this patient's condition?

A. Anxiety
B. Smoking
C. Occupation
D. Activity level

43. The nurse knows that chronic bronchitis is classified as COPD because of which pathogenic occurrence?

A. Increased goblet cell production and disappearance of cilia
B. Hyperplasia of bronchiolar mucus-secreting glands
C. Hyperplasia and inflammation of goblet cells and increased production of thick mucus
D. Increased production and stimulation of neutrophils and macrophages

44. The nurse would expect the physician to order all of the following treatments for a patient with COPD except:

A. Fluid restriction
B. Bronchodilator therapy
C. Chest physiotherapy
D. Diuretic therapy

45. The patient wonders aloud whether it is too late to quit smoking. The nurse correctly explains that if the patient stops smoking now:

A. His symptoms will disappear and he will be cured
B. His cough and sputum production will decrease and his pulmonary function tests will improve
C. His symptoms will not improve because too much damage has been done
D. He will suffer much stress because of his illness

46. Which term best describes the condition of a patient with the above medical history and evidence of alveolar destruction?

A. Pink puffer
B. Blue bloater
C. Hyperreactive airway
D. None of the above

47. The nurse knows that cor pulmonale is a complication of COPD secondary to:

A. Atrophy of the right ventricle caused by heart failure
B. Stimulation of erythropoiesis, which decreases blood viscosity
C. Decreased intravascular blood volume with arterial congestion
D. Pulmonary hypertension caused by vasoconstriction in response to hypoxia

48. When assessing a patient with cor pulmonale resulting from COPD:

A. Bibasilar crackles
B. Capillary refill time of 4 seconds
C. Poor skin turgor
D. Jugular vein distention

49. In which condition is small-airway obstruction usually irreversible?

A. Asthma
B. Atelectasis
C. Pneumonia
D. Emphysema

50. Which information should the nurse plan to include in the discharge instructions for this patient?

A. The importance of an annual chest X-ray and spirometry testing
B. The need for weight control and vitamin supplements
C. The need for influenza and pneumonia vaccines
D. The benefits of living in a warm, dry climate with air conditioning

51. Nursing assessment of a patient with emphysema typically reveals barrel chest, which results from:

A. Hyperinflation and overdistension of alveoli
B. Distention and destruction of the primary lobules
C. Hyperventilation in response to hypoxemia and hypocapnia
D. Hypoventilation in response to hypoxemia and hypercapnia

52. Which nursing intervention is useful early in the management of a patient with dyspnea caused by emphysema?

A. Inspiratory muscle training
B. Postural drainage
C. Pursed-lip breathing exercises
D. Chest percussion and vibration

53. Chronic cough is common in COPD. When planning the discharge instructions for a patient with COPD, the nurse should remember to advise the patient to avoid:

A. Hydration and aerosol humidification
B. Spicy foods
C. Cough suppressants and self-medication with antihistamines
D. Chest physiotherapy and postural drainage

54. Which nursing diagnostic category would be appropriate for a patient with COPD?

A. Altered nutrition: More than body requirements
B. Ineffective individual coping
C. Potential for injury
D. Fluid volume excess

55. At 3 am, a 13-year-old girl is brought to the ED by her mother because of coughing and severe dyspnea. Her medical history reveals allergic rhinitis and eczema since early childhood. The nurse notes that the patient is wheezing and talking with effort. When questioned about precipitating factors, the mother states that her daughter had put on a new acrylic sweater to go to a makeup demonstration at a friend's house the previous evening and that she also had worn a new down jacket, which she is wearing now. The physician diagnoses acute asthmatic attack. Which term best describes the type of asthma precipitated by a known allergen?

A. Intrinsic
B. Extrinsic
C. Mixed
D. Idiopathic

56. Which of the following is likely to contribute to the onset of acute extrinsic asthma attack?

A. Season
B. Makeup
C. Acrylic sweater
D. Down jacket

57. The patient complains of increased dyspnea and tightness in her chest. The nurse knows that these symptoms of asthma may result from all of the following except:

A. Bronchospasm
B. Mucus production in response to mucosal edema
C. Bronchiolar constriction during expiration
D. Alveolar constriction during respiration

58. At 3 am, a 13-year-old girl is brought to the ED by her mother because of coughing and severe dyspnea. The physician diagnoses acute asthma attack. Which additional findings would the nurse expect to note during assessment of this patient?

A. Rhonchi and labored inspiratory breathing
B. Coughing and pursed-lip breathing
C. Prolonged wheezing on expiration with a nonproductive cough
D. Shallow wheezing on inspiration with a productive cough

59. The physician diagnoses a 19-year-old male with acute asthma attack. Which early treatment is likely to improve this patient's condition most rapidly?

A. Administration of prednisone (Deltasone) orally and terbutaline sulfate (Brethine) orally
B. Administration of cromolyn sodium (Intal) by inhalation and terbutaline sulfate SC
C. Administration of albuterol
D. Administration of oxygen via a facemask and Lactated Ringer's solution IV

60. At 3 am, a 13-year-old girl is brought to the ED by her mother because of coughing and severe dyspnea. Her medical history reveals allergic rhinitis and eczema since early childhood. The nurse notes that the patient is wheezing and talking with effort. When questioned about precipitating factors, the mother states that her daughter had put on a new acrylic sweater to go to a makeup demonstration at a friend's house the previous evening and that she also had worn a new down jacket, which she is wearing now. The physician diagnoses acute asthmatic attack. Which nursing intervention would be most appropriate when treating this patient's asthma attack?

A. Maintaining a calm, reassuring attitude while with the patient
B. Teaching the patient about measures to prevent future attacks
C. Keeping the patient's mother away from the bedside
D. Providing diversional therapy to avoid panic or anxiety

61. When writing discharge instructions for a patient diagnosed with an acute asthmatic episode, the nurse should include information on the importance of:

A. Obtaining prompt treatment for all upper respiratory tract infections
B. Attending an aerobic exercise program on a regular basis
C. Participating in outdoor activities to improve respiratory aeration
D. Eliminating any exercise regimen to prevent undue exertion

62. The nurse knows that the most common type of bacterial pneumonia is caused by:

A. Staphylococcus aureus
B. Streptococcus pneumoniae
C. Streptococcus pyogenes
D. Bacillus anthracis

63. The nurse is examining a 21-year-old man in the ED. His temperature is 103.6°F (39.8°C) rectally, pulse rate 88 beats/minute, and respiratory rate 28 breaths/minute. He complains of chills and a productive cough with rust-colored sputum. The physician diagnoses bacterial pneumonia. Which diagnostic studies would the nurse expect the physician to order for this patient?

A. Bronchoscopy and electrolyte studies
B. Pulmonary function tests and arterial blood gas
   measurements
C. Gram stain of sputum and chest X-rays
D. Lung scan and sputum cultures

64. Which assessment findings are commonly associated with epiglottitis?

A. Cherry red, edematous epiglottis and muffled voice sounds
B. Cyanotic, edematous epiglottis and muffled voice sounds
C. Grayish, edematous epiglottis and muffled voice sounds
D. Pink, edematous epiglottis and aphonia

65. When a child in the acute stage of epiglottitis begins to exhibit airway obstruction, the nurse's main priority would be to:

A. Request the parents to leave the room
B. Secure intubation and tracheotomy equipment
C. Obtain the parents' consent to perform a tracheotomy
D. Administer oxygen via a facemask

66. A 4-year-old boy is brought to the ED because of dysphagia, excessive salivation, mild respiratory distress, orthopnea, and fever. The child's father reports an abrupt onset of symptoms, with the child refusing to lie down for a nap. The physician diagnoses epiglottitis and arranges for the child to be admitted to the pediatric unit. Which factor should the nurse consider when planning this patient's care?

A. The possibility of agitation and combative behavior
B. Bacteremia, which occurs in almost all cases of epiglottitis
C. The possibility of a productive cough and vomiting
D. Laryngospasm, which may occur upon attempted visualization of the child's epiglottis

67. Which is the primary reason for administering chloral hydrate to an intubated child with epiglottitis?

A. To produce mild sedation and prevent seizure activity from fever
B. To produce mild sedation without drying respiratory secretions
C. To promote rest through respiratory muscle paralysis
D. To reduce epiglottic edema and promote rest

68. The physician diagnoses a 14-month-old female with laryngotracheobronchitis (croup). Upon assessment, the nurse would expect to note which early signs of hypoxemia in this patient?

A. Use of accessory respiratory muscles and development of a resonant cough
B. Expiratory stridor and cyanosis
C. Lethargy and tachypnea
D. Restlessness and a rapidly increasing heart rate

69. The ED nurse is examining a 19-month-old boy with respiratory distress. The child's mother reports that he has had a temperature of 101°F (38.3°C), fatigue, and hoarseness for the past 2 days, during which time the hoarseness and fatigue have progressively increased. The patient developed a barking cough during the night. The physician diagnoses laryngotracheobronchitis (croup). The nurse knows that management of a child with croup is primarily directed toward:

A. Maintaining the patient's airway and adequate respiratory exchange
B. Maintaining acid-base balance
C. Increasing the humidification of inspired air
D. Liquefying respiratory secretions

70. The nurse's care plan for a patient diagnosed with laryngotracheobronchitis should include a notation to inform the parents about the importance of avoiding the administration of:

A. Antitussives
B. Acetaminophen
C. Acetylsalicylic acid
D. Decongestants

71. The nurse knows that, to ensure adequate respiratory exchange of a child with croup should be placed in:

A. Semi-Fowler's position with the neck slightly extended
B. Semi-Fowler's position with the neck slightly flexed
C. Supine position
D. Prone position

72. The patient developed a barking cough during the night. The physician diagnoses laryngotracheobronchitis (croup). The nurse initiates IV therapy, as ordered, and monitors the child's hydration status by assessing:

A. Weight, fluid intake and output, and serum electrolyte levels
B. Weight, fluid intake and output, and fontanelle tension
C. Skin turgor, fluid intake and output, and fontanelle tension
D. Skin turgor, fluid intake and output, and urine specific gravity

73. A 64-year-old man with emphysema is admitted to the ED because of a sudden attack of dyspnea. Auscultation reveals no breath sounds over the right lung. The physician diagnoses spontaneous pneumothorax and inserts a chest tube. The patient's chest tube is ordered to be on suction, at -20 cm of water pressure. When checking the chest tube drainage system at the start of the shift, the nurse notices continuous bubbling in the suction chamber. The nurse correctly interprets this to mean:

A. The tubing or system is leaking
B. Bronchial disruption has developed
C. Esophageal fistula has developed
D. The system is functioning normally

74. A patient is status post insertion of a chest tube for pneumothorax, now has a well expanded lung, and the chest tube is positioned to allow for water-seal drainage without suction. The nurse should anticipate that the water-seal level would:

A. No longer be needed
B. Rise upon spontaneous inspiration
C. Rise with positive-pressure ventilation
D. Fall during forceful coughing

75. A 26-year-old man diagnosed with spontaneous pneumothorax is being monitored in the holding room overnight. Because the patient had limited symptoms and lung involvement, decompression of the pleural cavity was not initiated. Which assessment finding should the nurse report immediately to the physician?

A. Pain on deep inspiration
B. Expanding hyperresonance on lung percussion
C. Respiratory rate of 20 breaths/minute, moderate depth, and easy arousal
D. Heart rate of 64 beats/minute

76. Which finding would be least useful in evaluating recurrence of a pneumothorax?

A. Activity intolerance
B. Fever and chills
C. Sudden, sharp chest pain
D. Diaphoresis and dyspnea

77. A paramedic radios data to the base station regarding the status of a 64-year-old man who is showing signs and symptoms of an acute tension pneumothorax after involvement in an automobile accident. The paramedics are instructed to perform a needle thoracotomy. The nurse anticipates that the paramedic will correctly insert the needle:

A. Under the fourth rib at the anterior axillary line
B. Over the third rib at the midclavicular line
C. On the side toward which the trachea deviates
D. On the right side to avoid puncturing the heart

78. Which signs and symptoms are characteristic of tension pneumothorax?

A. Cyanosis, chest pain, and vasodilation
B. Tachycardia, subcutaneous emphysema, and dullness on percussion
C. Paradoxical chest movement, bradycardia, and high cardiac output
D. Dyspnea, jugular vein distention, hypotension, and tracheal deviation

79. After thoracotomy for a tension pneumothorax, the patient's condition does not improve despite assisted ventilation with 100% oxygen and rapid infusion of crystalloids. Which other condition causes similar symptoms?

A. Large diaphragmatic hernia
B. Cardiac contusion
C. COPD
D. 10% hemothorax

80. When the patient arrives in the ED, a chest tube is inserted. The tube is connected to a water-seal bottle that has a moderate air and fluid leak seen on expiration. When the patient is taken to the radiology department, the bottle is accidently broken. Which nursing action should be taken?

A. Remove the chest tube immediately to prevent aspiration of glass particles
B. Apply a clamp to the chest tube near the insertion site, and instruct the patient to exhale deeply
C. Pinch the chest tube, place the end of the tube in a bottle of sterile saline solution or water, and encourage the patient to cough and breathe deeply
D. Use the phone in radiology to order a new bottle, and do not manipulate the chest tube

81. The pregnant patient's respiratory status changes during gestation; her ABG would reveal:

A. Increased PO_2.
B. Increased bicarbonate.
C. Decreased $PaCO_2$.
D. Decreased pH.

82. Which of the following may be an early assessment finding of pneumonia in an elderly patient?

A. Acute onset of confusion.
B. Hyperresonance found on percussion.
C. High fever.
D. Increased heart rate.

83. Which of the following is the most common cause of airway obstruction in the elderly?

A. Displaced Dentures
B. Goiter
C. Tongue
D. Epiglottic Inflammation

84. The nurse would define anatomic dead space (VD) as:

A. The entire area from the nose to the terminal bronchioles
B. The area from the pharynx to the posterior nares
C. The tracheal tree and its branches
D. Bad lung areas of the chest

85. The nurse would assess the following ABG: pH 7.38, PaO_2 83, SaO_2 96%, CO_2 37, HCO_3 25 as:

A. Abnormal because the pH shows acidemia
B. Abnormal because the O_2 demonstrates hypoxemia
C. Normal
D. Abnormal because the patient needs bicarbonate

RESPIRATORY EMERGENCIES: RATIONALE

1. **B** Atelectasis is indicated when bronchial breath sounds are heard over the right middle lung lobe. Bronchial sounds normally are heard only over the manubrium of the sternum and along the sternal borders, which are located over the trachea. They are characteristically high-pitched, loud, and harsh in quality, with a pause between the inspiratory and expiratory phases. Bronchial breath sounds heard over the lung periphery may indicate abnormal sound transmission because of consolidated lung tissue, as in atelectasis.

2. **B** Consolidated lung areas typically produce a flat or dull sound on percussion because of the increased mass. Percussion over a normal lung produces a resonant or hollow sound that is of low pitch and intensity. An overinflated lung, such as in emphysema, typically produces a sustained hyperresonant sound. Tympanic sounds are high-pitched and are produced by air-containing organs, such as the stomach.

3. **A** Bronchovesicular breath sounds normally are auscultated over the large bronchi, below the clavicles and between the scapulae. These sounds are of moderate amplitude and medium to high in pitch, representing a mixture of bronchial and vesicular sounds. In other lung areas, bronchovesicular sounds may indicate consolidation or other abnormalities. Bronchial sounds, which typically are loud and high-pitched, normally are auscultated over the trachea.

4. **D** Any condition that produces disruption of alveolar function, consolidation, or compression (such as pulmonary fibrosis, pleural effusion, or chronic obstructive pulmonary disease [COPD]) may result in decreased or absent vesicular sounds. Vesicular sounds, produced by the opening of alveoli

on inspiration and the movement of air through the larynx (glottic hiss) during expiration, are of low amplitude and medium to low pitch; they may be described as swishing or rustling.

5. **C** Palpation is commonly used in respiratory assessment to determine the degree of respiratory excursion as well as to identify areas of tenderness, to assess for abnormalities, and to elicit fremitus. The nurse assesses respiratory excursion by determining if each lung expands to the same degree at different chest locations. This is accomplished by placing the hands, with thumbs together and fingers spread, over the center of the chest. As the patient takes a deep breath, the nurse notes if the fingers and thumbs move apart to an equal degree. Each lung lobe, or its equivalent area on the chest wall, should be assessed in this manner. Unequal excursion may be caused by such conditions as atelectasis or pneumothorax.

6. **D** A relaxed tongue is the most common cause of upper airway obstruction in the unconscious adult. Because of insufficient muscle tone, the relaxed tongue can fall over the back of the throat, obstructing the pharynx and larynx. Since the tongue is attached to the lower jaw, moving the lower jaw forward (as in the head-tilt-chin-lift maneuver) lifts the tongue away from the back of the throat and opens the airway. Performing this maneuver may restore spontaneous respirations in an apneic patient.

7. **B** Complete airway obstruction is marked by the absence of air movement and coughing and by the inability to speak. Partial airway obstruction may produce good or poor air exchange. A patient with good air exchange typically is able to cough forcefully but may experience wheezing between coughs.

A patient with poor air exchange typically has an ineffective, weak cough, inspiratory stridor, and cyanosis.

8. **B** The American Heart Association recommends administering abdominal thrusts (the Heimlich maneuver) as the initial management for relieving foreign-body airway obstruction in a conscious adult patient. This procedure involves the delivery of repeated sub-diaphragmatic thrusts, each one delivered with enough force to remove a sufficient volume of air from the lungs and produce an artificial cough capable of expelling a foreign body from the airway. The procedure should be repeated, as necessary, until the object is expelled from the victim. The efficacy of back blows in relieving airway obstruction is not well documented. An adult with complete airway obstruction would be unable to cough to expel a foreign body. Administering artificial respiration would be of no help in ventilating the victim if the obstruction has not been relieved.

9. **D** If a patient suddenly goes into respiratory arrest, the nurse's highest priority would be to open the patient's airway. In an emergency, the nurse should always follow the ABCs of airway management, ensuring the patient's Airway, Breathing, and Circulation sequentially. Without spinal trauma, the airway may be opened using a head-tilt-chin-lift or jaw-thrust maneuver. This action allows the victim to resume spontaneous respirations without the need for further intervention. For a patient going into cardiac arrest the American Heart Association (AHA) recommends C-A-B (not ABC). Being that the patient's carotid pulse (adult/child)—or brachial pulse for an infant—is the point of pulse check. A radial pulse check is not recommended in determining the presence of a pulse with regards to resuscitation.

10. **C** Although intubation will likely be a definitive airway, endotracheal intubation should be attempted only after other oxygenation methods have failed; it should never be used as the initial procedure for ventilation in respiratory arrest. The lungs should be well oxygenated before any intubation attempt; adequate ventilation can be provided with the use of a bag-valve-mask device. Intubation requires the skill of a trained individual who can efficiently complete the procedure in 20 to 30 seconds.

11. **D** Esophageal obturator airway removal commonly is followed by immediate regurgitation of stomach contents; therefore, suction equipment must be readily available. The patient who does not have an endotracheal tube in place should be turned on the left side before removal of the esophageal obturator airway to prevent aspiration of stomach contents. The esophageal obturator airway consists of a tube approximately 14½" (37 cm) long that is open at the top and has a blind end at the bottom. The blind end is inserted into the esophagus; the airway is not visualized. An inflatable cuff is located just above the blind end, and several side holes located near the upper end allow passage of air from the interior of the tube into the pharynx. Possible hazards associated with the use of this airway include laceration and rupture of the esophagus, not the trachea. Performing endotracheal intubation with an esophageal obturator airway in place is possible.

12. **C** Cyanosis is not an early sign of respiratory failure. Restlessness, tachycardia, and tachypnea are early signs of hypoxia and hypoxemia that occur in respiratory failure. Cyanosis, which occurs secondary to un-oxygenation of hemoglobin in the capillaries, is imperceptible until 5 g of un-oxygenated hemoglobin/100 mL of blood is detected. Therefore, cyanosis is a later sign of respiratory failure.

Cyanosis may not present in a patient with a decreased hematocrit.

13. **B** Acute respiratory failure resulting from impaired ventilation initially produces hypoxia and hypercapnia. Ventilation impairment (such as occurs in atelectasis, emphysema and the late states of asthma) prevents gas exchange, leading to decreased oxygen and carbon dioxide retention in the blood. Oxygenation impairment (such as occurs in lung tumors and pulmonary edema) initially produces only hypoxia. Although oxygen reaches the alveoli, it is either not absorbed or not used. Carbon dioxide is not retained because it is 20 times more diffusable then oxygen. Hypocapnia and hypoxia are seen in the early states of asthma because of the blowing off of carbon dioxide that results from tachypnea.

14. **C** In a patient with no underlying lung disease and essentially normal lung tissue, respiratory failure usually is indicated by a $PaCO_2$, greater than 50 mmHg and a PaO_2 less than 50 mmHg (oxygen saturation below 85%). Respiratory failure is defined as any condition in which the blood oxygen content is insufficient to fulfill tissue demands for oxygen secondary to decreased lung function. A diagnosis of respiratory failure must be based on the patient's history, clinical appearance, and changes in serial arterial blood gas (ABG) studies. A patient with an obstructive disorder, such as COPD, will function with abnormal blood gas levels, such as those indicative of hypoxia and hypercapnia.

15. **D** When given too quickly patients can projectile vomit. Therefore, ensure you push naloxone SLOWLY. The other options are assessment findings you may encounter for a narcotic overdose.

16. **D** Aspiration of gastric contents commonly results from attempts to ventilate an obstructed airway. Excessive air pressure is needed to inflate a partially or completely obstructed airway. Since air follows the path of least resistance, a large volume of air travels down the esophagus and into the stomach, resulting in gastric distention and a high risk of regurgitation and aspiration. To decrease the risk of distention, the American Heart Association has issued new basic life support guidelines that alter the recommended speed of airflow delivery during mouth-to-mouth or mouth-to-mask resuscitation. An unconscious patient is at high risk for aspiration because of depressed or absent gag and cough reflexes. Aspiration of gastric contents is more common in children than adults. Children have a greater tendency for aerophagia (air swallowing) when crying or frightened; this increases the risk of gastric distention and aspiration. Adult respiratory distress syndrome (ARDS) can occur as a result of aspiration because of the low pH of gastric contents.

17. **A** Level of consciousness should be the nurse's most important consideration when determining a patient's risk of aspiration. An alert, cooperative patient with intact cerebral, brain stem, and spinal input typically can swallow with concurrent glottic closure while maintaining cough and gag reflexes; such a patient is at decreased risk for aspiration. A sedated or unconscious patient, however, has reduced protective reflex mechanisms and therefore is at increased risk for aspiration. Appropriate nursing interventions for preventing aspiration include ensuring proper positioning (semi-Fowler's or side-lying), including the positioning of the alert patient who is immobilized for spinal precautions; ensuring that suction equipment is accessible; and monitoring for gastric distention and patency of nasogastric tubes. The cardiac sphincter is the

lower esophageal sphincter near the opening of the stomach; its integrity cannot be assessed easily in the clinical setting.

18. **D** In this situation, the nurse would expect the physician to order dextrose administration because the patient's symptoms suggest severe hypoglycemia. Because neurons, which are glucose-dependent, become irreversibly damaged when deprived of glucose, administering dextrose IV can help prevent any further damage. If possible, the nurse should draw a blood specimen before administering dextrose to document the serum glucose level. After administration, the nurse should observe the patient's reaction to the drug. Usually, naloxone is given along with dextrose early in therapy to reverse possible respiratory depression from a drug overdose. However, since the patient's airway is not being maintained, administering this medication is not the highest priority. Lidocaine and epinephrine are not indicated because the patient has no lethal arrhythmias.

19. **D** The carina is the landmark by which proper depth of endotracheal intubation should be measured. Placement of the tip of the endotracheal tube too near or below the carina can result in right main-stem bronchus intubation or atelectasis of the left lung. Placement too far above the carina increases the risk of vocal cord damage or inadvertent extubation. Nasotracheal intubation is not necessarily a logical choice in a patient with a maxillofacial injury. Despite the association of facial injury with spinal cord injury and the fact that nasotracheal intubation is safer than endotracheal intubation in a patient with a suspected spinal cord injury (it requires less extension and manipulation of the patient's neck), nasotracheal intubation is hazardous because of the risk of nasal fracture, frontal skull and cribriform plate damage, and sinus or intracranial infection. Cricothyroidotomy is an emergency

procedure involving the formation of an opening for an artificial airway in the cricothyroid membrane, which is below the thyroid cartilage (Adam's apple) and above the cricoid cartilage. The vocal cords are above these landmarks. Because cricothyroidotomy involves catheterization with a needle, it is less invasive and traumatic than a tracheostomy. It is reported that the most difficult aspect of performing a cricothyroidotomy is making the decision to do it. Regardless, the decision should become clear when there are futile attempts to secure the airway.

20. **C** Pulmonary contusion is the most common cause of impaired gas exchange after blunt thoracic trauma. Blunt or penetrating trauma to the lung characteristically results in the accumulation of blood and fluid in the involved interstitial tissue, alveoli, and small bronchi. The reduced vital capacity and pulmonary compliance together with increased secretions from the injured lung produce increasing atelectasis. This combination of atelectasis, disrupted tissue, and extravasated blood results in impaired gas exchange. Flail chest is a type of penetrating chest trauma. Apnea, hypopnea, and phrenic nerve paralysis may occur after spinal cord injury.

21. **C** During the emergent phase of care, pulmonary contusion is best indicated by radiographic studies. Pulmonary contusion, a bruise on the lung that causes interstitial edema and hemorrhage, may appear as patchy infiltrates initially on chest X-ray; later X-rays typically show consolidation. Auscultation may not initially reveal abnormalities unless other injuries are present. ABG test results, although checked serially, may not demonstrate intrapulmonary shunting in the emergent phase. Hypoxemia may be delayed; therefore, dyspnea may not be evident. Signs and symptoms depend on the severity of

contusion and associated injuries. Pulmonary contusion may evolve into ARDS.

22. **A** Changes in level of consciousness, such as restlessness, confusion, irritability, and decreased responsiveness, indicate serious hypoxia. Peripheral vasoconstriction, changes in urine output, and delayed capillary refill are related primarily to reduced vascular volume and inadequate perfusion.

23. **C** An increase in negative pressure inside the pleural space results in normal inspiration. Airflow into the lungs normally travels from an area of higher pressure to an area of lower pressure. As the diaphragm contracts, the thorax enlarges and the visceral and parietal pleura move with it. Healthy lungs will recoil and pull away from the chest wall, which pulls the parietal pleural layer, creating negative (sub atmospheric) pressure within the intrapleural space. The more the thorax enlarges, the more the lung stretches and tries to recoil, creating more and more negative pressure. Outside air at atmospheric pressure flows into the lungs during this inspiratory process. Positive pleural pressure will collapse the lung, resulting in a pneumothorax.

24. **D** Dyspnea in this situation is most likely caused by an associated chest injury. The lungs extend to the sixth rib anteriorly and the eighth rib laterally, and may descend to the twelfth rib posteriorly on deep inspiration. The nurse should suspect a chest injury in any patient with a blunt or penetrating injury to the upper abdomen or a gunshot wound in the same area because of the possible trajectory of the knife or bullet.

25. **B** These finings are indicative of a mediastinal air leak. Subcutaneous emphysema may occur in pneumothorax or any condition that causes a sudden increase in intrathoracic pressure

that results in alveolar rupture. Air dissects to the loose mediastinal tissues and gravitates up to the neck, face, and supraclavicular area, where it may be first detected. A mediastinal air leak, which may arise from the esophagus or lungs, can be heard during auscultation of the apical rate as the air is compressed by the contraction of the heart with each beat (Hamman's sign).

26. **A** These symptoms may indicate pneumonia (inflammation or infection of the lung) or costochondritis (inflammation of the cartilage surrounding the ribs). Pneumothorax, a rare occurrence after a rib contusion or rib fracture, usually is associated with all of the symptoms except fever and sputum production. Empyema may develop after penetrating chest trauma. Pulmonary hypertension does not develop after a rib fracture.

27. **C** A large chest tube, with or without a trocar, is used to evacuate blood from the chest cavity to prevent obstruction from clots. The typical size used is a #36 French or #40 French for a hemothorax, a #28 French for pneumothorax.

28. **A** Hemothorax is the most common reason for autotransfusion in an emergency setting. Most basic autotransfusion devices are attached to the chest tube, which evacuates accumulated blood. Evacuating blood from other sites, such as the liver or thigh, places the patient at increased risk for bacterial contamination and development of clotting and particulate matter; autotransfusing blood from these sites would not be advantageous unless the patient were exsanguinating and blood products were unavailable. Hypotension from a spinal cord injury does not result from hemorrhage; therefore, transfusion is not required.

29. **B** Hypocapnia, which may result from aggressive ventilation, would be of least concern because this results in a mild respiratory alkalosis that is offset by metabolic acidosis. Ventilatory efforts will prevent hypoxia. Other contributing factors, such as pericardial tamponade, volume deficit, or pneumothorax, will seriously hinder resuscitation but can be rapidly corrected.

30. **C** Positioning the patient on his injured (right) side would cause great pain and might cause further internal injury. Placing him on his left side would be optimal. This position would allow for insertion of chest tubes, as necessary, while providing the best ventilation and perfusion to the uninjured lung, since pulmonary blood flow follows gravity, and ventilation (per unit of lung volume) is greater in the dependent area of the lung. Positioning the patient on his left side also would help to drain secretions from his affected side.

31. **D** Flail chest is defined as two or more ribs fractured in two or more places, or with one fracture plus costochondral separation, or a fractured sternum. A flail segment or free-floating piece of thoracic cage must be present. This piece causes the chest wall to move paradoxically because of the defect in thoracic skeletal structure. The chest wall is pulled toward the negative intrapleural pressure during inspiration and pushed away from positive intrapleural pressure on expiration. Changes in ventilation and perfusion are most closely linked with underlying pulmonary damage rather than paradoxical motion.

32. **B** Flail chest is easiest to assess when the thoracic fracture segments occur anteriorly, as anterior thoracic structures are least supported by muscle and easiest to visualize. Flail chest is most difficult to visualize in a muscular patient or a patient with

posterior thoracic fracture segments because contracted muscle splints the area. Flail chest is moderately easy to assess when segments occur laterally. An alert patient typically splints the area to relieve the pain, making the flail less evident until fatigue sets in. Because an unconscious patient does not react to discomfort and does not splint the area, flail chest is typically easy to detect.

33. **A** Although advanced age and obesity can contribute to reduced ventilatory reserve; they do not necessarily indicate the need for ventilatory support in a patient with a massive flail chest. A patient with flail chest may need assisted ventilation if breathing fatigue progressively worsens and if signs and symptoms of inadequate oxygen and carbon dioxide exchange (hypercapnia, hypoxia, and dyspnea) are evident. All trauma patients are intubated and ventilated during surgery. When associated injuries are present, assisted ventilation may be provided on a temporary basis to ensure proper oxygenation.

34. **B** The appropriate nursing intervention in this situation would be to frequently administer low-dose narcotics, as ordered. This will relieve the patient's pain without causing significant respiratory depression. The most effective method of pain control is through physician-initiated intercostal nerve blocks or thoracic epidural analgesia. These allow for optimal chest wall movement and ventilation; then incentive spirometry may be used. The other interventions are inappropriate in the early stages of injury because the patient will be unable to tolerate chest percussion or postural drainage because of his pain and unstable condition. Also, binding and taping the chest wall will limit chest excursion and air exchange.

35. **A** A decreased oxygen tension or room air (PaO_2 less than 80 mmHg) and elevated lactic dehydrogenase (LDH) levels are

the most common laboratory findings in pulmonary embolism. The white blood cell (WBC) count may be elevated or normal (normal is 5,000 to 10,000/mm^3). A PaO$_2$ greater than 80 mmHg is inconsistent with pulmonary embolism. Elevated LDH levels are common in many diseases; this finding alone is not specifically diagnostic for pulmonary embolus.

36. **D** The priority nursing diagnosis would be impaired gas exchange related to altered pulmonary tissue perfusion because, at this time, the patient is at highest risk for complications from pulmonary embolism. Although anxiety related to hypoxia and pain and pain related to pulmonary ischemia are important diagnoses, they are not the priority at this time. Potential for injury related to hemorrhage from anticoagulant therapy would not be a concern because heparin therapy has not yet been started.

37. **B** Calf pain on dorsiflexion of the foot is considered a positive Homans' sign, which could indicative deep vein thrombosis; however, this is not reliable. Trousseau's sign is a carpal spasm elicited by compressing the upper arm, causing ischemia of the distal nerves; a positive sign is indicative of tetany. Babinski's reflex is dorsiflexion of the great toe and fanning of the smaller toes in response to a strong stimulus on the sole of the foot. A positive Babinski's sign in a patient over age 2 indicates an upper motor neuron lesion. Kehr's sign, radiating shoulder pain that occurs when the diaphragm is irritated from blood loss in the peritoneum, usually is seen in a patient with a ruptured spleen.

38. **A** Pulmonary embolism rarely causes specific electrocardiographic (EKG) changes. However, sinus tachycardia caused by apprehension, pain, and a decreased PO$_2$ is the most common EKG finding. Some EKG findings that

may suggest a pulmonary embolus include enlarged P waves, depressed ST segments, inverted T waves, and atrial fibrillation. If a massive pulmonary embolism has occurred, the EKG may show right axis deviation, indicating right ventricular failure.

39. **B** Heparin impedes clotting by preventing thrombi formation. It does not act on existing clots. Because adequate anticoagulation is based on the partial thromboplastin time (PTT), the dosage is adjusted to achieve a PTT from 55 to 85 seconds (this range varies slightly between facilities). Continuous IV heparin administration is preferred for a high-risk patient because it maintains a steady therapeutic blood level. Heparin bolus administration produces peak levels for a short time, but subtherapeutic levels are evident before the next dose is due.

40. **A** The initial emergency treatment for a patient in acute respiratory distress secondary to chronic obstructive pulmonary disease (COPD) includes administering 30% oxygen via face mask and bronchodilator therapy. Unless the patient has severe acidosis or is obtunded, a conservative approach to treatment is initially recommended. Most patients with COPD are dependent on the hypoxic drive to maintain adequate ventilation. Uncontrolled or high-flow oxygen therapy may precipitate severe carbon dioxide narcosis and respiratory arrest. Precise oxygen therapy delivered by facemask may allow time for use of other therapeutic measures, such as bronchodilator therapy, thereby avoiding the need for intubation and mechanical ventilation. Morphine sulfate would be inappropriate in this situation because of its ensuing respiratory depressant effects.

41. **B** An appropriate intervention for a patient in acute respiratory distress secondary to COPD would be to place the patient in a high-Fowler's position or leaning upright over bedside table to ensure optimal ventilation. In a less acutely ill patient, having the patient sit in a chair is also beneficial. All these positions assist in lowering the diaphragm, thereby increasing respiratory excursion. Placing the patient in a supine position would diminish optimal ventilation and worsen the respiratory failure. Endotracheal intubation is not indicated at this time. Respiratory depressants, such as morphine sulfate, are not indicated at this time, as they will further inhibit the stimulus to breathe.

42. **B** Cigarette smoking appears to be the single most important factor leading to chronic airway obstruction. In most cases, cigarette smoking also interacts with virtually every other contributing factor. Anxiety may affect breathing patterns, typically by causing hyperventilation and exacerbation of dyspnea during respiratory distress. In certain occupational groups, such as auto mechanics and miners, the incidence of COPD is high; however, this is not the case with the patient in this situation. Although increased activity in a patient with lung disease may exacerbate symptoms, the patient in this situation had been sedentary during that attack.

43. **C** Chronic bronchitis is classified as COPD because of hyperplasia and inflammation of goblet cells and increased production of thick mucus. The constant irritation of the bronchioles leads to hypertrophy of mucus-secreting glands, goblet cell hyperplasia, and increased mucus production, which leads to bronchial plugging and narrowing and diminished airflow.

44. **A** The nurse would not expect the physician to order fluid restriction for a patient with COPD. Instead, intake should be encouraged to help mobilize secretions.

45. **B** In the early stages of COPD, cessation of cigarette smoking is probably the most significant factor in halting the disease's progression. After discontinuation of smoking, the accelerated decline in pulmonary function slows and the patient's pulmonary function returns to a more normal level, i.e. that of a nonsmoker. Therefore, if the patient stops smoking now, his cough and sputum production will decrease and his pulmonary function tests will improve.

46. **B** A patient with severe bronchial abnormalities and mild emphysema is commonly labeled a blue bloater. In this condition, hypoventilation leads to hypoxemia and hypercapnia. A patient with severe emphysema and mild bronchitis is commonly labeled a pink puffer. In this condition, hyperventilation assists in adequate oxygenation; therefore, cyanosis is absent. Asthmatic symptoms are caused by a hyperreactive airway.

47. **D** Cor pulmonale is a complication of COPD secondary to pulmonary hypertension caused by vasoconstriction in response to hypoxia; acidosis further potentiates the ability to vasoconstrict. Chronic alveolar hypoxia causes ventricular hypertrophy and stimulates erythropoiesis, which increases the blood viscosity. Clinical manifestations are related to dilation and failure of the right ventricle, with subsequent intravascular volume expansion and systemic venous congestion.

48. **D** A patient with cor pulmonale resulting from COPD typically develops pulmonary hypertension and signs of right-sided heart failure, including jugular vein distention,

hepatosplenomegaly, and edema. Bibasilar crackles are typically seen in left-sided heart failure. A capillary refill of 4 seconds indicates impaired circulation or an inadequate circulatory volume. Poor skin turgor indicates a fluid volume deficit.

49. **D** Small-airway obstruction usually is irreversible in such chronic diseases as emphysema and bronchitis; however, this same obstruction usually is reversible in asthma. Pneumonia is an inflammation of the lung, not of the small airways. Improving ventilation can reverse atelectasis.

50. **C** The nurse should plan to include information on the importance of receiving influenza vaccines at the prescribed times and to seek medical advice about receiving a vaccine against streptococcal pneumonia. A patient with COPD is more prone to respiratory infections, which subsequently intensify the pathologic destruction of lung tissue and the progression of COPD. The most common causative organisms are Haemophilus influenzae and Streptococcus pneumoniae. Retained secretions provide a good medium for the proliferation of these organisms. Chest X-rays are not recommended annually. Vitamin supplements are not usually recommended unless the patient also has a vitamin deficiency or poor dietary intake. Dry climates could be harmful for a patient who is expectorating sputum that is not liquefied.

51. **A** Barrel chest results from hyperinflation and over-distention of alveoli. In a patient with emphysema, elastin and collagen, the supporting structures of the lung, are destroyed. Without this support, the bronchiolar walls tend to collapse and air becomes trapped in the distal alveoli, resulting in hyperinflation and over-distention of the alveoli. This trapped air gives the patient a barrel chested appearance.

52. **C** Pursed-lip breathing slows expiration and prevents collapse of lung units by helping to increase PEEP (positive end expiratory pressure). It also helps the patient to control the rate and depth of respirations and to relax, which decreases dyspnea and feelings of panic. Use of inspiratory muscle training devices must be judiciously monitored by a health care professional. Indiscriminate use can produce inspiratory muscle exhaustion and acute ventilator failure. Postural drainage, chest percussion, and vibration are indicated for patients with increased sputum production.

53. **C** Although the use of expectorants is not uniformly recommended for a patient with COPD, cough suppressants must be avoided. Antihistamines cause drying of the respiratory mucosa, which can result in mucus thickening and possible airway obstruction. Hydration, aerosol humidification, chest physiotherapy, and postural drainage loosen and remove thick secretions. The patient with COPD does not need to avoid spicy foods.

54. **B** Ineffective individual coping is a common diagnostic category used by nurses caring for patients with COPD. Developing healthy psychological coping mechanisms is perhaps the most difficult task the patient must master. Because a patient with COPD typically must learn to cope with and manage various life-style changes, he may find himself in a vicious cycle of emotional entrapment. The nurse may need to help him learn to communicate honestly with supportive family and friends and to avoid anxiety-producing situations. Learning these skills is more difficult than learning facts about the nutritional and therapeutic aspects of COPD.

55. **B** Extrinsic asthma is precipitated by a known allergen or allergy. Patients with extrinsic asthma usually have a family

history of allergies and a medical history of infantile eczema or allergic rhinitis. Intrinsic asthma is exacerbated by cold air, air pollution, and primary infection. Mixed asthma is associated with some allergic tendencies. Idiopathic asthma has unknown causative factors.

56. **D** Because extrinsic asthma attacks are precipitated by exposure to certain allergens, such as pollen, dander, feathers, mold, dust, and some foods, the nurse would suspect that the down jacket precipitated the attack. The other answer choices are not likely to be respiratory allergens.

57. **C** Normally, the bronchioles constrict during expiration. However, expiration becomes more difficult when the bronchioles are already constricted, edematous, and filled with mucus. Bronchospasm and mucus production typically occur during asthma attacks.

58. **C** Besides the dyspnea and chest tightness, the nurse would expect to note the characteristic clinical manifestations of asthma—wheezing and coughing. Expiration is more difficult than inspiration; therefore, prolonged, wheezing expirations are characteristic. The cough may be nonproductive, possibly indicating widespread bronchiolar plugging. Production of thick, tenacious, white, gelatinous mucus also may occur, typically only after treatment has begun.

59. **C** Administration of albuterol should improve the patient's condition most rapidly. To relieve bronchospasm, treatment is aimed at decreasing mucosal edema and facilitating secretion removal. Beta-adrenergic agents and bronchodilators, such as albuterol, epinephrine, and terbutaline, offer rapid relief. Corticosteroids usually are effective 6 to 9 hours after administration. Cromolyn sodium is an old medication and was

used prophylactically, if still used it should not be used for an acute attack. Oxygen and IV fluids will not reverse bronchospasm.

60. **A** An important nursing goal during an acute asthma attack is to decrease the patient's sense of panic. The best approach would be to maintain a calm, quiet, reassuring attitude to help the patient relax. Staying with the patient and being available provides additional comfort. Teaching is most effective after the attack subsides. Although visitors should be restricted, a parent may be helpful in alleviating anxiety in an adolescent. Although diversional therapy is a commonly used tactic, it would be inappropriate in this situation because the patient is having difficulty breathing and probably would not be able to concentrate on the diversion.

61. **A** Prompt diagnosis and treatment of upper respiratory tract infections may prevent exacerbations. Physical exercise within the patient's tolerance level is beneficial. Staying indoors when the air pollution index is high is helpful.

62. **B** The most common type of pneumonia is pneumococcal, caused by Streptococcus pneumoniae. Staphylococcus pneumonia occurs more commonly in hospitalized patients than in people in the community. Bacillus pneumonia is associated with agricultural or industrial exposure to Bacillus microorganisms. Pneumonia caused by Streptococcus pyogenes is known to occur in military populations after influenza epidemics.

63. **C** The nurse would expect the physician to order a Gram stain of the patient's sputum and chest X-rays. A Gram stain of sputum provides the information on which the initial therapy is based. Immediate identification of the infecting organism

permits the institution of appropriate antimicrobial therapy. Sputum and blood cultures take 24 to 72 hours. Chest X-rays frequently show a pattern characteristic of the infecting organisms; lung scans do not show this. Bronchoscopy may be necessary if the patient cannot voluntarily produce a sputum specimen. Arterial blood gas measurements and electrolyte studies, although helpful, usually are not critical unless the patient is tachypneic and diaphoretic.

64. **A** Epiglottitis, which typically occurs between ages 3 and 7, is associated with a large, cherry red, edematous epiglottis; muffled voice sounds or aphonia, dysphagia, drooling, and a croaking or froglike sound on inspiration. The patient may have a rapid onset of symptoms and complain of a sore throat. Typically, the patient will not struggle to breathe, but rather prefers to remain still for better air exchange. He may assume an upright position and lean with his chin thrust forward (tripod position). A younger child may protrude his tongue. Temperatures may range from 100° to 105° F (37.8° to 40.6° C).

65. **B** Intubation or tracheotomy equipment must be available whenever epiglottitis is suspected because complete airway obstruction can occur suddenly. Suction equipment and humidified oxygen also should be accessible. Epiglottitis requires immediate intervention, and the child should be admitted to the pediatric intensive care unit. He should never be left unattended. Separation from the parents may increase the child's anxiety and agitation, thereby increasing his oxygen need. The need for tracheotomy consent varies according to the institution. Usually, the physician is responsible for obtaining an informed consent for surgical procedures or medical care. Oxygen may not be needed once an airway is established.

66. **D** Attempts to directly visualize the epiglottis with a tongue blade can precipitate sudden laryngospasm and result in complete airway obstruction. A nurse should never attempt to visualize the epiglottis. Such visualization should occur within the operating room, with intubation or tracheotomy equipment available. An IV infusion should be started before the procedure. To prevent trauma, the endotracheal tube should be smaller than that normally used. To prevent laryngospasm, a throat culture should be obtained after the airway is established. Haemophilus influenzae is the most common bacterial agent found. Because bacteremia is present in 50% of cases, blood cultures should be obtained. The white blood cell count typically is greater than 15,000/mm^3. A child with epiglottitis typically is quiet because he has better air exchange with little activity. Coughing and vomiting do not occur with epiglottitis, although occasionally a child may have some retching.

67. **B** Chloral hydrate is commonly administered to produce mild sedation without respiratory depression or drying of secretions. Restlessness, agitation, or anxiety can increase the respiratory rate and oxygen demand. Sedation may be required to prevent the child from removing the artificial airway, as restraints typically produce increased agitation and are not used. Steroids may be administered to reduce epiglottal edema. Chloral hydrate has no anticonvulsant effect.

68. **D** The earliest signs of hypoxemia in children are restlessness, tachypnea, and a rapidly increasing heart rate. Accessory respiratory muscle use, retractions, and nasal flaring are intermediate signs of hypoxemia. Cyanosis and lethargy are late signs and require immediate intervention. The cough is brassy or barking and resonant. Inspiratory stridor is caused by partial upper airway obstruction. In a child, any increase in

metabolism will increase oxygen consumption, thereby increasing the respiratory rate (the normal respiratory rate for a 19-month-old is 24 to 40 breaths/minute). A fever can increase the respiratory rate by 4 breaths/minute for each fahrenheit-degree rise in temperature above normal.

69. **A** Management of a child with croup is primarily directed toward maintaining the patient's airway and adequate respiratory exchange.

70. **C** Acetylsalicylic acid (aspirin) should not be administered to a child with croup. Acetylsalicylic acid has been correlated with Reye's syndrome, which can cause fatal encephalopathy. Reye's syndrome commonly follows acute upper respiratory tract viral infections. Laryngotracheobronchitis, the most common form of croup, results from a viral infection and usually occurs in the fall and winter. It is more prevalent in males between ages 3 months and 3 years. The nurse should keep in mind that a child with potential respiratory distress should never be given a sedative because it may mask restlessness, an early indicator of hypoxemia.

71. **A** Placing the patient in a semi-Fowler's position with the neck slightly extended will ensure adequate respiratory exchange, as semi-Fowler's position aids in lung expansion, and slight neck extension opens a child's narrow airway. A prone position helps to compress distended lungs during expiration, but this is not a problem in croup. During auscultation, the child should be sitting to facilitate an accurate assessment. Auscultation of the entire chest is necessary; because the chest is small, breath sounds frequently are referred to other aspects of the chest.

72. **D** Skin turgor, fluid intake and output, and urine specific gravity are the most important measures of hydration status. Hydration is particularly important in infants and young children because their total water body composition differs from that of adults. The composition does not become similar to that of an adult until about age 2. Until that time, the child's weight is a more important parameter for hydration assessment. In a child over age 2, the other parameters are of greater importance. Skin turgor is a good indication of hydration in a child as well as an adult. A dehydrated child's skin turgor typically is poor. IV fluid replacement may be necessary to decrease the child's physical exertion, respiratory rate, and risk of aspiration. Fluid intake and output measurements are essential to monitor the hydration status, especially to prevent overhydration with IV therapy. Urine specific gravity is an excellent indicator of hydration because the kidneys' ability to concentrate and dilute urine increases with age (because an infant's kidneys are immature, specific gravity is not a good indicator of renal function at such an early age). Although serum electrolyte levels provide an indirect measurement of hydration status, they are more valuable as indicators of electrolyte status. Fontanelle tension would not be an appropriate indicator in this situation because the posterior fontanelle usually closes by age 2 to 3 months and the anterior fontanelle by age 12 to 18 months.

73. **D** The suction chamber should be bubbling constantly if connected to suction; this indicates that the system is functioning normally. Continuous bubbling in the water-seal chamber would indicate fluctuation with respiration or an air leak on expiration; the patient may have a significant air leak caused by bronchial damage, or a leak may have developed in the chest tube connection or in the drainage holes in the end of

the tube extending outside the chest wall. Gastric drainage in the chest drainage system may indicate an esophageal fistula.

74. **B** If there is no air leak, the water level should rise and fall with the patient's respirations, reflecting normal pressure changes in the pleural cavity. During spontaneous respirations, the water level should rise during inhalation and fall during exhalation. If the patient is receiving positive pressure ventilation, the oscillation will be just the opposite—the water level should fall with inhalation and rise with exhalation. This oscillation is called tidaling and is one indicator of an intact and patent pleural chest tube.

75. **B** The nurse should report expanding hyperresonance on lung percussion. Extension of the pneumothorax rather than the desired reabsorption would be detected by auscultation of diminished breath because the liver better protects the right side. Excursion of the bowel and other abdominal structures into the thorax creates excessive pressure that can also compress and shift the thoracic structures. A 10% hemothorax and chronic obstructive pulmonary disease will not cause such severe symptoms. Cardiac contusion does not produce respiratory symptoms.

76. **B** Fever and chills may indicate atelectasis; however, with full lung expansion and a short duration of pulmonary abnormality, atelectasis is unlikely. The patient's symptoms are more likely caused by a viral infection. The other symptoms listed are characteristic of pneumothorax and place the patient at a higher risk of recurrence.

77. **B** The nurse would anticipate insertion of the needle over the third rib at the midclavicular line. The needle should be inserted over the third rib because the intercostal artery and vein

are located under the rib. Placement at the superior border should avoid vascular trauma. The procedure may be done at the second intercostal space midclavicular line or the fourth or fifth intercostal space midaxillary line. Tension pneumothorax is caused by excessive pressure on the injured side. This will eventually shift the mediastinal contents to the uninjured side, affecting vascular flow and ventilation. Treatment should be aimed at the side of origin of injury, the side opposite the tracheal deviation. Needle thoracotomy can be performed correctly on the left side of the chest without inducing cardiac injury.

78. **D** Signs and symptoms of a tension pneumothorax include dyspnea, jugular vein distention, hypotension, and tracheal deviation. In tension pneumothorax, the injured lung is collapsed and the contralateral lung is partially collapsed. This creates severe dyspnea from ineffective gas exchange. The mediastinal contents (large vessels, trachea, and heart) are shifted or deviated and compressed, depending on the pressure created. This results in ineffective cardiac contraction and reduced venous return, resulting in jugular vein distention and low cardiac output. Tachycardia is a compensatory mechanism and hypotension would be present.

79. **A** A large diaphragmatic hernia caused by a rupture or laceration of the diaphragm allows abdominal contents to enter the thoracic cavity. Pressure within the abdominal cavity is higher than intrathoracic pressure. Diaphragmatic hernias occur most often on the left side.

80. **C** The best action is to pinch the tubing to prevent atmospheric air from entering the pleural space until a temporary water seal can be obtained. In this situation, the nurse may be creative in seeking a new form of water seal and

enlist the help of other personnel in the immediate area. Use of a clean urinal filled with water would be better than sustained clamping. Pinching is suggested rather than clamping because the nurse is less likely to forget to release the tube. This patient required a needle thoracotomy to relieve a tension pneumothorax. The current chest tube, if clamped, is ineffective in allowing escape of intrapleural air or fluid; it should not be removed or the tension will recur.

81. **C** The presence of progesterone contributes to increasing the respiratory rate, which in turn decreases PaO_2 (30 - 34 mmHg).

82. **A** Early signs in the elderly are: acute onset of confusion, deterioration in general health, and lethargy.

83. **A** A goiter is rarely seen, unless the goiter is iodine induced--and is treated with thyroid hormone. A displaced denture can cause airway obstruction. Objects should be removed that block that airway. In younger populations the tongue is more common to obstruct the airway. Inflammation is also more commonly seen in younger populations, such as children, infants and the intoxicated.

84. **A** The entire area from the nose to the terminal bronchioles, where gas flows but not exchanged, is called the anatomic dead space. The pharynx is posterior to the nasal cavities and the mouth; air passes through, but continues on to the terminal bronchioles. There is no such thing as the tracheal tree and its branches—the bronchial tree is an appropriate term. The trachea is a tubular structure that continues on to the major bronchi and bronchioles. Bad lung areas of the chest are not part of the anatomic structure of the airway system.

85. **C** All of the parameters of this blood gas are normal. The pH is normal because it falls within the range of 7.35-7.45. The PO2 is normal at 83; hypoxia is demonstrated if the PO2 is below 55 mmHg. The HCO3 is within the normal range of 22-26 mEq/L.

SHOCK

1. Which sign would the nurse expect to note in a patient who has undergone multiple blood transfusions?

A. Brudzinski's sign
B. Chvostek's sign
C. Cullen's sign
D. Babinski's sign

2. The nurse knows that administering a vasopressor, such as dopamine hydrochloride (Intropin), is least beneficial for a patient in

A. Cardiogenic shock
B. Distributive shock
C. Septic shock
D. Hypovolemic shock

3. The nurse would anticipate a patient with which condition to develop hypovolemic shock?

A. Drug overdose
B. Postpartum fever
C. Intestinal obstruction
D. Cardiac tamponade

4. Which patient is at lowest risk for developing cardiogenic shock?

A. A 24-year-old patient with cardiac tamponade from a stab wound to the heart
B. A 72-year-old patient with a history of heart disease who has developed an arrhythmia
C. A 55-year-old patient with acute pericarditis who underwent cardiac surgery 3 weeks ago
D. A 44-year-old patient with an anterolateral wall myocardial infarction (MI)

5. Clinical manifestations of cardiogenic shock include all of the following except

A. Distended neck veins
B. Pulmonary congestion
C. S_3 heart sounds
D. Low central venous pressure (CVP)

6. Which treatment for a patient in cardiogenic shock is least effective in protecting the myocardium from further damage?

A. Decreasing peripheral vascular resistance
B. Decreasing ventricular preload
C. Increasing left ventricular afterload
D. Increasing cardiac output

7. When caring for a patient with an acute MI, which early assessment finding may indicate the development of cardiogenic shock?

A. S₃ heart sounds
B. Bilateral crackles heard during inspiration
C. Warm, diaphoretic skin
D. Urine output of 30 mL/hour

8. The nurse knows that the evaluation of renal function in a patient with early circulatory failure does not reveal

A. An increased blood urea nitrogen (BUN) level
B. An increased serum creatinine level
C. A decreased urine specific gravity
D. A decreased urine sodium level

9. Which of the following is a beneficial effect of vasodilator therapy in a patient in cardiogenic shock?

A. Increased systemic vascular pressure
B. Reduced preload and afterload
C. Increased pulmonary vascular pressure
D. Increased peripheral vascular resistance

10. Which of the following is a therapeutic outcome following use of inotropic agents in a patient in cardiogenic shock?

A. Vasodilation
B. Improved tissue perfusion
C. Increased heart rate
D. Decreased force of myocardial contractility

11. While assessing a patient, the nurse notes a sharp decrease in systolic pressure, dyspnea, and bilateral crackles. Which nursing action holds the highest priority at this time?

A. Beginning a vasopressor drip
B. Rapidly infusing 0.45% saline solution to maintain the patient's blood pressure
C. Placing the patient in a supine position and elevating his legs to increase the blood pressure
D. Elevating the patient's head and administering oxygen

12. Based on the following admission histories, which patient is least likely to develop septic shock?

A. A patient with multiple sclerosis who has an indwelling urinary catheter in place and a temperature of 100° F (37.8° C)
B. A patient with a lung carcinoma who is receiving chemotherapy and radiation therapy
C. A patient with a permanent pacemaker that was inserted 1 week ago
D. A patient who severed two fingers while using garden machinery

13. During the initial treatment phase of a patient with septic shock, which nursing action holds the highest priority?

A. Obtaining an allergy history
B. Obtaining blood for cultures, then administering antibiotic therapy
C. Initiating antibiotic therapy after obtaining urine culture results
D. Inserting an indwelling urinary catheter to monitor urine output

14. The nurse would expect a patient who is admitted to the emergency department (ED) in the early stages of septic shock to present with

A. Weak-thready pulses and low blood pressure
B. Decreased urine output and an elevated serum creatinine level
C. Warm, flushed, and moist skin
D. Hyperventilation and pulmonary congestion

15. In a patient with early septic shock, which respiratory symptom would the nurse expect to note?

A. Increased mucus production
B. Bilateral crackles
C. Hyperpnea
D. Respiratory acidosis

16. The nurse knows that a patient with septic shock typically is depleted of intravascular fluid (hypovolemia). Which factor does not cause hypovolemia in septic shock?

A. Leakage of fluid into tissues from an increase in vessel permeability
B. Fluid loss associated with infection, such as sweating during fever, and respiratory losses during hyperventilation
C. Sequestration of plasma fluid in extravascular spaces
D. Increased vascular resistance compromising blood flow to vital areas

17. Which of the following is least likely to introduce the pathogens responsible for septic shock?

A. Bladder instrumentation
B. Childbirth
C. Appendectomy
D. Gingival abscess

18. All of the following pharmacologic agents are appropriate treatments for a patient with septic shock except

A. Beta-adrenergic blockers
B. Corticosteroids
C. Salicylates
D. Vasopressors

19. Which of the following explains the cause of altered mental status during septic shock?

A. Increased cerebral perfusion resulting from the low flow state
B. Elevation of metabolic waste products, such as BUN and creatinine, because of decreased kidney perfusion
C. Alkalosis that results from hyperventilation, causing cerebrovascular constriction
D. Endotoxins acting directly on the central nervous system (CNS)

20. Which pathophysiologic alteration is responsible for the clinical manifestations of neurogenic shock?

A. Compression of the CNS within the spinal cord
B. Interruption of neural transmissions of the afferent spinal tracts
C. Inhibition of motor reflexes of the cerebral cortex
D. Disrupted transmission of the sympathetic nerve impulses from the vasomotor center

21. The nurse knows that all of the following conditions contribute to the development of neurogenic shock except

A. Encephalitis
B. General anesthesia
C. Head trauma
D. Spinal cord injury

22. Which assessment findings indicate neurogenic shock?

A. Increased heart rate and low blood pressure
B. Shallow breathing and diaphoresis
C. Warm, dry skin, and bradycardia
D. Weak, thready pulse, and hypotension

23. Which nursing action is inappropriate during the management of a patient with neurogenic shock resulting from a spinal cord injury?

A. Elevating the head of the bed 20 degrees to promote oxygenation
B. Inserting a nasogastric tube to prevent aspiration caused by paralytic ileus
C. Keeping the patient supine at all times
D. Inserting an indwelling urinary catheter to prevent urine retention

24. A 26-year-old man was involved in an automobile accident. Approximately 20 minutes elapsed between the time of the accident and the arrival of the paramedics. He sustained severe abdominal injuries, spinal cord injury, and multiple fractures. On arrival at the ED, the patient's vital signs are blood pressure 80/50 mmHg, heart rate 120 beats/minute, and respiratory rate 30 breaths/minute. Which nursing action is inappropriate during the initial stabilization of this patient?

A. Administering oxygen therapy
B. Applying medical antishock trousers (MAST, or pneumatic antishock garment)
C. Placing the patient in the Trendelenburg (head-down) position
D. Infusing Lactated Ringer's solution via a large-bore IV line

25. At the time of admission, which assessment finding may be indicative of hypovolemic shock?

A. Pulsus paradoxus
B. A hemoglobin of 10 mg/dL and a hematocrit of 38%
C. A widening pulse pressure
D. A central venous pressure (CVP) of 4 mmHg

26. Which of the following assessment findings suggests that hypovolemia may be a cause of shock?

A. A decreased CVP and distended neck veins only while the patient is prone
B. An increased urine sodium level and a urine specific gravity of 1.010
C. A positive tilt-test result and a decreasing pulse pressure
D. Tachycardia with ventricular gallop (S_3 heart sounds)

27. Which statement best describes shock?

A. It is the inability of the body to excrete metabolic waste products
B. It refers to the collapse of the respiratory system
C. It refers to the collapse of the sympathetic nervous system
D. It is a state of inadequate tissue perfusion

28. The nurse would expect a patient in early shock to have

A. Metabolic acidosis
B. Metabolic alkalosis
C. Respiratory acidosis
D. Respiratory alkalosis

29. Which assessment finding indicates that the compensatory response mechanisms for shock are failing?

A. An increase in capillary refill time
B. Cool, clammy skin
C. Pale, moist skin
D. Mottled skin

30. An 18-year-old man sustained musculoskeletal and abdominal injuries when he crashed into a tree and was thrown from his motorcycle. Paramedics bring him to the ED with MAST in place. Which statement about MAST is false?

A. It is a single-unit apparatus with three compartments
B. Each compartment may be pressurized and deflated individually or in combination
C. When inflated, it achieves pressures ranging from 0 to 160 mmHg
D. Once optimal pressure is achieved, automatic release valves prevent further pressure increases

31. The therapeutic effects of MAST on a hypovolemic patient include:

A. Augmentation of preload to increase stroke volume
B. Increased peripheral vascular resistance in unpressurized areas
C. Decreased functional residual capacity and tidal volume
D. Decreased cerebral perfusion pressure

32. MAST would be least beneficial for a patient with:

A. Spinal shock
B. Pelvic fractures
C. Severe intra-abdominal bleeding
D. Bilateral hemothorax

33. Which procedure is correct when using MAST to stabilize a patient?

A. Inflate it to the highest pressure, then slowly deflate it until the desired response is obtained
B. When deflation is indicated, the leg segments should be depressurized one at a time followed by the abdominal segment
C. During deflation, if the patient's systolic blood pressure drops more than 5 mmHg, stop deflating and infuse fluids
D. If cyanosis of the feet occurs, even though dorsalis pedis pulses are palpable, decrease the MAST pressure by 10 mmHg

34. Paramedics are transporting a 32-year-old woman with a severe anaphylactic reaction. The estimated time of arrival in the ED is 11 minutes. The nurse knows that anaphylaxis most commonly is precipitated by:

A. Insect venom
B. Food ingestion
C. Antibiotic use
D. Blood transfusions

35. After exposure to an allergen, a patient typically develops symptoms of anaphylaxis within:

A. 2 to 20 minutes
B. 20 to 60 minutes
C. 48 hours
D. 3 days

36. Which anaphylactic manifestation is the nurse's lowest priority when treating a patient with altered gas exchange?

A. Inspiratory wheezing
B. Stridor
C. Hoarseness
D. Angioneurotic edema

37. All of the following treatments are used in the initial management of anaphylaxis except:

A. Corticosteroids
B. IV fluids
C. Epinephrine (Adrenalin)
D. Diphenhydramine hydrochloride (Benadryl)

38. Which pharmacologic agent is least likely to be used to treat a patient with anaphylaxis?

A. Hydrocortisone (Cortef)
B. Dobutamine hydrochloride
C. IV Epinephrine
D. Antihistamine

39. Which principle holds the highest priority when caring for a patient with a history of allergies?

A. Avoid known allergens and unnecessary patient exposure by administering drugs only when indicated
B. Observe any patient who receives penicillin in the ED for at least 30 minutes before discharge
C. Initiate current skin-testing procedures to identify allergens
D. Obtain an accurate and thorough drug history, which includes identifying and describing previous drug reactions

40. Which of the following uncrossed matched blood should be administered for volume resuscitation secondary to hemorrhagic shock?

A. O Rh -
B. O Rh +
C. A Rh -
D. B Rh +

41. A 54-year-old male is brought to the ED in neurogenic shock, which of the following findings would the nurse anticipate?

A. Hypotension, bradycardia, and poikilothermia.
B. Tachycardia, hypothermia, vasoconstriction
C. Fever, hypoxia, and shortness of breath.
D. Pruritus, flushing, and bronchospasm.

42. A patient is bleeding and entering hypovolemic shock. The blood pressure is 88/50 mmHg and the HR is 66 beats/minute, which of the following medications would the nurse anticipate would inhibit the body's ability to compensate in shock?

A. Warfarin
B. Albuterol
C. Metoprolol
D. Vitamin B

43. Which of the following is not a sign that a patient is going into shock?

A. Decreased urinary output
B. Hypertension
C. Hypotension
D. Tachycardia

44. A patient known to be in hypovolemic shock has lost approximately 1,800 mL of fluid. How would this shock be classified?

A. Class I
B. Class II
C. Class III
D. Class IV

45. Which of the following is not a cause of distributive shock?

A. Hypovolemic shock
B. Neurogenic shock
C. Drug ingestion
D. Anaphylaxis

46. Which of the following lab results would you expect to see in a patient who is in septic shock?

A. Increased BU N
B. Elevated platelets
C. Decreased lactic acid
D. Decrease in bilirubin

47. Which of the following should be administered if IV fluids are insufficient in correcting hypotension?

A. Dobutamine
B. Atropine
C. Epinephrine
D. Dopamine

48. A patient has been diagnosed with septic shock and is being treated in the ED. In addition to IV fluids, antibiotics, and airway support, which of the following would most likely be indicated to treat your patient's hypotension?

A. Dopamine (Intropin)
B. Diltiazem (Cardizem)
C. Amiodarone (Pacerone)
D. Adenosine (Adenocard)

49. A four-year-old patient requires a large amount of fluid replacement for hemorrhagic shock. What is the best site for infusion of fluids if a peripheral IV cannot be performed?

A. Internal jugular central line
B. Subclavian central line
C. Femoral central line
D. Interosseous line

50. A 45-year-old patient, who sustained a neck injury from a fall off a ladder, complains of decreased sensation in his whole body. His HR is 54 and BP is 82/34. Which kind of shock is this client likely experiencing?

A. Cardiogenic
B. Hemorrhagic
C. Neurogenic
D. Respiratory

SHOCK: RATIONALE

1. **B** The nurse would expect to note Chvostek's sign in a patient who has undergone multiple transfusions. Hypocalcemia is a potential problem during massive transfusions because citrate preservatives may bind ionized calcium. In fact, alkalosis may develop after multiple transfusions, as sodium citrate is converted to sodium bicarbonate. A patient with these electrolyte and acid-base imbalances may demonstrate Chvostek's sign, a facial twitching that occurs when the side of the face is tapped. Brudzinski's sign indicates meningeal irritation; both the upper legs at the hips and the lower legs at the knees are flexed in response to the path of flexion of the head and the neck on the chest. Babinski's sign, which is the dorsiflexion of the big toe upon scratching the bottom of the foot, indicates upper motor neuron dysfunction. Cullen's sign, which is ecchymosis around the umbilicus, usually is seen in hemorrhagic pancreatitis.

2. **D** The administration of a vasopressor, such as dopamine, would be least beneficial to a patient in hypovolemic shock. Natural vasoconstriction compensates for a hypovolemic state during the early shock phase. Giving a vasopressor in early shock increases vasoconstriction, possibly closing arterioles and further halting blood flow. Hypovolemia must be treated before dopamine can be given. For the patient in cardiogenic shock or septic shock (distributive shock), a vasopressor is appropriate because it increases myocardial contractility and raises cardiac output and systolic blood pressure; however, for cardiogenic shock, in addition to pressors, other medications (inotropes) may be required, such as, dobutamine, milrinone, etc.

3. **C** This question asks the reader to define the classification of shock for the various disease states. The nurse should anticipate

manifestations of hypovolemic shock in a patient admitted to the emergency department (ED) with an intestinal obstruction. Such an obstruction could cause altered fluid movement, resulting in the trapping of fluid in the interstitial space within the intestinal lumen and the depletion of intravascular volume (third-space fluid shift). The nurse should suspect neurogenic shock in a patient with a drug overdose; septic shock in a postpartum patient with a fever; and cardiogenic shock in a patient with cardiac tamponade.

4. **C** A postoperative cardiac patient with acute pericarditis is least likely to develop cardiogenic shock. Cardiogenic shock is a vicious cycle that involves loss of myocardial contractility; resultant hemodynamic and metabolic reflex mechanisms cause further ischemia and the deterioration of contractility. Acute pericarditis, inflammation of the pericardium, has a self-limiting, short-term clinical course when related to an acute myocardial infarction (MI) or cardiac surgery. The cause is not irritation but, rather, an autoimmune response that lasts 2 to 6 weeks. Pericardial effusion usually does not develop. Leaning forward usually can alleviate pain, the most characteristic symptom of acute pericarditis. Pericardial friction rub is the most important physical finding in this condition. Most commonly, cardiogenic shock occurs as a complication of an MI, especially when at least 40% of the left ventricle is necrotic and ischemic. When the heart's ability to pump blood declines, the risk of cardiogenic shock increases. This occurs in conditions that produce deficient cardiac filling, such as cardiac tamponade and arrhythmias in a compromised patient.

5. **D** Low central venous pressure (CVP) is not one of the manifestations of cardiogenic shock. The clinical manifestations of cardiogenic shock result from impaired contractility of the heart, which decreases cardiac output and

elevates left ventricular end-diastolic pressure (LVEDP). The reduced cardiac output impairs perfusion to the vital organs and peripheral tissues. Thus, the patient exhibits changes in sensorium, such as restlessness, anxiety, or confusion. The skin is cold and clammy because of peripheral vasoconstriction. As the cardiac output declines, the pulse pressure narrows; peripheral pulses are rapid and thready. Systemic arterial pressure drops and hypotension ensues. Urine output decreases as kidney perfusion declines. A rise in LVEDP increases left atrial and pulmonary pressures, resulting in pulmonary congestion. Tachypnea, dyspnea, and pulmonary edema develop; S_3 heart sounds can be heard as the left ventricle fails and becomes over distended during diastole. Increased pressure on the left side of the heart progresses back through the pulmonary venous system into the right side of the heart. This increase in pulmonary pressure decreases right ventricular performance and may result in right ventricular failure, which in turn produces an elevated CVP and jugular vein distention with hepatomegaly.

6. **C** The treatment that is least effective in protecting the myocardium from further damage in a patient in cardiogenic shock involves increasing left ventricular afterload. The goals of therapy in this situation are to improve myocardial contractility, increase cardiac output, and reduce the myocardial demand for oxygen. Improvement of cardiovascular function is primarily managed by pharmacologic therapies. Nitroprusside sodium (Nipride) and nitroglycerin (Tridil) are commonly used to decrease both preload (ventricular end-diastolic pressure) and afterload (vascular resistance). These vasodilators reduce blood return to the heart and decrease systemic peripheral vascular resistance. Cardiac output is further increased by a decrease in cardiac workload and oxygen demand and by complete emptying of the ventricles during systole. Vasodilator therapy is

used with sympathomimetic drugs, such as dopamine hydrochloride and dobutamine hydrochloride (Dobutrex). These vasopressors have an inotropic effect that enhances myocardial contractility and increases cardiac output.

7. **A** S_3 heart sounds are an early assessment finding that may indicate the development of cardiogenic shock in a patient with an acute MI. The patient with an acute MI is at high risk for developing cardiogenic shock because of a decrease in the contractile function of the left ventricle. Early recognition of signs and symptoms of left ventricular failure, which may lead to shock, are vital. Initially, the failing ventricle causes a decrease in cardiac output. The body compensates by increasing sympathetic stimulation to increase the heart rate and to shunt blood to vital organs via peripheral vasoconstriction. The skin is typically cool and clammy. Tachycardia and increased afterload from vasoconstriction increase the cardiac workload and oxygen consumption. Decreased ventricular emptying during systole occurs, preload increases, and S_3 sounds may be heard. Pulmonary congestion then follows from the backward transmission of left-sided pressure, resulting in dyspnea, orthopnea, and bilateral crackles. As left ventricular failure progresses, pulmonary congestion increases and cardiogenic shock ensues.

8. **C** An evaluation of renal function in a patient with early circulatory failure typically does not reveal a decreased urine specific gravity. In the context of shock, the kidneys are peripheral organs. Thus, their perfusion declines from the onset of shock. Renal vessels are initially among the most constricted. As renal perfusion declines, the kidneys respond by conserving water; concentrating urine causes an increase in the urine specific gravity. Also, when the blood supply to the kidneys is decreased, the tubules respond by reabsorbing sodium. This

results in a decreased urine sodium level. An increase in blood urea nitrogen (BUN) level and serum creatinine levels occurs because of a decrease in the rate at which the kidneys clear metabolic end products, such as urea and creatinine, from plasma.

9. **B** A beneficial effect of vasodilator therapy in the management of cardiogenic shock is reduced preload and afterload. Vasodilator therapy reduces venous tone and increases venous capacitance. This decreases blood return to the heart, thereby lowering LVEDP. Vasodilator therapy also reduces arterial vascular tone, which results in decreased impedance to left ventricular ejection (afterload); cardiac workload is decreased, and cardiac output is increased.

10. **B** Inotropic agents improve tissue perfusion in a patient with cardiogenic shock. They increase the force of myocardial contraction, resulting in increased cardiac output from enhanced contractility. Dopamine, a sympathomimetic drug, has positive inotropic properties. Its vasopressor effects result in increased coronary blood flow, which improves tissue perfusion. Dopamine's positive chronotropic effects result in an increased heart rate; this potential adverse effect may limit dopamine's use because tachycardia increases myocardial oxygen consumption.

11. **D** Initial nursing measures in this situation include positioning the patient with his shoulders and head elevated to decrease pulmonary congestion and administering oxygen to increase the myocardial oxygen supply. This will protect the myocardium from further damage. After implementing necessary measures to ensure improvement in airway and breathing, the nurse should help to stabilize the patient's arterial pressure. Any infusion of IV fluids or vasopressor drips

requires a physician's order. The rapid infusion of a hypotonic solution, such as 0.45% saline solution, may result in a sudden decrease in serum osmolarity. This can cause a shift of fluid into the cells, resulting in intravascular depletion and symptoms of increased intracranial pressure. Dextran, glucose, normal saline, and albumin solutions can be used in patients with cardiogenic shock.

12. **D** A patient who severed two fingers while using garden machinery is least likely to develop septic shock. Factors that increase a patient's risk include any invasive procedure or foreign body insertion, such as an IV line, an indwelling catheter line, or a pacemaker; diseases affecting the reticuloendothelial system (RES), such as leukemia; and any therapy that suppresses the RES, such as radiation therapy and cytotoxic or immunosuppressant drug therapy.

13. **A** Obtaining an allergy history holds the highest priority in this situation because antibiotics, which are essential in treating septic shock, cause anaphylaxis more often than any other substance. Afterward, the nurse should obtain blood for cultures before administering the first antibiotic dose. Initiating antibiotics before collecting cultures is a serious error. Accurately identifying the infecting organism is essential to provide optimal antibiotic treatment. A switch to a more appropriate therapy can help ensure patient survival.

14. **C** The nurse would expect a patient who is admitted in the early (hyperdynamic) stages of septic shock to present with warm-flushed-moist skin, tachycardia—with full bounding pulses, tachypnea, confusion, normal or slightly increased urine output, and normal or slightly decreased blood pressure.

15. **C** Hyperpnea is common in early sepsis. Sometimes bordering on respiratory alkalosis, this symptom is caused by the respiratory response to lactic acidosis as well as by stimulation of the medullary respiratory control center by the release of endotoxins. Advanced shock is characterized by pulmonary edema, which produces bilateral crackles. Also, adult respiratory distress syndrome has been associated with gram-negative sepsis.

16. **D** Several factors account for the hypovolemia that occurs in septic shock; however, increased vascular resistance compromising blood flow to vital areas is not among them. Fluid and electrolytes can leave the body through events associated with infection, such as sweating during fever, diarrhea, vomiting, and respiratory losses during tachypnea. Also, plasma fluid can be sequestered in the extravascular spaces because of a local or generalized increase in vessel permeability secondary to the production of histamine, bradykinin, and other agents. Vessel permeability is increased in septic shock; thus there is an increased tendency for fluid leakage into tissues.

17. **D** Gingival abscess is least likely to introduce the pathogens responsible for septic shock. Septic shock is more common in women than men because of the greater number of urinary tract infections and genitourinary procedures. Women are most vulnerable to septic shock after pregnancy. The ED nurse must determine whether the patient has undergone a recent pelvic examination, appendectomy, or catheterization, especially during childbirth. These procedures are common methods for induction of causative organisms. Indwelling urinary tubes, intrauterine devices, instrumented abortions, and peritonitis from a ruptured appendix are additional ways in which gram-negative bacilli may be introduced.

18. **A** Beta-adrenergic blockers are used rarely in septic shock because they depress myocardial function. The use of steroids is still controversial, although studies have shown that, overall, pharmacologic doses of steroids appear to be efficacious in the treatment of septic shock. Multiple mechanisms of action have been proposed to explain their reported therapeutic effects. The most common explanations involve the intracellular action of steroids in stabilizing lysosomal membranes. Stabilization of lysosomal membranes decreases the release of vasoactive substances and interrupts the pathogenesis of the shock syndrome. Vasopressors, such as vasopressin, dopamine hydrochloride, and norepinephrine (Levophed) are also used during shock because of their ability to improve the patient's hemodynamic status. Salicylates are used to decrease body temperature.

19. **D** Endotoxins acting directly on the central nervous system are responsible for the altered mental status that occurs in septic shock. Early in septic shock, a patient's sensorium may change from awake, alert, and oriented to confused, agitated, and restless. This results from decreased cerebral perfusion caused by the low flow state produced by endotoxin-induced vasodilation, which increases pooling of blood within the venous system. The elevated BUN and creatinine levels and respiratory alkalosis seen in septic shock are not responsible for changes in mental status.

20. **D** The primary problem in neurogenic shock is altered blood vessel capacity caused by disrupted transmission of sympathetic nerve impulses from the brain's vasomotor center. The unopposed parasympathetic stimulation causes a loss of vasomotor tone, resulting in massive vasodilation. The result is relative hypovolemia, decreased venous return, and decreased cardiac output.

21. **A** Encephalitis does not contribute to the development of neurogenic shock. Neurogenic shock may result from any condition that shuts down the entire vasomotor system, including spinal anesthesia, the most common cause of neurogenic shock; deep general anesthesia, which may severely depress the brain's vasomotor center and lead to vasomotor collapse; head trauma; and spinal trauma.

22. **C** Assessment findings indicative of neurogenic shock include warm, dry, flushed skin, normal to low blood pressure, full and regular pulses, profound bradycardia, and an increased respiratory rate. These result from blocked sympathetic vasomotor regulation.

23. **A** Elevating the head is inappropriate for a patient with neurogenic shock resulting from a spinal cord injury. Such a patient should be maintained in a supine position to avoid further spinal cord damage and prevent orthostatic hypotension, which may result from relative hypovolemia caused by increased vascular capacity. IV fluids should be instituted to expand the intravascular volume. Fluids must be administered cautiously, as they may cause fluid overload when vasomotor tone is restored. An indwelling urinary catheter should be inserted to permit frequent measurement of urine output. Catheterization also helps prevent urine retention if the patient has a spinal cord injury that has paralyzed the bladder.

24. **C** Placing the patient in the Trendelenburg (head-down) position would be inappropriate during the initial stabilization of this patient. The initial management of a patient in shock involves ensuring an adequate airway and ventilation, maintaining blood volume, pressure, circulation, and maintaining cellular oxygen consumption. Specific measures include administering oxygen and IV fluids, preferably

Lactated Ringer's solution via a large-bore IV line, as ordered. Although rarely use in the civilian setting, Medical Anti-shock Shock Trousers (MAST, or pneumatic antishock garment) also may be used on a patient with lower-extremity or abdominal injuries who has signs and symptoms of hypovolemic shock. This will redirect approximately 1,000 mL of blood, reduce blood loss by application of direct pressure, and immobilize injuries of the lower extremities. The patient in shock should lie flat with only the legs elevated. The Trendelenburg position, once favored, has been abandoned because it allows the diaphragm to migrate upward, thus compromising ventilation. Also, this position may cause a reflex inhibition of the baroreceptor activity, thereby decreasing sympathetic stimulation and further compromising arterial blood pressure.

25. **A** Pulsus paradoxus is indicative of hypovolemic shock. It is characterized by an abnormal drop (greater than 10 mmHg) in systolic blood pressure during inspiration. The systolic sound disappears during inspiration because of pulmonary vascular pooling caused by increased lung expansion and increased intrathoracic negative pressure. When intravascular depletion is present, such as in hypovolemic shock, the drop in systolic blood pressure during inspiration is exaggerated when venous blood return to the heart is compromised. The patient also may demonstrate a narrowing pulse pressure, indicating a fall in cardiac output, and a central venous pressure (CVP) reading below 4 mmHg, indicating intravascular depletion. A single hematocrit or hemoglobin value is an unreliable indicator of the patient's condition. Either an increase or a decrease in hemoglobin values may signal hypovolemia; dropping values suggest whole blood loss, whereas rising values suggest plasma loss. Acute blood loss may cause a significant drop in hemoglobin over 1 to 2 hours; however, in older patients, acute

blood loss may not cause a significant drop for at least 12 hours.

26. **C** An abnormal tilt-test result and a decreasing pulse pressure may suggest that hypovolemia is the cause of shock in this patient. The tilt test is an assessment tool that indicates circulating blood volume loss by measuring blood pressure and pulse rate changes during patient position changes. Abnormal tilt-test findings include improved blood pressure levels when the patient's legs are raised above heart level or a 10mmHg or greater drop in systolic blood pressure between supine and sitting positions. Pulse pressure is a far better indicator of early shock than is blood pressure. Pulse pressure is related to cardiac stroke volume; thus, changes provide a good indication of blood flow. During the early stages of shock, the systolic pressure usually drops faster than the diastolic pressure, thereby narrowing or decreasing the pulse pressure. A hypovolemic patient typically has flat neck veins when prone, a low CVP, a decreased urine sodium level, and a high urine specific gravity. S_3 heart sounds are heard when the patient experiences an increase in left-ventricular end-diastolic pressure, as occurs in congestive heart failure or cardiogenic shock. Tachycardia, which occurs in all forms of shock, results from the heart's attempt to increase cardiac output.

27. **D** Shock is a complex clinical syndrome characterized by impaired cellular metabolism from decreased blood flow. It is a state of inadequate tissue perfusion. The major pathophysiologic problem occurs in the microcirculation at the capillary level. Inadequate tissue perfusion and decreased oxygen delivery result in a constellation of physiologic responses. As shock develops, a fall in cardiac output triggers compensatory mechanisms as vasoreceptors are stimulated to cause vasoconstriction. The net effect is an increase in mean

arterial pressure and a restriction of peripheral blood flow. The available circulating volume is shunted to perfuse vital organs. As peripheral vasoconstriction progresses, a marked reduction in oxygen delivery to the cells forces a switch from aerobic to anaerobic metabolism. Increased lactic acid is produced, resulting in respiratory compensation. Acid load can be reduced by blowing off carbon dioxide. As a shock state continues, respiratory compensation fails and the progressive decline in pH from excessive lactate levels ensues. Metabolic acidosis causes impaired cellular function and impaired capillary permeability. Intravascular volume is further decreased as blood flows into capillary beds. At this point, the patient is in a progressive state of shock as compensatory mechanisms fail to maintain an adequate cardiac output.

28. **D** Respiratory alkalosis develops in the initial phase of shock. A compensatory mechanism of tachypnea is initiated as a decrease in peripheral tissue perfusion occurs, resulting in hypoxia. In early shock, the patient hyperventilates to increase oxygenation, thus blowing off carbon dioxide. During progressive stages, excessive and prolonged vasoconstriction causes lactic acid levels to increase within the body, producing systemic acidosis.

29. **D** Mottled skin would indicate that compensatory mechanisms for shock are failing. During the compensatory stage of shock, the skin is typically cool, pale, and clammy as a result of peripheral vasoconstriction and increased sweat gland activity. If the cause of shock is not corrected and compensatory mechanisms continue, the same physiologic events that were initiated to compensate for decreased cardiac output will lead to detrimental effects. Impaired cellular function leads to acidosis; the resultant is a decrease in cardiac

contractility and loss of vasomotor tone, to produce mottled skin. The capillary refill time decreases in shock.

30. **C** MAST is a single-unit device with three compartments: an abdominal compartment and two individual leg compartments. It may achieve pressures ranging from 0 to 104 mmHg. Each of the three compartments may be pressurized and deflated individually or in combination. Once a pressure of 104 mmHg is achieved, automatic release (or pop-off) valves prevent further pressure increases.

31. **A** The therapeutic effects of MAST on a hypovolemic patient include augmentation of preload, thereby increasing blood return to the heart. This results in a greater cardiac output because of increased contractility and stroke volume. MAST increases peripheral vascular resistance in pressurized areas, decreases peripheral vascular resistance in the remainder of the body, and increases cerebral perfusion pressure. Although use of MAST also decreases the patient's functional residual capacity and tidal volume, these effects are not considered therapeutic.

32. **D** MAST would be least beneficial for a patient with a bilateral hemothorax, as this device is contraindicated in shock secondary to hemorrhage above the diaphragm. Indications for MAST use include hypotension secondary to hypovolemia, as occurs in acute trauma, nontraumatic bleeding and non-hemorrhagic hypovolemia, hypotension secondary to volume mal distribution, as occurs in spinal shock, drug effects, and septic shock, and hypotension secondary to low cardiac output, as occurs in cardiac tamponade and cardiogenic shock. MAST is beneficial in stabilizing patients with pelvic and lower-extremity fractures. MAST not only supports the fracture site and decreases unwanted movement, but it also decreases

bleeding. It is useful in lower-extremity hemorrhage and intra-abdominal bleeding.

33. **C** At no time should suit deflation continue if the patient's systolic blood pressure drops more than 5 mmHg. Such a drop implies an inadequate circulating volume, and IV fluids should be administered until the patient's vital signs are stable. After MAST is applied, the leg segments are inflated, followed by the abdominal segment, if needed. The end point of pressurization is determined in all instances by the stabilization of the patient's blood pressure, which must be continuously monitored. When desired blood pressure is achieved and maintained, inflation stops. During inflation, the patient's feet may turn bluish. The suit's maximum pressure, 104 mmHg, usually is not sufficient to totally occlude perfusion; however, routine palpation of the dorsalis pedis pulses is mandatory. When deflation of the garment is indicated, the abdominal segment is depressurized first, followed by the leg segments.

34. **C** Anaphylaxis is most commonly precipitated by antibiotics, although a variety of agents have been reported to precipitate this severe reaction. Essentially, any compound capable of acting as an allergen may cause an anaphylactic reaction. The most common examples of such compounds include antibiotics, especially penicillin (300 fatal anaphylactic reactions to penicillin occur each year in the United States), followed by medicines derived from animal sources, insect bites and stings, and iodinated radioactive contrast media.

35. **A** After exposure to an allergen, a patient typically develops symptoms of anaphylaxis within 2 to 20 minutes. The immediate reaction is usually life threatening and displays the symptoms characteristic of anaphylaxis. The classic manifestations of anaphylaxis include the triad of urticaria,

laryngeal edema with bronchospasm, and hypotension. The initial signs typically are cutaneous, consisting of diffuse erythema, pruritus, urticaria, or angioneurotic edema. These are frequently followed by pulmonary insufficiency from bronchospasm, laryngeal edema, or both. The patient typically demonstrates stridor and wheezing. Airway obstruction may progress rapidly and lead to severe respiratory distress. Cardiovascular collapse may occur either before or after the cutaneous and pulmonary manifestations. An accelerated reaction, which occurs 20 minutes to 48 hours after exposure, is rarely life threatening. Typically, This type of reaction manifests as urticaria and occasionally laryngeal edema. A delayed reaction may develop 3 or more days after drug administration is initiated and typically consists of a rash.

36. **D** Angioneurotic edema, a cutaneous manifestation seen initially in anaphylaxis, would be the nurse's lowest priority when treating a patient with altered gas exchange. Stridor, hoarseness, and inspiratory wheezing indicate respiratory compromise; treating these symptoms is the nurse's highest priority because airway obstruction and severe respiratory distress may follow quickly.

37. **A** Corticosteroids are not used in the initial management of anaphylaxis. These drugs are used only in protracted cases and then only after IV fluids, epinephrine, and antihistamines have been administered. Epinephrine is regarded as the drug of choice; it can reverse all signs and symptoms of anaphylaxis. Its beta-adrenergic properties decrease histamine and bradykinin release and cause bronchodilation. Its alpha-adrenergic activity affects vasoconstriction, reversing hypotension.

38. **B** Dobutamine hydrochloride is least likely to be used to treat anaphylaxis. During anaphylaxis, vasodilation due to the

release of histamine, rather than a primary loss of myocardial contractility is thought to be responsible for the hypotension. Thus, an agent with principally vasoconstrictive effects would be desirable. Dobutamine does not have enough vasoconstrictive effect to be useful in this situation, whereas epinephrine is indicated in instances of bronchospasm and hypotension. Antihistamines are useful as adjunctive measures in relieving urticaria. Hydrocortisone, a steroid, decreases inflammation.

39. **D** The most important principle that should be considered when caring for a patient with a history of allergies is to obtain an accurate and thorough drug history, which includes identifying and describing previous drug reactions. All of the other choices are important, but the drug history has the highest priority.

40. **A** O Rh - is the universal donor. However, the patients specific type is preferred, but when unavailable O Rh - will suffice. O Rh + can be administered for those beyond childrearing age.

41. **A** In neurogenic shock there is a loss of sympathetic vasomotor regulation. Because of this loss there is a bradycardia, the ability to generate heat, via piloerection (poikilothermia), is lost. Hypotension results from the inability to vasoconstrict, which is due to the loss of sympathetic stimulation. Pruritus and bronchospasm is commonly seen in allergic reaction. Fever, hypoxia, and shortness of breath may suggest pneumonia.

42. **D** Beta-Blockers, such as metoprolol, inhibit (or block) the heart's ability to increase its rate. Therefore, inhibiting the body's ability to compensate. Vitamins may be useful in

correcting anemia, or other vitamin deficiencies. Anticoagulants, such as, warfarin, would make bleeding more difficult to stop. Albuterol would not inhibit the body's compensatory mechanism.

43. **B** When a patient goes into shock, regardless of the cause, symptoms include hypotension, tachycardia, decreased urinary output, increase or decrease in respiratory rate, hypoxemia, and change in mental status. Low blood pressure reduces tissue perfusion, thus less oxygen being delivered to the tissues Hypertension does not occur in any type of shock.

44. **C** Classification of hypovolemic shock is based on the amount of fluid lost. Class I would be considered when 750 mL or less (or 15% or less of total circulating volume) is lost. Class II is determined when there is a loss of 750 to 1,000 mL (15% to 30% blood volume loss). When 1,500 to 2,000 mL of fluid is lost (30% to 40% blood volume loss), the patient is said to be in class III. Class IV occurs when over 2,000 mL (or more than 40% blood volume loss) of fluid is lost. Hypovolemic shock can occur for a number of reasons. Common causes include blood loss, severe diarrhea or vomiting, internal fluid shifts, or a severe injury in which the integrity of large blood vessels is compromised.

45. **A** Hypovolemic shock is not a cause of distributive shock. Hypovolemic shock occurs when a large amount of blood volume is lost and the loss of volume is the cause of the shock. In distributive shock, the volume of blood is sufficient but an underlying condition causes the vasculature to dilate abnormally. The over-dilated blood vessels lose their ability to effectively move blood throughout the body leading to hypoperfusion.

46. **A** A patient in septic shock may experience a multitude of systemic complications, including liver and renal failure. Patients in acute renal failure have elevated BUN levels and decreased urinary output. A patient in liver failure would have increased bilirubin and liver enzymes, not decreased. Lactic acid is increased, not decreased when a patient is in septic shock due to excess lactic acid production in times of tissue hypoperfusion. Hemodynamic changes can cause platelet levels to decrease, not increase.

47. **D** Dopamine is a potent vasopressor and the drug of choice given to correct hypotension. It is administered IV at a rate of 0.5 to 5 mcg/kg/min. Dobutamine increases cardiac output and contractility, and is administered at a rate of 2 to 20 mcg/kg/min. Systolic blood pressure may or may not increase as a result of the increased cardiac output. Atropine is an antiarrhythmic used to treat bradycardia and is not used in the treatment of hypotension. Epinephrine is also a vasopressor, but is indicated in the treatment of cardiac arrest.

48. **A** Dopamine is a vasopressor and can be used to maintain effective blood pressure while undergoing additional treatment for septic shock.

49. **D** An interosseous line is best to provide rapid infusion of fluids in a trauma situation in young children. Central lines are not ideal in rapid fluid infusion due to the length of the line and size of the cannula.

50. **C** Having a positive history of recent trauma and a HR, which does not compensate for a low BP is indicative of neurogenic shock. An additional finding in patients with neurogenic shock would be a finding of decreased rectal sphincter tone.

TOXICOLOGY EMERGENCIES

1. A 23-year-old man who had been hiking is brought to the emergency department (ED) after having sustained a snakebite to his lower left leg 20 minutes ago. The most appropriate nursing intervention for this patient would be to:

A. Accurately identify the snake type
B. Immobilize and elevate the affected leg
C. Immobilize the affected extremity below heart level and apply a lightly constrictive tourniquet
D. Apply ice to the skin over the snakebite wound

2. Which incident is the most common cause of death from acute alcohol intoxication?

A. Respiratory depression or arrest
B. Aspiration of vomitus
C. GI bleeding
D. Accidental injury

3. Which condition commonly mimics the signs and symptoms of alcohol intoxication?

A. Diabetic reactions
B. Head injury
C. Drug overdose
D. All of the above

4. The nurse would expect the management of a patient with acute alcohol intoxication to include administration of all of the following except:

A. Thiamine 100 mg IM.
B. Chlordiazepoxide (Librium) 100 mg IM every 2 to 4 hours as needed
C. Diazepam (Valium) 5 to 10 mg IV bolus for seizure management
D. Normal saline solution IV

5. When planning the care of a patient with alcohol intoxication, the nurse should keep in mind that alcohol withdrawal syndrome:

A. Does not cause death
B. Typically starts 6 to 72 hours after the last alcohol ingestion
C. Lasts up to 12 hours after withdrawal
D. Is best managed by restricting fluid intake

6. Many patients undergoing therapy for alcohol abuse use disulfiram (Antabuse). The nurse would anticipate the emergency management of a disulfiram-alcohol reaction to include:

A. Initiation of an infusion of normal saline solution
B. Administration of diphenhydramine hydrochloride (Benadryl) 50 mg
C. Administration of chlorpheniramine maleate (Chlor-Trimeton) or a similar drug
D. All of the above

7. A 19-year-old man arrives at the ED exhibiting signs of confusion, lethargy, dysarthria, and emotional instability. Which drug is most likely to produce these symptoms?

A. Phencyclidine (PCP)
B. Barbiturates
C. Amphetamines
D. Cocaine

8. A 22-year-old man arrives at the ED for treatment of phencyclidine (PCP) ingestion. Which of the following would be an important concern when planning the care of this patient?

A. Offering the patient constant verbal reassurance
B. Administering phenothiazines
C. Providing tactile stimulation
D. Placing the patient in a dimly lit room

9. The nurse who is assessing a patient with a methadone addiction knows that withdrawal symptoms typically appear within:

A. 8 to 10 hours
B. 12 to 24 hours
C. 24 to 36 hours
D. 36 to 48 hours

10. The correct procedure for gastric lavage in the initial management of the unconscious patient who has a substance overdose includes:

A. Instillation of 200 mL of warmed saline solution via a nasogastric or orogastric tube by gravity
B. Instillation of iced normal saline solution
C. Performing the lavage before endotracheal intubation
D. Performing the lavage using 50% normal saline solution and 50% magnesium sulfate solution

11. The nurse would anticipate the absorption of methyl salicylate to continue how long after ingestion?

A. 2 hours
B. 3 hours
C. 6 hours
D. 10 hours

12. The nurse would expect to note signs of acute salicylate intoxication in a patient who has taken a single dose greater than:

A. 50 mg/kg
B. 100 mg/kg
C. 150 mg/kg
D. 200 mg/kg

13. Which sign of salicylate poisoning (salicylism) should the nurse assess for?

A. Tetany
B. Coma
C. Hypernatremia
D. Hypothermia

14. A 75-year-old woman with a long history of rheumatoid arthritis is brought to the ED in a convulsive state. About 4 hours earlier, she complained to her primary physician that her arthritis was very painful. Her physician ordered methyl salicylate (wintergreen oil) to be applied topically. The patient's son tells the nurse that his mother may have taken the drug orally (1 tsp. = 5 mL = 160 mg). The nurse would anticipate emergency treatment for this patient to include all of the following except:

A. Gastric lavage with activated charcoal
B. Administration of ipecac syrup
C. Administration of sodium bicarbonate
D. Hemodialysis

15. Which statement about salicylate intoxication after ingestion of enteric-coated aspirins is true?

A. Because of the drug's enteric coating, symptoms will not be as severe
B. Hospitalization probably will not be required
C. Toxic effects will be delayed because of delayed absorption
D. Early blood levels are a reliable guide to prognosis

16. How long after ingestion of acetaminophen would the nurse expect to note signs and symptoms of overdose in a patient?

A. 1 to 3 hours
B. 4 to 6 hours
C. 12 to 24 hours
D. 24 to 48 hours

17. A 3-year-old girl weighing 35 lb (15.9 kg) is brought to the ED. She is alert but has been nauseated, vomiting, and diaphoretic since this morning. Last night an open bottle of pediatric acetaminophen (Children's Tylenol) was found in a bathroom at the patient's home. The nurse knows that, if treatment is unsuccessful for this patient, all of the following complications may occur except:

A. Liver necrosis
B. Liver failure
C. Impaired renal function
D. Arrhythmias

18. Which laboratory value is characteristically abnormal in acetaminophen toxicity?

A. Creatinine phosphokinase level
B. Alkaline phosphatase level
C. Prothrombin time
D. Direct Coombs' test

19. The nurse is aware that the antidote for acetaminophen overdose consists of administering:

A. Activated charcoal
B. Physostigmine (Antilirium)
C. Acetylcysteine (Mucomyst)
D. Naloxone (Narcan)

20. A 3-year-old girl weighing 35 lb (15.9 kg) is brought to the ED. She is alert but has been nauseated, vomiting, and diaphoretic since this morning. Last night an open bottle of pediatric acetaminophen (Children's Tylenol) was found in a bathroom at the patient's home. Which nursing diagnosis is most appropriate for this patient?

A. Decreased cardiac output related to bleeding secondary to impaired coagulation
B. Decreased cardiac output related to bleeding from irritated GI mucosa
C. Potential for injury related to seizures
D. Impaired gas exchange related to respiratory depression

21. Which statement regarding iron poisoning is true?

A. Toxicity depends on the amount of iron salt ingested
B. Ingestion of 50 to 100 ferrous sulfate tablets is not considered fatal
C. Acute iron poisoning occurs primarily in elderly people
D. Shock is the most common cause of death in iron poisoning

22. The nurse knows that iron ingestion may be confirmed by:

A. Gastric fluid analysis
B. Serum triiodothyronine (T_3) and thyroxine (T_4) levels
C. Serum hemoglobin levels
D. Abdominal X-rays 72 hours after ingestion

23. If iron toxicity were suspected, the nurse would expect the physician to order which procedure first?

A. Administration of a saline cathartic
B. Administration of ipecac syrup or gastric lavage
C. Abdominal X-rays
D. Serum iron level analysis

24. Which assessment finding may indicate iron toxicity?

A. Metabolic alkalosis
B. Abdominal pain and hemorrhagic gastroenteritis
C. Seizures
D. Renal failure

25. A woman arrives at the pediatric clinic with her 5-year-old son, who she thinks has swallowed 5 to 10 iron supplement tablets. The child is vomiting and complaining of severe abdominal pain. The nurse would expect supportive care for this patient to consist of:

A. Maintaining the patient's body temperature
B. Administering antihypertensives
C. Administering diuretics
D. Dialysis

26. Which statement concerning caustic substances is true?

A. Acidic substances have the same effect as alkaline substances
B. The severity of an alkaline burn depends on the pH of the substance and the duration of contact with the mucosa
C. Oropharyngeal and esophageal damage is more common with liquids than with solids
D. The absence of oral burns excludes the possibility of esophageal burns

27. Of the following, which symptom of caustic ingestion should the nurse assess for?

A. Tinnitus
B. Hyperthermia
C. Drooling
D. Dyspnea

28. The nurse would anticipate treatment for caustic ingestion to include:

A. Dilution with 8 oz. (240 mL) of milk or water
B. Administration of activated charcoal
C. Administration of a cathartic
D. Induction of emesis or gastric lavage

29. Which dose of a concentrated acid or alkali is considered lethal to an adult?

A. 5 mL
B. 10 mL
C. 15 mL
D. 30 mL

30. Which statement about the nursing management of a patient who has ingested or been exposed to a caustic substance is true?

A. Dermal and ocular decontamination should be carried out
B. Antibiotics may be administered prophylactically
C. Steroids should never be administered
D. Barium swallow is contraindicated

31. A 21-year-old woman arrives at the ED, complaining of blurred vision, sore throat, dizziness, and nausea. She reports to the nurse that her sister has similar symptoms. Both women ordered the same meal at a restaurant yesterday. The physician suspects that the patient has botulism. Which statement about botulism is true?

A. Ingestion of improperly home-processed vegetables, fruits, and meats is responsible for most cases of botulism
B. Botulism is not caused by fresh vegetables that have been grown in the ground
C. Danger arises when cooked foods remain at room temperature for more than 2 hours
D. The spores of Clostridium botulinum cannot withstand boiling for more than 30 minutes

32. Botulism is caused by a neurotoxin that blocks release of acetylcholine at peripheral nerve endings. The nurse is aware that botulism produces signs and symptoms similar to those of:

A. Guillain-Barre syndrome
B. Brown-Sequard syndrome
C. Salmonella poisoning
D. Acetaminophen overdose

33. The nurse is aware that eight serologically different toxins of C. botulinum exist, but types A, B, and E most commonly affect humans. Which statement about toxin types is true?

A. Identification of the type of toxin requires serum or stool analysis
B. The incubation period for Type A is longer than that for Types B and E
C. Patient care is the same, regardless of toxin type
D. Respiratory insufficiency occurs with the same frequency, regardless of toxin type

34. The nurse would anticipate treatment of botulism to include

A. Administration of magnesium salts (Milk of Magnesia)
B. Administration of acetylcysteine
C. Exchange transfusion
D. Hemofiltration

35. A 51-year-old woman was admitted to the ED about 2 hours ago. She has a history of asthma, and her admitting diagnosis is pneumonia. She is now complaining of breathing difficulty. The nurse notes an audible wheeze and an erythematous rash over the patient's entire body; the rash was not noted on admission. The patient received an initial dose of penicillin by IV piggyback 1 hour ago but has no history of allergies to antibiotics. Which sign of anaphylaxis would the nurse expect to find while assessing this patient?

A. Bradyarrhythmias
B. Cheyne-Stokes respirations
C. Laryngeal edema
D. Hypertension

36. Which statement concerning allergic drug reactions is true?

A. A drug reaction typically begins as a macular eruption on the head and proximal extremities that spreads in a symmetrical pattern
B. Initial episodes of an exanthematous-type hypersensitivity drug reaction always occur within 1 week after the drug is started
C. If a patient has received a drug many times without a reaction, the nurse can safely presume that a reaction will never develop
D. The morphology of the erupted rash provides clues to the causative agent

37. The nurse would expect immediate treatment of a severe allergic drug reaction to include administration of:

A. Oxygen
B. Norepinephrine (Levophed)
C. Furosemide (Lasix)
D. Prednisone (Deltasone)

38. Which nursing intervention is appropriate for a patient in anaphylactic shock?

A. Place a tourniquet on the patient's arm above the IV site
B. Place the patient in high-Fowler's position
C. Administer atropine sulfate to reverse bradycardia
D. Place the patient in Trendelenburg's position

39. A 15-year-old boy is brought to the ED by his father for evaluation of a painful, erythemic lesion on his right leg. The patient, who had been walking through a wooded area earlier in the day, thinks that he may have been stung or bitten. Which nursing intervention is appropriate when treating a patient with an insect bite or sting?

A. Carefully place a tourniquet proximal to the sting or bite
B. Ensure that emergency equipment is available in the event of respiratory failure
C. Ensure that antivenom is available for IV administration
D. No intervention is necessary because serious complications typically do not occur

40. Which therapy would the nurse expect the physician to order for a patient who incurred any bite, regardless of the type?

A. Antibiotic
B. Antipruritic
C. Calcium gluconate
D. Tetanus toxoid

41. When advising a patient about how to reduce the risk of future bites or stings, the nurse instructs him to:

A. Wear protective clothing when hiking or working outdoors near sheds or woodpiles, and check the protective clothing before each use
B. Spray insect repellent in the yard, on himself, and on his clothing
C. Take no special precautions, as nothing can prevent bites
D. None of the above

42. The nurse's discharge instructions for a patient who suffered an insect-related allergic reaction should include information on all of the following except:

A. The necessity of wearing a medical alert bracelet or necklace to indicate an allergy
B. If the patient is allergic to bee stings, the importance of carrying an anaphylaxis kit and knowing its proper use
C. Avoiding the use of perfumes, sprays, and brightly colored clothing because these attract insects
D. The possibility of serum sickness, which may occur 2 to 3 days after being stung

43. The nurse knows that, unlike other bites, the bite of the brown recluse spider:

A. Can occur any time of the year, but usually between September and March
B. Can occur any time of the year, but usually between April and October
C. Can be disfiguring, sometimes requiring skin grafting to close the wound
D. Has no particular differentiating characteristics

44. A 24-year-old man is brought to the ED by family members, who found him slumped over in a chair at home. An empty prescription bottle for 30 x 100mg amitriptyline (Elavil) tablets, with an issue date of 5 days ago, was found near the patient. He is unresponsive except to deep pain, which elicits purposeful movements. The patient has clear lung sounds. His vital signs are blood pressure 160/96 mmHg, pulse rate 140 beats/minute, and respiratory rate 14 breaths/minute. Considering the patient's prescription for amitriptyline, the nurse should elicit from the family whether the patient has a history of:

A. Psychotic disorders
B. Anxiety-related neurosis
C. Chronic paranoia
D. Depression

45. Which action is the nurse's highest priority during the initial management of a patient with a tricyclic antidepressant overdose?

A. Instituting cardiac monitoring
B. Performing a neurologic assessment
C. Instituting measures to prevent aspiration
D. Beginning an infusion of normal saline solution

46. During the initial phase, of a patient with a tricyclic antidepressant overdose, the nurse should anticipate the need for:

A. Evacuation of gastric contents
B. Insertion of an indwelling urinary catheter
C. Parenteral infusion of physostigmine salicylate
D. Administration of quinidine sulfate (Quinidine) for arrhythmia control

47. Which assessment finding is not typically seen in the early manifestation of tricyclic antidepressant overdose?

A. Agitation
B. Diaphoresis
C. Dilated pupils
D. Exaggerated reflexes

48. The nurse would expect the most effective and conservative treatment for the patient who has overdosed on a tricyclic antidepressant and develops severe tachycardia to include the administration of:

A. Sodium bicarbonate
B. Magnesium sulfate
C. Diazepam
D. Phenytoin (Dilantin)

49. Upon evaluation of the effectiveness of therapy for a patient who has taken an overdose of tricyclic antidepressants, which assessment finding indicates the need for further treatment?

A. Cardiac arrhythmias
B. Miosis
C. Urinary incontinence
D. Hypothermia

50. Which symptoms of cocaine abuse would the nurse expect to detect during a patient assessment?

A. Lethargy and obtundation
B. Constricted pupils
C. Hypothermia and tiredness
D. Euphoria and restlessness

51. A 22-year-old man is brought to the ED by his friends, who tell inform the nurse that they think he has overdosed on cocaine. Further assessment of this patient is likely to reveal which cardiovascular effect?

A. Hypotension
B. Myocardial ischemia
C. Atrioventricular block
D. Sinus bradycardia

52. Which treatment would the nurse expect the physician to order for a patient with a suspected cocaine overdose?

A. Oxygen
B. Naloxone
C. Physostigmine
D. Activated charcoal

53. When documenting suspected cocaine use, the nurse must keep in mind that cocaine can be detected in the urine for up to:

A. 12 hours
B. 36 hours
C. 5 days
D. 10 to 14 days

54. A 22-year-old man is brought to the ED by his friends, who inform the nurse that they think he has overdosed on cocaine. After the patient has been in the ED for some time, the nurse begins to evaluate him for signs of withdrawal. Which symptom is characteristic of cocaine withdrawal?

A. Euphoria
B. Hunger
C. Suicidal ideation
D. Lengthy sleep periods

55. A patient presents with isopropanol poisoning. The nurse anticipates?

A. Elevated BUN
B. Ketosis without acidosis
C. Elevated Anion Gap
D. Ocular accumulation causing blindness

56. A 43-year-old male has been stung by a stingray on his right foot. How long should his foot be submerged?

A. When the bleeding stops.
B. When the swelling decreases.
C. After 8 hours.
D. Cessation of pain.

57. A patient has taken an overdose of tricyclic antidepressants (TCA), it is most important to monitor which of the following body systems?

A. Urine output
B. Cardiovascular status
C. Pulmonary function
D. Neurological status

58. A family of 5 present to the ED all with altered mental status, severe headache, weakness, dizziness, and reddened complexion. What is the likely cause of their condition?

A. Carbon monoxide (CO) poisoning
B. Organophosphate poisoning
C. Influenza
D. Food poisoning

59. Mr. Jones, a 44-year-old, presents to your emergency department with nausea, vomiting, bradycardia, salivation, and lacrimation. He reports he was out hiking and ate grapes from a local farm. Which treatment should the nurse anticipate?

A. Adenosine
B. Atropine
C. Epinephrine
D. Dopamine

60. A 15-year-old female is admitted to the ER following a Tylenol overdose. She admits to drinking 8 beers and swallowing 20 tablets after a fight with her boyfriend, 3 hours ago. The toxicology screen results are reviewed and the MD and orders Mucomyst. Before the administration of the Mucomyst, the ER nurse evaluates the following medications, which were given during the prior ER shift. Why is this information important?

A. Narcan binds up Mucomyst, rendering it ineffective
B. Syrup of Ipecac will cause patient to vomit the Mucomyst
C. Activated charcoal binds up Mucomyst, rendering it ineffective
D. Sodium bicarbonate reverses the effects of Mucomyst

61. A 75-year-old male is admitted to the ED and is has a narrow complex bradycardiac and is hypotensive. He is suspected to have taken an overdose of his medications. Upon reviewing the list of medications which of the following is likely contributing to his bradycardiac and hypotension.

A. Metoprolol
B. Aspirin
C. Folic Acid
D. Potassium supplement

62. A patient who is receiving flumazenil, and has overdosed on benzodiazepines and tricyclic antidepressants, should be monitored carefully for:

A. Ventricular dysrhythmias
B. Seizures
C. Hypertensive crisis
D. Pancreatitis

63. What additional laboratory tests would the nurse expect to be drawn on the patient with acetaminophen overdose?

A. Amylase, lipase, PT, PTT, LDH_1 and LDH_2
B. CBC with differential, bleeding times, amylase
C. AST, ALT, PT, bilirubin, CK, APAP, myoglobinuria
D. Lipase, CK, CK-MB, Troponin I

64. In caring for this 15-year-old patient recovering from an overdose, the ER nurse would:

A. Address concerns about her future
B. Let the patient know that her behavior has devastated her parents
C. Encourage the patient to talk about her life experiences
D. Allow the patient's peers to visit

65. The nurse knows that the definition of the DONT mnemonic is:

A. Dictate, Orders, Now, Today
B. Dextrose, Oxygen, Narcan, Thiamine
C. Dextrose, Oxygen, Nardil, Tridil
D. Dexamethasone, Oxygen, Narcan, Thiamine

TOXICOLOGY EMERGENCIES: RATIONALE

1. **C** If less than 30 minutes has elapsed since the snakebite, the nurse should promptly initiate treatment, beginning with immobilization of the affected extremity below heart level and the immediate application of a lightly constrictive tourniquet. The skin should be washed, but ice should not be applied to the bite. Snakebites involving the head or trunk are the most dangerous; however, most snakebites occur below the elbow or knee. The nurse must remember to avoid elevating the affected extremity because this action increases envenomation. In the United States, rattlesnakes, water moccasins, copperheads, and coral snakes are the most common poisonous snakes. Identifying the type of snake that inflicted the bite is helpful, although valuable treatment time must not be wasted in doing so.

2. **A** The most common cause of death from acute alcohol intoxication is respiratory depression. Such depression begins to occur at alcohol blood levels of 0.20%; death occurs at approximately 0.40% to 0.50%. Death also commonly results from aspiration of vomitus and accidental injury, especially from automobile accidents. GI bleeding occurs most commonly in patients who chronically abuse alcohol.

3. **D** Head injury, drug overdose, and diabetic reactions can all mimic acute alcohol intoxication. Other disorders also should be considered, such as acute brain syndrome, meningitis, and psychiatric disorders. An accurate history and physical examination and appropriate diagnostic studies are necessary to arrive at the correct diagnosis.

4. **D** Normal saline solution would not be included in the management of a patient with acute alcohol intoxication. The

appropriate IV solution for treating an intoxicated patient contains dextrose (dextrose 5% in water or dextrose 10% in water) to facilitate the metabolism of the alcohol. Diazepam and chlordiazepoxide are tranquilizers that may be helpful in controlling behavior. Strong sedatives should not be used because they increase the risk of respiratory depression. Diazepam also is indicated for seizure control. Thiamine maintains or restores neurologic function that may be impaired from malnutrition and vitamin deficiency.

5. **B** Alcohol withdrawal syndrome typically begins 72 hours after alcohol is last ingested, and may continue for several days. However, its onset is unpredictable; it may begin as early as 6 hours after alcohol is withdrawn. The cause of a significant number of deaths, alcohol withdrawal syndrome has a mortality rate of 10% to 15%. Adequate hydration and proper electrolyte balance are critical to maintaining multisystem functioning.

6. **D** Disulfiram-alcohol reactions mimic anaphylactic shock and should be managed in basically the same manner. This includes initiating an infusion of normal saline solution and administering diphenhydramine hydrochloride and chlorpheniramine maleate (Chlor-Trimeton). Reactions may last up to several hours or as long as alcohol is in the bloodstream. Reaction also may occur from up to 14 days after discontinuation of disulfiram because of the drug's slow elimination from the body.

7. **B** Barbiturates are known to cause symptoms of central nervous system depression such as confusion, lethargy, and dysarthria, along with emotional instability. Phencyclidine (PCP), amphetamines, and cocaine usually produce euphoria and increased activity.

8. **D** Due to the dissociative and potentially volatile effects of PCP, a patient under its influence typically responds better to the least amount of stimulation. Therefore, the patient should be placed in a dimly lit, quiet room and should be cared for by only one nurse. Phenothiazines are clinically similar to PCP; their administration may produce an anticholinergic crisis or potentiate the effects of PCP.

9. **C** Methadone typically remains in a patient's system for approximately 48 hours. Depending on the patient's metabolism and drug history, withdrawal symptoms may become evident in 24 to 36 hours after the last dose.

10. **A** The correct procedure for gastric lavage for a patient with a substance overdose involves the instillation of 200 mL increments of warmed normal saline solution, which is instilled then drained, by gravity, intermittently. Instillation of iced normal saline solution, which causes local venous constriction, is effective for a patient with a GI hemorrhage. The airway of an unconscious patient must be protected before gastric lavage; therefore, endotracheal intubation must be performed first. Magnesium sulfate or citrate is administered after the lavage is completed to enhance excretion. Activated charcoal may also be given at this time to increase adsorption of the toxin.

11. **C** The nurse would anticipate the absorption of methyl salicylate to continue for 4 to 6 hours after ingestion, with peak levels occurring in about 6 hours. The nurse should keep in mind that absorption may be delayed if the patient has ingested food. The absorption of regular baby aspirin tablets is nearly complete within 2 hours.

12. **C** Signs of salicylate intoxication occur when more than 150 mg/kg is ingested at one time.

13. **B** Salicylate poisoning may result in a variable degree of central nervous system depression, producing such signs as lethargy, coma, and seizures. Dehydration, hyponatremia, and hypokalemia are signs of acute salicylism, along with the hallmark signs and symptoms of tinnitus, vomiting, hyperthermia, and hyperpnea.

14. **B** Emergency treatment for this patient would not include administration of ipecac syrup, as emesis should not be induced in a patient experiencing convulsions or an altered level of consciousness. Activated charcoal binds salicylates and prevents further absorption; it may be given via a nasogastric tube, if necessary. Sodium bicarbonate corrects metabolic acidosis and shifts salicylates from the tissues into the plasma. Indications for hemodialysis include a potentially lethal salicylate blood level (greater than 100 mg/dL), a deteriorating condition despite conservative therapy, or an inability to affect alkaline diuresis.

15. **C** If the aspirin or salicylate product ingested had an enteric coating, the toxic effects could be delayed because absorption of these products occurs more slowly. The patient must be kept under observation for at least 24 hours because enteric-coated salicylates may not reach their highest concentration until 24 hours or more after the overdose. Since absorption occurs more slowly, early levels may be an unreliable guide to prognosis.

16. **C** Initial signs and symptoms of acetaminophen overdose - nausea, vomiting, lethargy, and diaphoresis - usually occur within 12 to 24 hours after ingestion. Elevated serum aspartate aminotransferase (AST), serum alanine aminotransferase (ALT), and serum bilirubin levels, as well as a prolonged prothrombin time (PT) and tenderness in the right upper abdominal quadrant over the liver, usually occur after 24 to 48

hours. About 3 to 5 days after ingestion, the patient may experience jaundice, hepatic coma, hypoglycemia, oliguria, or a severely prolonged PT.

17. **D** Acetaminophen overdose does not produce arrhythmias. The hepatotoxicity of acetaminophen is related to depleted glutathione stores and the accumulation of a toxic metabolite of acetaminophen. Liver necrosis, liver failure, and impaired renal function may occur. Renal failure, a less common occurrence, is typically mild, although severe tubular necrosis may ensue.

18. **C** The PT is characteristically abnormal in acetaminophen overdose, with a prolonged bleeding time. Other hepatotoxic effects of acetaminophen include elevated AST, ALT, and bilirubin levels.

19. **C** The antidote for acetaminophen overdose consists of administering acetylcysteine. Within the first 12 hours, initial treatment begins with clearing residual acetaminophen from the patient's GI tract using emesis or lavage and saline cathartics. However, if the patient is at high risk for developing hepatic damage, the currently recommended treatment is to administer acetylcysteine within 12 to 16 hours of ingestion. Activated charcoal binds acetylcysteine and should not be given. Oxygen is not indicated as an emergency treatment. Peritoneal dialysis or hemodialysis is indicated in severe cases when early treatment is not administered.

20. **A** The most appropriate nursing diagnosis for this patient is decreased cardiac output related to bleeding secondary to impaired coagulation, as the patient may have altered hepatic function and impaired coagulation from decreased production of clotting factors by the liver. This may predispose the patient to decreased cardiac output from hypovolemia and hemorrhage.

21. **D** Shock is the most common cause of death in iron poisoning. Toxicity is based on the amount of elemental iron ingested, not on the amount of iron salt ingested. Ferrous fumarate (Ferranol) has 33% elemental iron; ferrous sulfate (Irospan), 20%; and ferrous gluconate (Ferralet), 11.5%. The ingestion of fewer than 10 tablets of ferrous sulfate can be fatal. Acute iron poisoning is most common in young children and usually results from accidental ingestion.

22. **A** Iron ingestion may be confirmed in several ways. Gastric fluid may be analyzed qualitatively by the deferoxamine color test. Plain X-rays of the abdomen may demonstrate radiopaque particles; however, iron tablets may dissolve after 4 hours and iron solutions are not radiopaque. While serum hemoglobin levels may be decreased secondary to bleeding, the test does not confirm iron ingestion in and of itself. The provocative chelation test, which uses 50 mg/kg of intramuscular deferoxamine mesylate (Desferal), requires significant iron absorption before the urine appears pinkish red. Serum iron levels and iron-binding capacity should be determined in any patient who has ingested an unknown or potentially toxic amount of iron.

23. **B** In cases of suspected iron toxicity, the nurse would expect the physician to order administration of ipecac syrup or gastric lavage, as the patient's stomach should be emptied as soon as possible. Ipecac syrup is the method of choice. However, if the patient has an altered sensorium or if hematemesis has occurred, gastric lavage is indicated.

24. **B** Abdominal pain and hemorrhagic gastroenteritis are common assessment findings in iron toxicity, as iron has a corrosive effect on the mucosa of the GI tract. GI symptoms resulting from direct irritation of the GI mucosa occur within 1

to 6 hours of ingestion. Severity ranges from mild epigastric distress and vomiting to marked abdominal pain and hemorrhagic gastroenteritis. In patients who have taken a severe overdose, the serum iron level exceeds the iron-binding capacity and results in free-circulating iron. Free iron causes systemic symptoms to develop over 24 to 48 hours. Metabolic acidosis and shock are common early features of severe overdose. Coagulation defects and hepatic damage are variable and inconsistent.

25. **A** Supportive care for this patient would consist of maintaining body temperature, administering parenteral fluids to maintain hydration, and correcting hypotension with vascular expanders and vasopressors, if necessary. Hypoxia may be treated with oxygen therapy; metabolic acidosis may be initially treated with sodium bicarbonate.

26. **B** The severity of an alkaline burn depends on the pH of the substance and the duration of contact with the mucosa. Strong alkaline products produce a liquefactive necrosis, penetrate deeply and rapidly, and result in esophageal stricture. Acidic substances cause a coagulation necrosis and thus do not penetrate as deeply as alkalis. Oropharyngeal and esophageal damage is more common with solids than with liquids. In 10% to 15% of cases, esophageal burns are present despite the absence of oral burns.

27. **C** Drooling occurs as a result of dysphagia combined with an outpouring of saliva. Although local pain or burning is almost always present, severe burns may damage nerve endings, resulting in anesthesia. Dysphagia is common. A physical examination may reveal mucosal burns, appearing as whitish gray or red patches. Unless there is aspiration of the caustic substance then dyspnea may not be seen.

28. **A** Dilution of the ingested acid or alkaline substance with 6 to 8 oz. (180 to 240 mL) of milk or water is the preferred treatment, providing the patient can tolerate oral fluid. After that, the patient should take nothing by mouth. Induced emesis, gastric lavage, and administration of activated charcoal and cathartics are inappropriate. Airway management, adequate fluid replacement, and careful monitoring for perforation and hemorrhage are essential.

29. **A** In adults, 5 mL of a concentrated strong acid or alkali is considered lethal.

30. **A** Dermal and ocular decontamination should be carried out, when appropriate, for any patient who has ingested or been exposed to a caustic substance. Antibiotics are not useful prophylactically. A barium swallow 10 days to 3 weeks after the incident may help determine the severity of damage. Steroid use is very controversial for caustic ingestion, but there is some evidence to suggest that they may reduce the incidence of esophageal stricture formation in some patients, so they are sometimes prescribed.

31. **A** Most cases of botulism result from improperly home-processed vegetables, fruits, and meats. The spores of Clostridium botulinum can withstand boiling temperatures for several hours; after cooling to room temperature, they can germinate and begin to produce toxin. Danger arises when cooked food remains at room temperature for more than 16 hours. Fresh vegetables grown in the ground also can produce botulism.

32. **A** Botulism produces signs and symptoms similar to those of Guillain-Barre syndrome, such as muscle weakness and sudden onset of paralysis. Other differential diagnoses for

botulism include hypermagnesemia, basilar artery stroke, chemical intoxication, tick-borne paralysis, trichinosis, and various neuropsychiatric syndromes.

33. **A** Identification of the specific type of C. botulinum toxin requires serum or stool analysis. Type A toxin is more dangerous than Types B and E because of its prolonged morbidity and increased mortality. The incubation period is shorter in Type A, with the onset of symptoms ranging from 12 hours to 8 days after ingestion of the toxin. Acute onset of respiratory insufficiency, requiring prolonged mechanical ventilation, occurs more commonly with Type A.

34. **A** Medical therapy for botulism can include administration of magnesium salts, saline solution enemas, equine antitoxin, and plasmapheresis. Medical therapy is aimed at preventing progression of toxic effects and complications by eliminating any unabsorbed toxin and neutralizing unfixed toxin. Subsequent supportive care is directed toward maintaining body functions to allow for metabolism of the fixed toxin.

35. **C** The nurse would expect a patient with anaphylaxis to have signs of tachycardia, tachypnea, laryngeal edema, and hypotension. Depending on the severity of the reaction, other findings may include urticaria, airway obstruction, altered level of consciousness, or cardiovascular collapse.

36. **A** An allergic drug reaction typically begins as a macular eruption on the head and proximal extremities, and then spreads in a symmetrical pattern. Initial episodes of an exanthematous-type reaction usually occur within 1 week after the patient has started taking the drug; however, occasionally, the rash appears as long as 14 days after the drug has been discontinued. A patient may be treated with a drug many times before

developing a reaction. The morphology of the eruption gives no clue to the specific causative agent; therefore, a careful history of all medications and other substances that have entered the body via any route is essential to making the proper diagnosis.

37. **A** Immediate treatment of a severe allergic drug reaction includes the administration of oxygen. The patient in this situation has signs of systemic anaphylaxis. Because she is a known asthmatic, she has a greater risk of bronchoconstriction than a non-asthmatic person. Anaphylaxis is a life-threatening condition that requires immediate treatment. Treatment is directed toward impairing absorption of the antigen, enhancing oxygenation, and treating or preventing hypotension. Besides oxygen therapy, other emergency measures include the administration of epinephrine (Adrenalin), aminophylline (Phyllocontin), and hydrocortisone (Cortef). Prednisone may take 4 to 6 hours to start working.

38. **B** The most appropriate measure in this situation would be to place the patient in high-Fowler's position to optimize ventilation. The Trendelenburg position may be dangerous because it impairs ventilation, especially in a hypotensive patient or a patient with dyspnea and bronchospasm. Since the antibiotic was given an hour ago, it has already been distributed to the bloodstream and tissues; therefore, applying a tourniquet above the IV site would be of little value. Tachycardia is seen in anaphylactic shock, so atropine sulfate is not indicated.

39. **B** Respiratory failure is always a possibility after insect stings and bites; therefore, emergency equipment must be readily available in the event of a severe allergic reaction or anaphylaxis resulting in respiratory failure. Antivenom IV is recommended for scorpion and black widow spider bites, not

insect bites. Tourniquet application is used for scorpion bites and snakebites.

40. **D** Tetanus toxoid should be administered to any patient who has incurred a bite, regardless of the type of bite, unless the patient has received a tetanus toxoid booster within the past 5 years. Prophylactic antibiotics may be prescribed. Calcium gluconate controls muscle spasms associated with black widow spider and scorpion bites. Antipruritics reduce itching associated with tick bites.

41. **A** Wearing protective clothing when hiking or working outdoors or near sheds or woodpiles and checking the condition of protective clothing before each use are recommended to reduce the risk of infestation and to prevent bites.

42. **D** Before the patient is discharged, the nurse should inform the patient who was treated for an insect-related allergic reaction that he may experience serum sickness 10 to 14 days after the sting. The nurse also should stress the necessity of wearing a medical alert bracelet or necklace indicating the patient's allergy. Other important discharge instructions include information on the importance of carrying an anaphylaxis kit and knowing its proper use and on the need to avoid using perfumes, sprays, and brightly colored clothing, which attract insects.

43. **C** The bite from a brown recluse spider can be quite disfiguring; sometimes, skin grafting is required to close the wound. Ulcers form and, with a graft, can take 6 to 8 weeks to heal. Brown recluse spiders are found in the South, Southwest, and Pacific Northwest. Like other spiders' bites, these bites occur throughout the year but most commonly in summer or fall.

44. **D** Tricyclic antidepressants, such as amitriptyline, are primarily used to treat depression, which typically manifests as mixed clinical signs of lethargy, insomnia, anorexia, and agitation. Although tricyclic antidepressants are highly effective in treating nonorganic depression, these drugs should be used cautiously; patients with nonorganic depression are prone to self-destructive behavior, such as life-threatening overdoses.

45. **C** Instituting measures to prevent aspiration is the nurse's highest priority because it deals with airway maintenance. Definitive treatment for any overdose always begins with the ABCs of emergency care: airway, breathing, and circulation. All supportive care is based on the assessment and maintenance of these factors.

46. **A** We need to stop the ingestion while simultaneously managing the patients ABCs and hemodynamics; therefore, the nurse should anticipate the need for evacuation of gastric contents. Tricyclic antidepressants slow peristalsis; significant amounts of ingested drugs can be found in the stomach several hours after intake. Gastric aspiration ensures removal of stomach contents; repeated lavage removes tricyclic antidepressant metabolites that are periodically released from the liver and gallbladder. Repeated charcoal administration has been recommended in cases involving tricyclic antidepressant overdosage. Such administration allows for the continued absorption of any ingested drug that may remain in the stomach. Administering quinidine sulfate would worsen the already toxic effects, which result in prolonged QRS complexes and QT intervals. Physostigmine administration may be required, but only if anticholinergic symptoms develop. An indwelling urinary catheter may then be warranted to measure urine output.

47. **B** The clinical manifestations of tricyclic antidepressant overdose do not include diaphoresis. These drugs mimic anticholinergic drugs and produce fever, agitation, dilated pupils, tachycardia, and dry mucous membranes. Many patients who overdose experience twitching that progresses to tonic-clonic seizures.

48. **A** The most effective and conservative treatment is to administer sodium bicarbonate to alkalize the blood to a pH of 7.5; studies indicate that tachycardia usually disappears at this pH, breaking the tricyclic antidepressant bonding with body protein is the proposed mechanism by which this occurs. Magnesium sulfate speeds the slowed peristalsis and hastens the elimination of drugs absorbed by charcoal. Diazepam and phenytoin are used to treat seizure activity associated with overdosage.

49. **A** Tricyclic antidepressant overdose causes arrhythmias, fever, mydriasis, and urine retention from the anticholinergic effects of the drug. Assessment of such symptoms indicates that further treatment is necessary.

50. **D** Symptoms of cocaine abuse include euphoria, restlessness, excitability, hyperthermia, and pupil dilation.

51. **B** Further assessment would likely reveal myocardial ischemia in this situation. Cocaine produces vasoconstrictive effects on the cardiovascular system similar to sympathetic nervous stimulation. Tachycardia and hypertension are the most common effects. Myocardial ischemia, infarction, and ventricular arrhythmias are also common.

52. **A** Because no antidote for cocaine overdose exists, the nurse would expect the physician to order oxygen

administration to prevent some of the cardiovascular effects caused by vasoconstriction.

53. **B** Cocaine can be detected in the urine for up to 36 hours after ingestion.

54. **C** Suicidal ideation and depression are signs of cocaine withdrawal, along with sleep disturbances, lethargy, and fatigue.

55. **B** Isopropanolol is converted to acetone by hepatic alcohol dehydrogenase. Acetone is a ketone body, but is not acidic or charged, and does not contribute to the anion gap. Serum creatinine, not BUN maybe falsely elevated. Dialysis may be indicated if the poisoning is severe.

56. **D** A stingray's venom is in deactivated when in hot water. Therefore, upon the cessation of pain would be the indication to cease hot water therapy. The other options are not appropriate for this type of emergency.

57. **B** TCA are cardiotoxic and if left untreated often will cause death. A profound hypotension, prolonged PR, prolonged QT, widened QTS, and V-Tach are early indicators of the cardiotoxic effects of TCAs. Neurological decline is a sign of TCA toxicity, however, it is a late indicator of TCA overdose. The patient may require intubation and aggressive pulmonary management, however, the system that can be most effected is the cardiovascular system. Monitoring cardiovascular status is key in detecting hemodynamic compromise.

58. **A** The signs and symptoms presented here are classic findings for carbon monoxide poisoning. Additionally, the number of people affected by this exposure also is a key

suspicion to CO exposure. A general rule of thumb is that when multiple patients are found to have the same signs and symptoms that some from of environmental exposure should be ruled out. The signs and symptoms presented do not fully support the other options.

59. **B** This patient has presented with signs and symptoms of nerve agent poisoning (from the grapes). Atropine is one medication that can assist with reversing the symptoms of this poisoning. The mnemonic SLUDGE is often applied to assist with identifying the signs and symptoms (Salivation, Lacrimation, Urination, Defecation, Gastrointestinal distress, Emesis). The other medications listed are not indicated for this type of emergency. The 4 Bs can also be used to assess effect: Bronchial edema, Bronchospasm, Blurred vision, and Bradycardia.

60. **C** Activated charcoal is given within 2-4 hours of toxic ingestion of Tylenol to bind up the metabolites of Tylenol and prevent hepatic failure. Activated charcoal will also bind up Mucomyst and render it ineffective. Narcan has no effect on Mucomyst. Syrup of Ipecac causes emesis of all stomach contents, and is usually not a recommended treatment in an alcohol and Tylenol overdose. Sodium bicarbonate does not reverse the therapeutic effect of Mucomyst.

61. **A** Metoprolol is likely to be the cause of his hypotension and bradycardia. Beta-blockers, along with calcium channel blockers can cause these signs. Aspirin overdose would not likely cause this problem. Folic acid, although can cause flushing wouldn't cause this problem. Potassium supplements would cause a widened PR, QRS, and QT interval. Hyperkalemia would likely contribute to cardiac arrest is the

dose taken was high enough and the ingestion of the overdose was permitted to progress.

62. **B** The risk of seizure increases with flumazenil administration following toxic ingestion of benzodiazepines and tricyclic antidepressants. This combination of medications is not known to produce ventricular dysrhythmias, hypertensive crisis, or pancreatitis.

63. **C** Tylenol overdose causes liver toxicity and may lead to hepatic failure and death. Liver function is assessed and monitored as frequently as every 4 hours, along with the serum APAP level. An overdose of an SSRI may cause serotonin syndrome. Monitoring cardiac rhythm, BP, and heart rate are an important part of nursing care following an overdose of Prozac (an SSRI). EKG changes guide further assessment of cardiac function. Lab work includes CK, CK-MB, and troponin levels.

64. **D** Adolescents in this phase of life are searching for answers to the question "Who am I?" Relationships with peers become more important than with adults. During this phase of life, an adolescent experiments with different roles. They achieve self-certainty as opposed to self-consciousness and self-doubt. They anticipate achievement or are "paralyzed" by feelings of inferiority or by inadequate time perspective. An adolescent seeks leadership and develops a set of ideals, if successful. Enforcing her parent's "devastation" equates to enforcing her parents disappointment in her behavior, furthering self-consciousness, and self-doubt. 15 year olds rarely, if ever, understand or can appreciate liver failure. They are in the hospital because they are sick. Surely, they will get better. Communication between patient and nurse in this setting should reinforce achievement of self-certainty and the development of a set of ideals.

65. **B** The DONT mnemonic is used to aid in recalling the medications to administer to an unresponsive patient. The other options, although maybe meaningful to some, are not relevant initial overdose troubleshooting.

SURFACE TRAUMA

1. After a traumatic injury, the nurse should continue to assess for signs and symptoms of compartment syndrome for up to:

A. 3 days
B. 6 days
C. 10 days
D. 14 days

2. The nurse knows that reliable signs and symptoms of increased compartment pressure include pain, weakness, hypoesthesia, and:

A. Prolonged capillary refill time
B. Cold extremity
C. Tenseness of the compartment on palpation
D. Pallor

3. A patient with a leg injury and developing compartment syndrome asks the nurse why his pain is so bad. The nurse correctly responds that the pain is most likely caused by:

A. Pressure on the nerves in the leg
B. Lack of blood flow to the muscles
C. Pressure on deep tendons
D. Bleeding into the leg

4. The nurse is aware that, in compartment syndrome, irreversible damage to nerves and muscles in the affected compartment typically occurs within how many hours after the onset of impaired perfusion?

A. 1 to 4
B. 4 to 12
C. 16 to 24
D. 24 to 48

5. Which assessment finding may be a late sign of compartment syndrome?

A. Pain upon flexion of the extremity
B. Paresthesia over the affected area
C. Loss of distal pulses
D. Edema formation

6. Surgical fasciotomy for decompression of compartment pressure is indicated when compartment pressure exceeds:

A. 5 mmHg
B. 15 mmHg
C. 25 mmHg
D. 40 mmHg

7. All of the following factors would contribute to compartment syndrome except:

A. Direct soft-tissue trauma, causing increased interstitial space pressure and edema
B. Tissue pressure within a fascial compartment that falls below the capillary hydrostatic pressure
C. Venous outflow obstruction
D. Superficial pressure sore formation

8. During triage, all of the following interventions are indicated for a severe soft-tissue injury except:

A. Wound culture
B. Traction
C. Sterile dressing
D. X-rays

9. A 43-year-old woman arrives at the emergency department (ED) accompanied by her husband, who states that she lost the first three fingers of her left hand while using a food processor. The husband has carried the amputated fingers in a plastic bag to the ED. The nurse is aware that, after amputation of body parts, the prognosis for successful reattachment is poor when warm muscle ischemia time has exceeded:

A. 1 hour
B. 2 hours
C. 4 hours
D. 6 hours

10. Which injury typically holds the best prognosis for successful reattachment of an amputated body part?

A. Guillotine injury
B. Localized crush injury
C. Diffuse crush or explosion injury
D. Avulsion injury

11. Which early nursing intervention is least desirable when caring for an amputation site?

A. Applying a dry sterile dressing to the wound
B. Applying a povidone-iodine (Betadine) dressing to the wound
C. Irrigating the wound with Lactated Ringer's solution
D. Irrigating the wound with normal saline solution

12. All of the following principles of caring for an amputated body part are correct except:

A. Debris should be washed away with irrigation using cool sterile water, normal saline solution, or Lactated Ringer's solution
B. The body part should be handled using sterile technique
C. The body part should be wrapped in sterile gauze and placed directly on ice
D. An X-ray of the body part should be obtained

13. A patient with a serious or contaminated amputation and who has no known or previous tetanus vaccination should undergo tetanus immunization. To complete the full series of tetanus immunization, how long after the first dose should the patient return to receive the second dose of tetanus toxoid?

A. 2 to 4 weeks
B. 4 to 6 weeks
C. 6 to 8 weeks
D. 8 to 10 weeks

14. A 45-year-old woman sustained an injury to her left thigh when she was run over by a bus after slipping off an icy curb. Paramedics who arrive at the scene describe the patient's condition as stable, and then transport her to the ED. Though the patient has no open wounds, her thigh is markedly swollen and tense. A tire tread mark is evident on the patient's thigh, and a large hematoma has formed. Distal pulses are strong, and distal sensory and motor examination is normal. No pain is noted with passive stretch of her foot. X-rays reveal no fractures. The nurse determines that the patient's findings are consistent with:

A. An arterial injury
B. A degloving injury
C. An occult fracture
D. A compartment syndrome

15. A 45-year-old woman sustained an injury to her left thigh when she was run over by a bus after slipping off an icy curb. Paramedics who arrive at the scene describe the patient's condition as stable, and then transport her to the ED. Though the patient has no open wounds, her thigh is markedly swollen and tense. A tire tread mark is evident on the patient's thigh, and a large hematoma has formed. Distal pulses are strong, and distal sensory and motor examination is normal. No pain is noted with passive stretch of her foot. X-rays reveal no fractures. Which nursing diagnosis holds the highest priority for this patient?

A. Altered peripheral tissue perfusion related to edema formation in the fascia
B. Potential for infection related to altered skin integrity
C. Altered patterns of urine elimination related to associated genitourinary trauma
D. Potential for injury related to possible spinal cord injury

16. A 31-year-old man had been cutting logs when the chain saw he was using struck a knot, then kicked back and struck him on the right side of his face and right upper arm. The nurse knows that facial damage sustained from this type of injury would least likely involve the:

A. Lacrimal duct
B. Facial nerve
C. Trigeminal nerve
D. Acoustic nerve

17. The patient complains of loss of sensation in his right index, second, and third fingers. Based on these findings, the nurse would suspect that the patient sustained damage to his:

A. Median nerve
B. Ulnar nerve
C. Radial nerve
D. Axillary nerve

18. The ED nurse is assessing a machinist who sustained an injury to his left hand when his ring finger became caught in a baling machine. The patient sustained multiple lacerations about the wrist and hand as well as significant loss of the skin, soft tissue, and tendons underlying the area. The skin torn from the patient's finger was transported to the ED in a plastic bag. The patient is right-handed. All of the following initial nursing actions would be appropriate except:

A. Wrapping the injured finger in sterile gauze
B. Mechanically removing large pieces of debris from the wound
C. Soaking the injured finger in povidone-iodine solution
D. Assessing the patient's distal neurovascular status

19. The ED nurse is assessing a machinist who sustained an injury to his left hand when his ring finger became caught in a baling machine. The patient sustained multiple lacerations about the wrist and hand as well as significant loss of the skin, soft tissue, and tendons underlying the area. The skin torn from the patient's finger was transported to the ED in a plastic bag. The patient is right-handed. The nurse would expect the likely outcome in this situation to include:

A. Replacement of avulsed skin and return of normal sensation
B. Replacement of avulsed skin, decreased sensation, and cold intolerance
C. Skin graft for coverage and limited range of motion
D. Amputation

20. A 32-year-old man is admitted to the ED with a crush injury to his lower legs after having been pinned under a bucket-loader for 4 hours. His vital signs are stable; he is alert, oriented, and complaining of extreme pain in his legs. Popliteal pulses are strong; pedal and posterior tibial pulses are weak. The ankles and feet appear dusky; the skin is tense, but the skin envelope is unbroken. X-rays reveal no broken bones. During assessment, the patient becomes semiconscious and continues to moan with pain. His blood pressure drops and his pulse rate increases. Which of the following is the most immediate life-threatening problem for this patient?

A. Arrhythmias
B. Hypovolemia
C. Respiratory depression from pain medication
D. Fat embolus to the lung

21. A patient has sustained a 4-hour crush injury. The nurse would anticipate the patient's arterial blood gas measurements to reveal which acid-base imbalance?

A. Metabolic acidosis
B. Respiratory acidosis
C. Metabolic alkalosis
D. Respiratory alkalosis

22. Which symptom is considered the classic sign of a developing compartment syndrome?

A. Tenseness of the compartment envelope
B. Weakness of the leg muscles
C. Pain that is out of proportion to the injury
D. Pain on passive stretch of the compartment muscles

23. The nurse knows that, if the patient's perfusion is compromised by compartment syndrome, the expected treatment involves:

A. Elevation of the affected leg
B. Application of cold packs
C. Application of warm packs
D. Fasciotomy

24. Which early major complication of a crush injury should the nurse assess for in this patient?

A. Adult respiratory distress syndrome
B. Acute renal failure
C. Hepatic failure
D. Paralytic ileus

25. The nurse should assess any patient admitted to the ED with a crush injury for possible:

A. Substance abuse
B. Gunshot wound
C. Stab injury
D. Infection

1. **B** Although compartment syndrome most commonly occurs within 12 to 72 hours after an injury, it may occur up to 6 days after the initial trauma. Compartment syndrome refers to the progressive vascular compromise of a portion of an extremity that, if left untreated, results in permanent death of muscle groups and nerves.

2. **C** Tenseness of the compartment upon palpation is a reliable sign of compartment syndrome. Pallor, a cold extremity, and prolonged capillary refill time are nonspecific signs seen in many states of hypoperfusion.

3. **B** The severe pain characteristic of compartment syndrome is caused by ischemia resulting from lack of blood flow to the patient's muscles.

4. **B** If compartment syndrome remains undetected, irreversible damage to nerves and muscles can occur within 4 to 12 hours of impaired perfusion.

5. **C** Loss of distal pulses is a relatively late sign of compartment syndrome, indicating complete disruption of arterial perfusion in the affected extremity.

6. **D** When pressure within the compartment exceeds 40 mmHg, surgical fasciotomy is indicated to relieve the pressure before irreversible necrosis develops in muscles and nerves.

7. **B** Tissue pressure within the fascial compartment that falls below the capillary hydrostatic pressure would not contribute to compartment syndrome. However, direct soft-tissue injury, causing increased interstitial pressure, may contribute to this

condition. When tissue pressure in a fascial compartment rises above the capillary hydrostatic pressure or mean arterial pressure, arterial inflow and venous outflow are obstructed. The prolonged inflow occlusion produces cellular ischemia, muscle necrosis, and pressure sore formation. These allow for bacterial invasion, infection, and rapid deterioration.

8. **B** Traction would not be indicated for a severe soft-tissue injury. Appropriate nursing interventions include collecting information about the mechanism of injury, contamination at the scene, and the patient's tetanus immunization status; thoroughly examining the wound area, particularly noting the underlying neurovascular structures; taking a culture specimen; bandaging the wound with sterile dressings; and obtaining appropriate X-rays. All patients should receive IV antibiotics. Surgical consultation may be necessary if the patient requires surgical debridement and possible reconstruction of associated nerves, blood vessels, or bones.

9. **D** A poor prognosis for successful reattachment is likely when warm muscle ischemia time has exceeded 6 hours. Because muscle tissue is most sensitive to anoxia, amputated parts that have not been cooled to decrease metabolism sustain damage. Connective tissue, bone, tendons, nerves, and skin can survive for up to 12 hours. Amputated parts that contain minimal muscle, such as fingers and thumbs, have reportedly remained viable for up to 30 hours at cold temperatures. Thus, immediate cooling of the amputated part and distal extremity is necessary to improve the prognosis for successful reattachment.

10. **A** A sharp guillotine injury, especially of the area beyond the proximal phalanx, holds the best prognosis for successful reattachment because minimal debridement is necessary. Such amputations typically result from accidents involving an object

with a sharp cutting edge, such as a knife, glass, meat cleaver, or band saw. Crush and avulsion injuries have poorer prognoses because extensive debridement and vein grafting usually are required.

11. **B** The least desirable nursing intervention in this situation would be applying a povidone-iodine dressing to the wound. Povidone-iodine is a desiccant solution, which can dry out subcutaneous tissue. Appropriate immediate care of the amputation site includes the removal of visible foreign bodies and irrigation with 2 liters of Lactated Ringer's solution, cool water, or normal saline solution. The area should be covered with sterile gauze, and the extremity should be supported and elevated on a board.

12. **C** Care of an amputated body part does not include wrapping the part in sterile gauze and placing it directly on ice. The emergency department (ED) nurse should always use sterile technique when handling an amputated part. The part should be irrigated with Lactated Ringer's solution, cool sterile water, or normal saline solution to remove debris; prolonged irrigation should be avoided. X-rays of the injured extremity and the amputated part should be done. Afterward, the amputated part should be wrapped in sterile gauze, put into a sterile container, and then placed on top of ice in a large container. Another acceptable method would involve wrapping the amputated part in a sterile sponge that has been moistened in a physiologic solution, placing it in a plastic bag or cup, and inserting it into an ice bath at 35°F to 39°F (2°C to 4° C). Placing the part directly on ice does not provide the homogeneous cooling that occurs with insertion in an ice bath. The specimen container must also be labeled with the patient's name.

13. **B** A full tetanus immunization series includes three doses of adult tetanus toxoid IM. The second dose is given 4 to 6 weeks after the first dose, the final dose is given 6 months to 1 year later. Obtaining the patient's tetanus immunization history and adhering to the established dosage schedule are important nursing considerations. Usually, the ED nurse administers 0.5 mL of absorbed tetanus toxoid IM and 250 units of tetanus immune globulin IM This dosage is appropriate for any patient with a serious, old, or contaminated wound or a wound involving destroyed tissue. It is also appropriate for a patient with an uncertain or no vaccination history and for a patient with major wounds who has received fewer than three doses of tetanus toxoid.

14. **B** The patient's findings are consistent with a degloving injury. Typically, large vehicles, such as trucks and buses, cause such extremity avulsion injuries. The large, broad double tires produce a tremendous shearing force over a large area, resulting in partial or circumferential avulsion of the skin and subcutaneous tissue. Characteristically, the patient sustaining such an injury also has an open wound. The avulsed area typically is severely crushed; damage to the underlying structures (muscles, nerves, blood vessels, and bone) is variable, possibly resulting in extensive disruption of the skin and subcutaneous tissue from the underlying structures. Fractures occur in about 80% of these injuries. In this case, the patient has an atypical degloving injury, which consists of a small traction-type wound on the skin and subcutaneous tissue. Most of the leg in this type of injury will appear normal; except for possible tire tread marks and a region of ecchymosis. A significant hematoma will probably occur in this area. The extent of avulsion at the fascial level is deceptive and can extend the entire length and circumference of the leg. The sequelae of such an injury are insidious because the extent is

grossly underestimated. Major skin loss or sepsis from extensive tissue necrosis may occur beneath the intact skin. Because X-rays confirm that the patient has no fracture and the patient has strong distal pulses, an arterial injury can be ruled out. Compartment syndrome, which typically occurs 12 to 72 hours after the initial injury, most commonly involves the lower leg beneath the knee.

15. **A** The priority nursing diagnosis for this patient would be altered peripheral tissue perfusion related to edema formation in the fascia, which could lead to compartment syndrome. Because the patient's skin is still intact, potential for infection related to altered skin integrity is inappropriate at this time. However, as necrosis and tissue destruction set in, the patient may succumb to infection. The situation reveals nothing about the patient's genitourinary status or the possibility of spinal cord injury.

16. **D** This type of injury is least likely to involve the acoustic nerve. A kickback injury, such as the one sustained by this patient, who results in facial damage usually involving the eye, nose, or mouth; therefore, the lacrimal duct and branches of the facial or trigeminal nerves are at risk. The acoustic nerve exits from the cranial vault through the internal acoustic meatus and is not located in a particularly hazardous position. Over the past several years, chain saw use has increased dramatically, along with a corresponding rise of associated injuries. Treatment of these devastating injuries should include neurovascular assessment based on anatomic location, as well as debridement, antibiotics, and tetanus prophylaxis.

17. **A** Loss of sensation in the index, second, and third fingers indicates damage to the median nerve. To test motor ability of the median nerve, the nurse should ask the patient to oppose his thumb by trying to touch his little finger.

18. **C** Soaking the injured finger in povidone-iodine solution would be inappropriate, as use of this desiccant agent can dry out subcutaneous tissue. Appropriate nursing actions during the initial management of this patient would include wrapping the injured finger in sterile gauze after removing pieces of debris and assessing distal neurovascular status.

19. **D** Amputation is the most likely outcome when the skin is completely detached and the finger is completely denuded. Skin replacement or grafting usually does not result in acceptable hand function in these situations. Industrial accidents commonly involve injuries to hands or fingers that become caught in moving machinery. Such injuries can range from crushing to degloving and even result in amputation. Parts of the hand may be torn or ground off and may not be suitable for salvage. A degloving injury, which is characterized by avulsion of skin, commonly leaves underlying tendons and bones intact. The primary problem in this injury is the viability of the skin. When the skin is still attached distally, vascularity is difficult to assess; however, skin replacement may be possible.

20. **B** Hypovolemia caused by extravasation of fluid into the patient's ischemic, crushed limbs is the most immediate, life-threatening problem in this situation. As much as 8 liters of fluid may extravasate into each limb. Arrhythmias may result from hypovolemia; therefore, the patient should be placed on a cardiac monitor. Since the patient has not yet received pain medication, respiratory depression would not be a problem. Development of a fat embolus, although a possibility, is inconsistent with the patient's signs and symptoms.

21. **A** The nurse would expect the patient's arterial blood gas measurements to reveal metabolic acidosis. Such an imbalance would occur when decreased tissue perfusion releases

metabolic ischemic by-products from crushed tissues, resulting in increased lactic acid production.

22. **C** Pain that is disproportional to the injury is a classic symptom of compartment syndrome. The patient in this situation is complaining of extreme pain and continues moaning while in a semiconscious state. Tenseness, muscle weakness, and pain on passive stretching are other symptoms of developing compartment syndrome.

23. **D** If the patient's perfusion is compromised by compartment syndrome, the expected treatment would involve a fasciotomy (a surgical incision made to release pressure) to minimize neurologic deficits and promptly restore local blood flow. If direct manometry of intramuscular pressures is available, fasciotomy is indicated when pressures exceed 45 cmH$_2$O. Elevating the affected leg would not produce quick enough results in this urgent situation. Applying cold packs is an early measure and of little help at this time. Applying warm packs would intensify the problem.

24. **B** The nurse should assess for acute renal failure. The initial hypovolemic insult causes peripheral and renal vasoconstriction. Compensatory mechanisms involving the circulation of catecholamines, aldosterone, antidiuretic hormone, and renin further decrease renal blood flow and glomerular filtration rate. Also, circulating myoglobin from rhabdomyolysis produce rapid rises of serum potassium, phosphate, and uric acid levels. Paralytic ileus may develop 3 to 5 days after the injury as a result of hypokalemia, which typically follows a crush injury.

25. **A** The nurse should assess any patient admitted with a crush injury involving trauma to the soft tissues for potential

substance abuse. Alcohol, heroin, analgesic, tranquilizer, sedative, or antidepressant drug abuse circumvents the protective effect of pain. During a period of excessive sedation, an addicted patient can sleep deeply with one or more limbs compressed by his full body weight for a prolonged period; this may cause tissue necrosis in the compromised limbs.

PROFESSIONAL ISSUES

1. In which circumstance may a nurse use force against a patient?

A. Under no circumstances
B. To help an emotionally distraught patient regain his senses
C. To assess an unconscious patient's level of reaction to physical stimuli
D. In self-defense, but only if the nurse has reasonable grounds to believe that he/she is being, or is about to be, attacked

2. Which statement about oral physician's orders is true?

A. Oral orders should be followed with written orders to ensure the nurse's legal protection
B. Oral orders are illegal in most states
C. Oral orders are valid only when witnessed by another person
D. Oral orders should be carried out only when verified and countersigned by another physician

3. If a patient does not understand the information just given by the physician during an informed consent, the nurse should:

A. Answer the patient's questions
B. Notify the supervisor
C. Notify the physician
D. Do nothing, as the consent is already signed

4. Administering a medication to a patient against his will is an example of:

A. False imprisonment
B. Negligence
C. Battery
D. Invasion of privacy

5. When witnessing an informed consent, the nurse is attesting that the:

A. Patient is informed about the procedure
B. Patient consents to the procedure
C. Patient is sufficiently alert and oriented to consent
D. Signature is that of the patient

6. In some hospitals, the nurse legally may obtain:

A. The informed consent
B. The patient's signature for an informed consent
C. Telephone consents from the next of kin
D. Administrative consent

7. If a patient has questions regarding the correctness of medical treatment, the nurse should:

A. Inform the physician
B. Discuss the possibility of other therapies
C. Refer the patient to other qualified physicians
D. Reinforce the appropriateness of the treatment

8. The nurse disagrees with the physician's judgment in ordering furosemide (Lasix) for a patient, feeling that, although furosemide is safe to give in this situation, dopamine (Intropin) would be more effective. If, after questioning the order, the nurse is told to administer furosemide, she should:

A. Refuse to administer the medication
B. Administer the medication, as ordered
C. Administer dopamine instead
D. Consult another physician

9. Which criterion is necessary for negligence to occur?

A. The wrong therapy must be given
B. Injury must be incurred
C. A change in the patient's condition must be overlooked
D. An error in judgment must be made

10. Which of the following is the most appropriate way to legally document patient teaching?

A. Referring to it in the nurses' notes
B. Providing the patient with written instructions
C. Conducting the patient-teaching session in the presence of a witness
D. Giving the patient a written examination

11. Which triage goal is considered the most important?

A. Giving priority care to the most critically ill patients
B. Performing a comprehensive patient assessment for each patient
C. Performing an immediate patient interview
D. Placing patients in appropriate treatment areas

12. Which nursing action would be inappropriate for the triage nurse to implement?

A. Initiating cardiopulmonary resuscitation
B. Intervening immediately in arterial bleeding
C. Splinting suspected or obvious fractures
D. Placing an adhesive closure over a minor laceration

13. All of the following are responsibilities of the triage nurse except:

A. Preventing cross-contamination of suspected infectious patients
B. Performing a complete and comprehensive patient assessment
C. Initiating patient or family education
D. Fostering good public relations

14. The objectives of quality assurance are to:

A. Monitor the quality of patient care
B. Identify actual or perceived patient problems
C. Identify educational or remedial needs
D. All of the above

15. Resources by which to identify patient care issues include:

A. Minutes of staff meetings and patient complaints
B. Staff suggestions and state regulations
C. Joint Commission on Accreditation of Healthcare Organizations (JCAHO) guidelines
D. All of the above

16. Components of quality assurance monitoring include:

A. Problem identification, study or survey, results reporting, and recommendations
B. Problem identification, study or survey, results reporting, recommendations, and noncompliance consequences
C. Retrospective problems, study or survey, recommendations, and noncompliance consequences
D. Concurrent problems, results reporting, and recommendations

17. The emergency department (ED) nurse receives a phone call from a hysterical, nearly incoherent woman who relays that she has just been sexually assaulted. She asks the nurse what she should do. The nurse correctly responds by:

A. Telling the woman to contact the police immediately
B. Telling the woman to contact the police and to come to the hospital immediately with a change of clothes
C. Referring the woman to a rape crisis center
D. Obtaining the woman's name, address, and phone number and telling her to call the police and come to the hospital immediately with a change of clothes

18. The ED nurse is speaking on the phone with a woman who states that she has just moved into the area and would like the name of a pediatrician. The nurse should:

A. Give her the name of a pediatrician on staff
B. Give her the name of a new pediatrician who is just starting a practice
C. Give her the number of the local medical society
D. Tell her to bring the child to the ED for evaluation and follow-up

19. Following hospital policy, the ED nurse places a follow-up phone call to a patient who has recently been discharged with a prescription for an antibiotic. The patient tells the nurse that he thinks he is having a drug reaction. The nurse should advise him to:

A. Decrease the dose and see if the reaction subsides
B. Continue taking the drug along with over-the-counter diphenhydramine (Benadryl)
C. Stop taking the drug
D. Stop taking the drug and return to the ED

20. The nurse knows that, in a police investigation, law enforcement agents are entitled to:

A. The patient's name, address, and age and the extent of injury
B. All patient information
C. A copy of the patient's medical record
D. No information without a court order

21. The ED nurse should know that the sequence of obtaining and securing evidence is known as:

A. The chain of evidence
B. Evidence integrity
C. Writ of evidence
D. Habeas corpus

22. Which term best describes an emergency consent?

A. Informed consent
B. Administrative consent
C. Implied consent
D. All of the above

23. The nurse knows that the parent or legal guardian of a minor, who is a suspected victim of child abuse or neglect, can:

A. Withdraw consent for treatment
B. Discharge the minor against medical advice
C. Be restrained by hospital personnel from taking the minor out of the hospital
D. Be restrained by police from taking the minor out of the hospital

24. The policy of an ED where most of the patient population is non-English speaking is to provide all discharge and patient instructions in English. For a patient who does not speak English but is accompanied by a friend who does, the nurse should:

A. Have the friend interpret the instructions for the patient
B. Determine the friend's ability to understand the instructions, and then have the friend interpret them for the patient, and document this in the patient report
C. Delay the patient's discharge until a hospital interpreter or translation service can be found
D. Advise the patient to take the instructions to his private physician, who will interpret them for him

25. One of the nurse's responsibilities is to determine whether the patient understands his discharge instructions. The best way to accomplish this is to:

A. Have the patient repeat the instructions verbatim
B. Have the patient sign the ED record, indicating that he received the instructions
C. Have the patient explain the instructions to the nurse
D. All of the above

26. The nurse is aware that patient education is necessary for:

A. Medical and legal reasons
B. JCAHO requirements
C. Professional responsibility
D. All of the above

27. When should the nurse begin discharge planning for a patient admitted to the ED?

A. As soon as a definitive diagnosis is made
B. When discharge is imminent
C. As soon as the patient arrives at the ED
D. When the patient shows signs of improvement and can participate in the planning

28. The goals of discharge planning are to:

A. Conform to JCAHO requirements, prevent readmission for the same problem, and provide patient or family education
B. Conform to JCAHO requirements, provide patient or family education, and enhance facility revenues
C. Prevent readmission and foster good public relations
D. Prevent the patient or family from using the ED as a primary care facility

29. Which statement regarding giving telephone advice is incorrect?

A. The nurse cannot be sued for advice given over the telephone
B. Before giving any advice, the nurse should determine whether professional liability insurance covers such activities
C. Any advice given must reflect current nursing practice
D. No fee should be charged for such advice

30. Which situation does not constitute the establishment of a nurse patient relationship?

A. A guest at a party discovers that he is speaking with a nurse and begins asking several health-related questions
B. The day after a neighbor inquires about her child's recent behavior, the nurse pays a visit to check on the child's condition
C. A patient who had been treated recently in the ED meets the nurse in a supermarket and asks about the adverse effects of a prescribed medication
D. A patient who had been treated recently in the ED phones for a re-explanation of discharge instructions

31. Which statement reflects the legally correct action a nurse should take when a person solicits medical advice?

A. The nurse must always refer the person to a physician
B. The nurse does not need to refer the person to a physician if she is convinced it is unnecessary
C. A nurse in private practice who operates without written physicians' protocols may diagnose and treat the person without a physician's referral
D. The nurse must always follow-up on the person's status 1 or 2 days later

32. A woman telephones the ED, stating that she is pregnant and bleeding vaginally. Which response by the nurse would be inappropriate?

A. Asking the woman how many months pregnant she is because the advice will vary, depending on the trimester
B. Asking the woman if she has had any prenatal care, if not, recommending that she come to the ED immediately to rule out placenta previa.
C. Advising the woman to go to the nearest ED without soliciting any further information
D. Asking the woman to describe the amount of bleeding, in terms of the number of pads used in the last hour, to determine the bleeding's severity

33. A man recently discharged from the ED telephones for advice about the adverse effects of a prescribed medication. Which nursing action is most appropriate?

A. Checking the potential adverse effects in a valid drug resource and reporting the effects to the patient
B. Referring the patient to his physician
C. Referring the patient to a pharmacist
D. Asking the patient why he is concerned, then relating the adverse effects and referring the patient, if necessary, to a physician

34. The ED is notified by emergency medical services (EMS) about a multiple casualty accident involving a school bus and a truck carrying radioactive waste. Because of the proximity of the accident to the ED, the ED personnel prepare to receive the bulk of casualties. The nurse's first priority in this situation would be to:

A. Designate a decontamination area
B. Notify the admitting office to clear five intensive care unit (ICU) beds
C. Clear the ED of all nonserious patients and move those awaiting admission to a holding area
D. Notify EMS about the number of casualties that the ED can accommodate

35. The ED is notified by emergency medical services (EMS) about a multiple casualty accident involving a school bus and a truck carrying radioactive waste. Because of the proximity of the accident to the ED, the ED personnel prepare to receive the bulk of casualties. Which support services would the nurse expect to be most useful in this situation?

A. Laboratory and blood bank
B. Operating room
C. Pharmacy
D. Radiology

36. A prominent member of the community is brought to the ED after an attempted suicide. The nurse receives a phone call from a newspaper reporter, who asks about the incident. Which nursing action is appropriate in this situation?

A. Give the reporter the information requested as stipulated by the Freedom of Information Act
B. Give the reporter the general patient information as dictated by hospital policy
C. Allow the reporter to interview the patient when his condition permits
D. Notify the hospital administrator or nursing supervisor

37. A nurse who allows a reporter to gain unauthorized access to a patient's chart is liable for:

A. Breach of patient confidentiality
B. Malpractice
C. Professional misconduct
D. None of the above

38. An 18-year-old man is brought to the ED unresponsive, with shallow breathing and a rapid, weak pulse; blood pressure is palpable at 80 mmHg systolic. The patient's friends state that he just slumped over. After ensuring that the patient is stabilized, the nurse searches the patient's pockets to confirm identification and discovers an envelope containing a white powdery substance. Which nursing action is appropriate in this situation?

A. Replace the envelope and say nothing
B. Inform the physician
C. Inform the physician and secure the envelope
D. Inform the physician and notify the police

39. An 18-year-old man is brought to the ED unresponsive, with shallow breathing and a rapid, weak pulse; blood pressure is palpable at 80 mmHg systolic. The patient's friends state that he just slumped over. After ensuring that the patient is stabilized, the nurse searches the patient's pockets to confirm identification and discovers an envelope containing a white powdery substance. The nurse may be civilly liable in this situation for:

A. Illegal search and seizure
B. Invasion of privacy
C. Violation of constitutional rights
D. Nothing, as no civil liability exists

40. Which of the following with regards to family presence during resuscitation is not appropriate?

A. There is an increased risk of litigation.
B. It may facility the family's grieving process.
C. When available a dedicated person should be assigned to the family as to ensure appropriate explanations can be afforded when asked by the family member.
D. A family may request a termination of resuscitation efforts.

41. Which of the following would not be appropriate to consider when delegating a nursing task in the ED?

A. Education
B. Experience
C. A nurse with 20 years in the department
D. Competency

42. The nurses' role as the advocate for the patient may include all of the following except:

A. Respect the values, beliefs, and rights of the patient
B. Monitor and safeguard the quality of care the patient receives.
C. Convince the patient that he or she should take advantage of the best science available at your hospital
D. Provide education and support to help the patient and the patient's family make informed decisions

43. Which of the following is not considered an outcome of patient-nurse synergy?

A. Subjective measures of satisfaction of patients, families, and nurses
B. Functional changes and quality of life
C. Presence or absence of preventable complications
D. Staffing patterns and patient assignments

44. Mr. D. is post-arrest. As part of the RN's assessment the RN determines that his right pedal pulse is much fainter than 2 hours earlier. The RN completes the assessment and notifies the physician, who orders Doppler studies. Results show a small clot in the artery leading to the foot. The nurse-driven outcomes described in this scenario include all of the following except:

A. Patient Satisfaction based on promoting comfort and alleviating suffering
B. Absence of preventable complications
C. Life-style behavior changes
D. Cost and resource utilization

45. Which of the following is not a core knowledge area for ethical consultation?

A. Moral reasoning and ethical theory
B. Bioethics
C. Clinical knowledge as it relates to the issue
D. Political hot buttons related to the issue

46. Once a task has been delegated to another caregiver, the next responsibility of the RN includes:

A. Providing directions and clear expectations of how the task is to be performed
B. Returning to other duties; the performance of the task is now the sole responsibility of the designee
C. Searching for other tasks that can be delegated, if this task is performed well
D. Documenting the task that was delegated, the person to whom it was delegated and the patient's response

47. Mrs. F. begins to show signs of withdrawal from alcohol. She is becoming confused, trying to pull out her IV lines, and urinary catheter. The nurse working in the next room says, "You are just going to have to tie her down. She's going to hurt one of us if you don't." Before the nurse applies restraints to a patient, all of the following conditions must be met *except*:

A. Alternative treatments such as toileting and distractions should be considered
B. Sedatives should be administered first to see if she would just sleep
C. There must be a physician's order
D. Determine that restraints would be applied for medical reasons

48. The patient confesses to the RN that although her daughter wants her to "keep fighting," she is tired and does not want any extraordinary means taken to prolong her life. What ethical principle underlies the patients' right to direct her self-care?

A. Autonomy
B. Justice
C. Advocacy
D. Non-maleficence

49. In cases involving organ donation, health care professionals who make the declaration of death should be:

A. Members of the transplant team
B. A member of the patient's family
C. A board certified Neurologist
D. A physician, even if there is malpractice charges pending related to the case

50. An ED RN is giving report to the Cath Lab on Mr. D., a 47-year-old, MI patient. She is rushed and cannot give the patient's past medical history, home medications, or whether there is family with him. You recognize that this RN's handoff communication violates the following Patient Safety Goals of JCAHO:

A. Report of critical test results and physician orders
B. Improve the effectiveness of communication among caregivers
C. Accurately and completely reconcile medications across the continuum of care
D. All of the above

PROFESSIONAL ISSUES: RATIONALE

1. **D** A nurse may legally use force against a patient in self-defense but only if the nurse has reasonable grounds to believe that she is being, or is about to be, attacked. Everyone, including the nurse, has the legal right to self-protection as well as the right to work in a safe environment. When attempting to manage a combative patient and the risk of danger is imminent, the nurse has the right to defend herself as long as the defense is justified and she uses a reasonable amount of force. This self-defense must cease, however, when the apparent danger has passed and the patient is no longer combative.

2. **A** An oral order given by a physician to a nurse is legally valid but should be covered with a written order to prevent any legal implications. Because a physician may deny issuing an oral order, the nurse should always strive to obtain an oral order in the presence of a witness and secure a written order as soon as possible. Being aware of hospital policy regarding oral orders is also important. Some hospitals prohibit nurses from following oral orders; negligence could be charged if injury to a patient resulted from a nurse following a prohibited oral order, because hospital policy was not followed.

3. **C** If a patient does not understand the information just given by the physician during an informed consent, the nurse should notify the physician, who should return and answer the patient's questions. If the physician does not do so, the supervisor may need to be called and the procedure delayed until further explanations are rendered. The nurse should not answer the patient's questions because this would constitute assuming the role and expertise of a physician. If the patient has questions that the nurse is not at liberty to answer, an informed consent probably was not obtained.

4. **C** Administering a medication to a patient against his will is a form of battery, the harmful or offensive touching of one person by another. Assault, or threatened battery, refers to any act that creates a conscious, unreasonable apprehension in an individual of immediate, harmful, or offensive touching by another person. Giving a person medication or even a back rub against his will is battery. Assault and battery are examples of legal wrongs, or torts. The nurse who commits a legal wrong may be liable for damages in a lawsuit brought by the wronged person. Preventing a patient from leaving the emergency department (ED) against medical advice is considered false imprisonment. Failing to secure the bedside rails of a confused patient who subsequently falls out of bed and fractures his leg is a form of negligence. Failing to maintain the confidentiality of a patient's record is invasion of privacy.

5. **D** When witnessing an informed consent, the nurse is attesting that the signature is that of the patient. Such witnessing does not signify that the nurse has observed any exchange of information between the physician and patient. The responsibility for obtaining consent lies with the physician and is part of the physician-patient relationship.

6. **B** Although only the physician can obtain an informed consent, in some hospitals the nurse may legally obtain the patient's signature after the patient has been informed about a procedure. If the patient has any questions about the procedure, the nurse should refrain from seeking the signature and notify the physician. The nurse must be aware of individual hospital policy regarding the nurse's role in obtaining the patient's signature; as such policies vary from institution to institution. A nurse may witness a telephone consent from next of kin. Two physicians' statements are required to obtain administrative consent when the patient and family cannot consent.

7. **A** If a patient has questions regarding the correctness of a particular medical treatment, the nurse should inform the physician, who should answer the question(s). Because the nurse's role as patient advocate in such situations is not clearly defined by state laws, the most appropriate action would be to seek out the physician. Discussing other therapies and referring the patient to other qualified physicians may interfere with the physician-patient relationship; depending on the hospital, this may be grounds for dismissal. Reinforcing the appropriateness of the treatment has no bearing on the patient's right to adequate information. Should a patient have a question regarding a nursing intervention then the nurse should assist the patient by answering the nursing related question.

8. **B** If the nurse disagrees with the physician's judgment in ordering a particular drug for a patient and thinks that another drug would be more effective, and if, after questioning the order, she is told to give the first drug, she should do so. A disagreement in judgment does not constitute grounds for allowing the nurse to assume the role of a physician, that is, one that prescribes one medication over another. In this situation, the nurse disagreed in theory with the physician's choice of furosemide but did not specifically question the safety of giving the medication, only the medication's appropriateness. Because the physician reaffirmed the order, the nurse should comply with the physician's wishes. If the nurse still feels uncomfortable giving the medication, she may ask the physician to administer it. Legally, however, the nurse cannot refuse to administer medication unless it is blatantly erroneous to do so.

9. **B** For negligence to occur, injury must be incurred. The breach of duty that occurs in the negligent act must be the proximate cause of the injury. The negligent act must have

occurred before and resulted in the patient's injury. An error in judgment that results in an injury does not necessarily constitute negligence. If the judgment was made after careful assessment of the patient's condition and would have been made by any reasonable, prudent nurse in a similar situation, the resulting error and injury is unfortunate but not negligent. Giving the wrong therapy and overlooking a change in condition do not necessarily lead to injury.

10. **B** The most appropriate way to legally document patient teaching is by providing the patient with written instructions. The patient may dispute receiving oral instructions even if the incident is documented in the nurses' notes. Nurses' notes are highly important, however, in legal actions. Written instructions should always accompany oral instructions; they should be detailed enough for the patient and family to refer to at home, if necessary. Conducting patient-teaching sessions in the presence of a witness and giving the patient a written examination are impractical.

11. **A** The most important goal of triage is giving priority care to the most critically ill patients. Triage, a means of sorting patients, involves categorizing patients according to their urgency of care and placing them in appropriate, designated treatment areas. Performing a comprehensive patient assessment is the responsibility of the care providers in the designated treatment areas.

12. **D** Placing an adhesive closure over a minor laceration is an inappropriate action for the triage nurse. All of the other choices are appropriate functions of the triage nurse, who is responsible for immediate care or intervention for life-threatening or potentially life-threatening injuries or illnesses.

13. **B** The triage nurse is not accountable for complete and comprehensive patient assessment. She is the first health care provider to identify potentially infectious patients and must take appropriate precautions in preventing contamination of other patients and personnel. The triage nurse also acts as a resource for patient or family education. Lastly, because the triage nurse is typically the first contact the patient or family has with hospital personnel, she is a significant representative of the hospital and thus plays an important role in fostering good public relations for the facility.

14. **D** The objectives of quality assurance are to monitor the quality of patient care, identify actual or perceived patient problems, and, as a result of monitoring activities, identify educational and remedial activities necessary to correct identified problems.

15. **D** All are potential resources by which to identify patient care issues. Additional resources include specific illnesses or injuries, the condition of patients upon arrival at the facility, and the response of support services to the ED. In short, anything having to do with the processing and care of patients in the ED can be developed into a quality assurance activity.

16. **A** Problem identification, study or survey, results reporting, and recommendations are the specific components of quality assurance monitoring as recommended by the Joint Commission on Accreditation of Healthcare Organizations (JCAHO). The absence of any one or more of these factors results in an incomplete quality assurance activity.

17. **D** The correct response would be to obtain the woman's name, address, and phone number and tell her to call the police and then come to the hospital immediately with a change of

clothes. The nurse should request the patient's demographic information (name, address, and phone number) in case the phone line becomes disconnected or the patient never arrives in the ED; the nurse would then have enough information to follow-up on the case. Besides telling the patient to bring a change of clothes, the nurse should instruct her not to change her physical appearance or clothing or to shower, bathe, douche, or urinate. Depending on the patient's emotional status, the nurse also may briefly explain the need for strict compliance with these requests to ensure that all evidence remains intact.

18. **C** The appropriate action would be to give the woman the number of the local medical society, which will provide the names, addresses, and phone numbers of pediatricians in her geographic area. This method is the most objective way of referring patients to physicians.

19. **D** The nurse should advise the patient to stop taking the drug and return to the ED. This is the only appropriate nursing action in this situation, as any other action could be construed as the prescribing of a medication, which is the physician's domain.

20. **A** A patient's name, address, and age and the extent of injury are considered public information. Law enforcement agents are entitled to this information only, unless they can provide a valid court order, search warrant, or subpoena for additional information.

21. **A** The sequence of obtaining and securing evidence, and the chain of evidence, is most important in a court of law. Maintaining the integrity of evidence is best assured by limiting the number of people who have access to it and by documenting

how the evidence was obtained, where it was sent, and who received it.

22. **C** Implied consent best describes an emergency consent. When a patient's condition requires immediate evaluation and intervention and the patient cannot give consent for treatment and a legal guardian or next of kin is unavailable, the implication that the patient would agree to treatment if he could give consent constitutes an implied consent. Consent also is implied whenever a patient presents to the ED; in this case, the implication that the patient came to the ED expressly for evaluation and treatment constitutes consent. Although an implied consent is valid, an informed consent should always be obtained, whenever possible, before treatment is rendered. Administrative consents involve an agreement between two physicians that a particular procedure is required for a patient who cannot consent because of his mental state.

23. **D** The parents or guardians of a minor, who is a suspected victim of child abuse or neglect, can be restrained by police from taking the minor out of the hospital. All states have laws mandating the reporting of suspected or known cases of child abuse or neglect. Such laws identify who must report cases of child abuse; responsible parties include registered nurses, licensed practical nurses, and other health care providers. Law enforcement agencies must investigate and, when necessary, place the minor in protective custody. Since hospital staff are not law enforcement agents, they do not have the power to restrain a parent or guardian. However, when a minor has been placed in protective custody, the hospital may not release the child to anyone other than a court-appointed guardian.

24. **C** In this situation, the nurse should not determine the friend's ability to understand the instructions and then have the

friend interpret them for the patient. Joint Commission recommends not using family/friends for translating documents based on the 2014 standards of care. Nurses must use a 'hospital designated' interpreter or translation service. Although B may seem to be the 'best choice' it may not be the right choice. . Therefore, the correct choice is to use a hospital designated interpreter or a translation service. The nurse also should document the name of the person who provided the interpretation. If this situation occurs frequently, the discharge instructions should be translated into the most commonly encountered languages. Delaying a patient's discharge until a hospital interpreter may seem impractical as an interpreter is already available, but the legal and health liabilities are much greater then waiting for an approved service.

25. **C** The best way to determine whether a patient understands his discharge instructions is to have the patient explain the instructions to the nurse. The nurse should then document the patient's understanding of the instructions in the patient report. Having the patient repeat the instructions verbatim or sign a form indicating that he understands the instructions does not demonstrate actual understanding.

26. **D** Patient education is a nurse's professional and legal responsibility. According to JCAHO standards, it is a primary concern of all nursing and medical staff. The goals of patient education are to improve patient well being, promote and foster good public relations, and reinforce the prescribed medical regimen.

27. **C** The nurse should begin discharge planning as soon as the patient arrives at the ED to facilitate the processing and actual discharge of the patient. When possible, the nurse should

include the patient in the discharge planning, doing so helps to enhance the patient's disposition and care while in the ED.

28. **A** The goals of discharge planning are to conform to JCAHO requirements, prevent readmission for the same problem, and provide patient or family education. Discharge planning also aims to identify individual patient needs and to incorporate a multidisciplinary approach to patient care. Discharge planning does not affect the use of the ED as a primary care facility.

29. **A** The nurse can be sued for giving advice over the phone. Although this rarely occurs, a nurse can be sued for giving incorrect information, especially when the information can be directly related to patient harm. The best way to prevent such lawsuits is to ensure that malpractice insurance covers advice (given both on and off the job), make sure that any advice given reflects current nursing practice, and avoid charging a fee for advice.

30. **A** The guest at a party who discovers that he is speaking with a nurse and begins asking several health-related questions shows no indication that he wishes to establish an ongoing nurse-patient relationship. In an established nurse-patient relationship, the nurse is obligated to give the best nursing advice possible, which may include referral to a physician. Any misinformation could be considered, in a court of law, a breach of contract. The issue of breach of contract may be a deciding factor in a malpractice lawsuit.

31. **B** A nurse does not need to refer a person soliciting medical advice to a physician if he/she is convinced that it is unnecessary. Nor does she need to follow-up on such advice, unless a nurse-patient relationship has been established. Even in

private practice, a nurse can diagnose and treat only nursing, not medical, problems unless she is following standard orders, or is a Nurse Practitioner.

32. **C** Advising the woman to go to the nearest ED without soliciting further information is inappropriate. Although recommending that the patient go to the hospital regardless of her prevailing condition is safe advice legally, soliciting further information about the patient's condition may prevent an unnecessary trip to the ED as well as unnecessary patient anxiety. By finding out how many months pregnant the woman is, whether the woman has had prenatal care, and how heavy her bleeding is (in terms of the number of pads used in the last hour) the nurse can determine the appropriate advice to give this patient. For example, if the patient is 9 months' pregnant with her first child, has had prenatal care, is spotting blood, and is having mild contractions every ½ hour, the nurse would advise her to go to the hospital when the contractions are 5 minutes apart and 45 to 60 seconds long, unless heavy bleeding begins. However, if the patient has not had prenatal care, the nurse would recommend that she go to the ED immediately to rule out placenta previa.

33. **D** The most appropriate nursing action would be to ask the patient why he is concerned; then relate the adverse effects and refer him, if necessary, to a physician. Merely supplying facts about the adverse effects of a medication may cause the patient to discontinue the medication needlessly. Investigating his concerns may prevent this.

34. **C** The nurse's priority in this situation would be to clear the ED of all non-serious patients and move those awaiting admission to a holding area. Upon receipt of such news, the ED is responsible for preparing to receive casualties. A

decontamination area should be established as soon as patient care areas become available. Requesting the admitting office to clear intensive care unit beds is inappropriate because the extent and number of casualties is unknown at this time. Notifying the emergency medical systems (EMS) about available accommodations would be appropriate only after preparing the ED.

35. **D** The radiology department and the hospital's radiation disaster planning coordinator would be most useful in this type of accident. Even if the hospital does not receive the driver of the truck carrying radioactive waste, the school bus victims and EMS personnel may be contaminated. The help of the radiology and radiation coordinating staff is especially important in planning the management of casualties and preventing further contamination. The laboratory, blood bank, operating room, and pharmacy would be helpful in providing supportive care.

36. **D** Notifying the hospital administrator or nursing supervisor would be the most appropriate action in this situation. Under normal circumstances, the media are entitled to public information; however, because of the sensitivity of the diagnosis and the patient's prominence in the community, the nurse's primary concern is to protect the patient's right to privacy.

37. **A** A nurse who allows a reporter to gain unauthorized access to a patient's chart is guilty of breach of confidentiality. The nurse is responsible for maintaining the confidentiality of a patient's chart and information. Failure to do so is a breach of patient confidentiality, regardless of how that breach occurred.

38. **C** The most appropriate action for the ED nurse to take would be to inform the physician and secure the envelope. The

nurse must inform the physician of her discovery because it may directly affect the care rendered to the patient. Securing the substance is within the nurse's purview because analysis of the contents may be necessary at a future time. An appropriate action for a staff nurse would be to inform the nursing supervisor or administrator at the hospital about the discovery.

39. **D** The nurse would not be held civilly liable because no civil liability has occurred. The nurse in this situation acted in good faith in attempting to secure a positive identification and obtain medical information necessary for patient care.

40. **A** The literature shows that there is not an increase in litigation/lawsuits when a family is permitted to be present in the resuscitation environment. Family who are not present may be more likely to force a lawsuit. Families have reported that they found being present to provide them with more closure when witnessing the a resuscitation attempt of their family member; as opposed to them sitting in a waiting room and not being able to see the extent of resuscitation attempt performed and being told their loved one has deceased. Families are becoming more present during procedures and resuscitation. Many facilities already have policies in place to facilitate family presence.

41. **C** Time in a department does not dictate that the individual is competent in that skill/task. Therefore, education, competency, and experience are all appropriate factors to consider when delegating a task to another nurse.

42. **C** The fact that technology exists does not mean that it must be brought to bear in all situations. "Convincing" a patient against his or her wishes amounts to paternalism, this in effect, negates autonomy. The registered nurse, as patient advocate,

has the responsibility to respect the patient's belief system and their choices. Even though choices have been made to withdraw or withhold some treatment, the basic elements of care are still in play. Comfort, pain control, and symptomatic relief continue to be paramount in the care of the patient. Education is a key element of the nurse's role, to ensure that the decisions the patient makes are based on fact and not fiction, reason, not emotion, and a solid understanding of the consequences of engaging in the treatment or foregoing treatment.

43. **D** Staffing patterns and patient assignments are precursors to, or elements of, nurse-patient synergy. They lead to the outcomes, quality of life, and work satisfaction for the nurse, which are indicative of goal achievement for patients and families. Satisfaction measures indicate greater patient trust in the caregivers, and a sense that patient and family expectations are clear and met. The constant vigilance of the nurse creates a safe environment in which complications are avoided by preventive measures, or identified early and minimized. This in turn leads to recovery of function, quality of life, and decreased morbidity in a time of unstable and unpredictable crisis.

44. **C** All of the choices given above are nurse-driven outcomes. Behavior change is based on the giving and receiving of information the patient needs in order to make a decision to take greater responsibility for his or her health. This is a nurse-driven outcome, but does not apply to this scenario. The ER nurse's constant vigilance and early identification of problems provides the greatest edge against preventable complications. By preventing complications in this case, the expense of permanent disability and even limb amputation was averted. The patient satisfaction in this case, not only the relief of pain and suffering, but also the safeguarding of quality of life is central to the patient's goals of healing and wellness.

45. **D** One of the core knowledge areas for ethical consultation is health law relevant to the issue being discussed. Political debates and media coverage of issues usually serve to cloud the issue, not clarify it. Moral reasoning theory and ethical principles is the framework upon which consultation is led. If the issue is concerning advanced technology, or new or experimental treatments, a foundation of bioethics is necessary. Clinical knowledge as it relates to the patient's condition will provide science of standards and interventions that have been, and can be brought to bear, as well as the statistical outcomes that could be reasonably expected.

46. **A** As the delegator, the nurse maintains the ultimate accountability for the performance of the task. The nurse must verify that the delegate accepts the responsibility for carrying out the task correctly. Clear directions and expectations of how and when the task is to be performed are necessary to ensure patient safety. Tasks are delegated as part of an overall plan of care, so that delegation is performed appropriately and safely. Looking for tasks to delegate is a random practice and does not meet the requirements of planning safe care. Documentation is done when the task has been completed; patient response is a component of this documentation.

47. **B** The application of restraints, even for the benefit of the patient's safety (non-maleficence) violates patient autonomy. Alternative treatments such as scheduled toileting, offering of food and drink, pain relief, and the presence of family should all be pursued before choosing to apply physical restraints. In the intensive care unit, restraints may be applied for maintaining necessary equipment and treatment, as in the case of IVs, urinary catheters, dressings, endotracheal tubes, nasogastric tubes, chest tubes, etc. There must be a physician's order for restraints, and it must be renewed within the policy of

the hospital only after an assessment has been made of the continued necessity for restraints. Sedation, to meet the patient's anxiety needs, is appropriate; however, over-sedation is considered a chemical restraint, and should never take the place of appropriate nursing assessment and appropriate intervention.

48. **A** Autonomy is the principle a competent adult patient has the right to make his or her own healthcare decisions. Autonomy should be clinically supported through the informed consent process, which facilitates decision-making based on the patient's own values. Justice is a principle everyone fundamentally deserves equal respect. In the healthcare system, this involves allocation of resources and cost-benefit analysis of treatments. In society, justice is a point of reference for health care policy. Advocacy is the duty to stand up, or speak up for, the patient and family's to protect and promote the best outcome based on the patient's wishes. Non-maleficence is the principle embraced in the commitment to "do no harm" to the patient whom one seeks to treat, or for who one is making decisions.

49. **C** Some states require that a Neurologist make the declaration of death. No one with any stake in the outcome of organ donation is eligible to declare the death of a heart-beating donor. This includes anyone with any special interest in the patient's death, i.e., stands to inherit according to the patient's will. No one who is caring for the recipient of the organ to be donated may take part in the death declaration. A physician with malpractice charges pending is open to a wrongful death suit, and must exhibit all caution. The nurse's responsibility is to the dignity of the patient, donor, and to the family during the process of consent and letting go.

50. **D** Patient safety is a significant responsibility for the ED nurse, particularly in light of the increasing number of deaths related to the healthcare service delivery processes. It is crucial that health care workers improve safety by standardizing "hand off" communication. Elements of this hand off include critical test results and values, patient allergies, physician orders, and any other data pertinent to the immediate and long-term care of the patient. Medication reconciliation involves implementing a process to obtain and document a complete list of the patient's current medications, comparing them to medications ordered and given while in the hospital, and by communicating these accurately to the next provider of service.

SELECTED REFERENCES

Bemis, P. (2011) Emergency Nursing Bible. 5th ed. CA: National Nurses in Business Association, Inc.

Cline, D. & Ma, O. Et. al. (2012) *Tintinalli's Emergency Medicine Manual*, 7th Edition. Philadelphia, PA: McGraw Hill

Emergency Nurses Association. (2008) *Emergency Nursing Core Curriculum*, 6th Edition. PA: Saunders

Emergency Nurses Association. (2010) *Sheehy's Emergency Nursing, Principles and Practice*. PA: Mosby

Emergency Nurses Association. (2014) *Trauma Nursing Core Course (Provider manual)*. 7th ed. Des Plaines, IL: Author

Gasparis Vonfrolio, L & Taylor-Vaughan, L. (2015) *Critical Care Examination Review*. Revised 4th ed. Staten Island, NY: Education Enterprises

Harrison, R. & Daly, L. (2011) *A Nurses Survival Guide to Acute Medical Emergencies*, 3rd Edition. Philadelphia, PA: Elsevier

Stone, C. & Humphries, R. (2011) *Current Diagnosis & Treatment Emergency Medicine*. 7th Edition. Philadelphia, PA: McGraw Hill

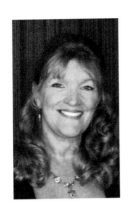

Dr. Gasparis Vonfrolio RN, an outstanding seminar leader, has held CCRN certification from AACN for 15 years and CEN Certification for 13 years. Through her highly-acclaimed CCRN and CEN Review Courses and educational products, such as the CCRN and CEN Review on DVD and CD, she has helped thousands of critical care nurses prepare for the CCRN and CEN exams. Laura has over 40 years experience as a critical care nurse, and has held the positions of Assistant Professor of Nursing with tenure, Nursing Educator, and Critical Care Staff Nurse.

She has an Associate degree from The College of Staten Island (1973), Bachelors degree in Nursing from Long Island University (1977), Masters in Nursing Education from New York University (1982) and a Ph.D. in Nursing Education (1994).

Dr. Gasparis Vonfrolio has written extensively on critical care topics in journals such as Nursing, RN, AJN and has authored, co-authored, and edited a total of 11 books. Dr. Vonfrolio was the organizer of the Nurses March on Washington DC, with over 35,000 nurses attending and has appeared on Good Morning America and Nightline with Ted Koppel.

Dr. Gasparis Vonfrolio is available for in-house presentations for hospitals, organizations, and associations. Please call her office at 1-800-331-6534 for information or visit **www.GREATNURSES.com**

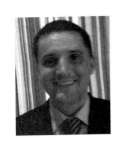

Mr. Lee Taylor-Vaughan, a native of Yorkshire England, began his health care career in 1995. He has completed programs for EMT, Paramedic, Registered Nurse, and Nurse Practitioner. He obtained his BS (Honors) and MS in Nursing from Rutgers University and he is currently earning his Doctorate in Law from Kaplan University. Lee's career has been strongly focused on Emergency and Critical Care, now as an Acute Care Nurse Practitioner with a specialty in Cardiothoracic Surgery and Critical Care.

He has been a successful business owner since 1991, both in the UK and the USA—owning 4 companies. Lee's current company employs over 75 staff, providing continuing education and certification review programs to nurses, physicians, and a wide variety of medical professionals.

Along with providing an enjoyable working environment, Lee has a great level of endurance and determination to see that patients are treated appropriately, which also flows into his personal life as he is an avid athlete, having completed multiple Ironman triathlons, several marathons, and endless specialty races.

Lee is a dynamic, an energetic, and an educational lecturer holding national and international speaking engagements.

Lee is available for in-house presentations for hospitals, organizations, and associations. Please call his office (732) 579-8690 for information or visit **www.CardiacEd.com**

If you are interested in working with Lee with regards to presenting, publishing, etc, please contact **Lee@CardiacEd.com**

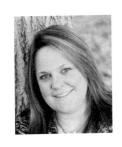

Mrs. Lauren Bohacik-Castillo is a 24 year emergency department and critical care veteran. Having worked in capacities from full-time staff, traveler, to per diem has allowed her the experience of over 30 different USA hospitals throughout her career. She received her BSN with honors from Seton Hall University in 1996. Prior to and throughout nursing school, Lauren worked as a prehospital emergency medical technician (EMT) and as a technician in the emergency department. Upon graduation, she began her nursing career directly in the emergency department.

After several years of staff and travel nursing assignments, Lauren transitioned to the cardiac catheterization lab, special procedures, nursing house supervisor, and recently to legal nurse consulting. She has consulted on thousands of cases ranging from personal injury, wrongful death, mass tort litigation, drug safety, expert witness location and has often, herself, acted as an emergency department nurse expert witness.

Through seminars, conferences, specialized nurse training events, and resume/career consulting services, Lauren provides fellow nurses with a wide range of educational opportunities and empowerment.

As part of her commitment to nursing excellence and support of nurses everywhere, Lauren is currently pursuing her own advancement in the form of a Doctorate in Law from Kaplan University. She hopes to use this degree to improve the field of nursing and support nurses nationwide.

Lauren can be reached via email **Lauren@TaylorCastillo.com** or through the office of CardiacEd at (732) 579-8690

For more information regarding educational products by Laura Gasparis Vonfrolio PhD, RN

Visit her website:

www.GREATNURSES.com

The website includes upcoming seminars, nursing symposiums, and educational vacation getaways—to places such as Bahamas, Cancun, Jamaica, Dominican Republic, and Costa Rica! Each held at All-Inclusive Resorts, which include contact hours for attending the nursing presentations.

Products on DVD and CD include:
CCRN Review Course
CEN Review Course
Hemodynamic Monitoring
12 Lead EKG Interpretation
Enhancing Your Critical Care Skills
Nursing Entrepreneurship

Call 1-800-331-6534 for a free Brochure!

PRODUCTS TO PASS THE CCRN® EXAMINATION

Prepare to successfully pass the CCRN® Certification Examination with the help of Laura Gasparis Vonfrolio RN, PhD, author of the best-selling book Critical Care Examination Review (this book!). Her comprehensive review materials cover the core curriculum and the most important content areas according to the new Certification Examination Blueprint. In addition to valuable test-taking strategies, you will gain the confidence you need to readily pass the exam. After watching or listening to these entertaining DVDs and CDs – you will understand why Dr Vonfrolio is such a popular and entertaining speaker. Laugh and Learn!

CCRN REVIEW COURSE ON CD OR DVD
This two-day program, 12-hour CCRN REVIEW COURSE was taped live at Dr. Vonfrolio's Seminar – Just like being there! Awards 12 contact hours. **TOPICS INCLUDE:**
CARDIAC: Acute myocardial infarction, angina, arrhythmias, CHF, hypertensive crisis, shock states, cardiac trauma, CABG

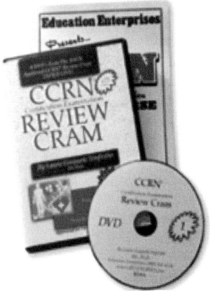

PULMONARY: ABG interpretation, respiratory assessment, acute respiratory failure, ARDS, status asthmaticus, pulmonary embolism, and thoracic trauma.
ENDOCRINE: Diabetes insipidus, SIADH, DKA, hyperosmolar coma, hypoglycemia
HEMATOLOGY: Disseminated intravascular coagulation, immunosuppression
NEUROLOGY: Neurological assessment, head trauma, increased intracranial pressure, aneurysm, acute spinal cord injury, seizures, intracerebral hemorrhage
GASTROINTESTINAL: GI Hemorrhage, hepatic failure, pancreatitis, abdominal trauma, bowel obstruction
MULTISYSTEM: Trauma, poisoning, MODS
RENAL: Renal anatomy, acute renal failure, electrolyte imbalances, renal trauma

PRICE: Individual use: $150 + Shipping & Handling
Institutional: $700, + Shipping & Handling (includes 20 booklets/post-test/CEUs)

To order visit **www.GREATNURSES.com** or call (800) 331-6534

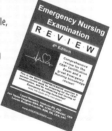